Erhard Meyer-Breiting · Arne Burkhardt

Tumours of the Larynx

Histopathology and Clinical Inferences

Foreword by J. Olofsson and H. Cottier

With 106 Figures

Springer-Verlag Berlin Heidelberg New York
London Paris Tokyo

Priv.-Doz. Dr. Erhard Meyer-Breiting
Zentrum der HNO-Heilkunde
Universitätsklinikum Frankfurt
Theodor-Stern-Kai 7
D-6000 Frankfurt am Main 70

Professor Dr. Arne Burkhardt
Pathologisches Institut der Universität Bern
Freiburg Str. 30
CH-3010 Bern

ISBN-13: 978-3-642-71102-2 e-ISBN: 978-3-642-71100-8
DOI: 10.1007/978-3-642-71100-8

Library of Congress Cataloging in Publication Data
Meyer-Breiting, E. (Erhard), Tumours of the larynx. Bibliography: p. Includes index. 1. Larynx-Tumours. 2. Larnyx-Tumours-Classification. 3. Histology, Pathological. I. Burkhardt, Arne. II. Title. [DNLM: 1. Laryngeal Neoplasms. WV 520 M613t] RC280.T5M49 1987 616.99'222 87-20633

Media conversion, printing and bookbinding: Appl, Wemding
2123/3145-543210

The authors dedicate this book to the two teachers who so decisively influenced the course of their scientific endeavours:

Professor Dr. KARL-HEINZ VOSTEEN
Head of the ENT Clinic
University of Düsseldorf
Federal Republic of Germany

Professor Dr. GERHARD SEIFERT
Head of the Institute of Pathology
University of Hamburg
Federal Republic of Germany

Foreword

There has been a marked development in laryngeal diagnosis during the latter two decades. The introduction of microlaryngoscopy made a more accurate endolaryngeal diagnosis possible and widened our possibilities to perform endoscopic surgery, which has been further enhanced by the use of the carbon dioxide laser.

Computed tomography (CT) and magnetic resonance imaging (MRI) enables a better assessment of deep tumour invasion and thereby a more correct classification av laryngeal cancer.

Photographic and video documentation has been made possible on an outpatient basis by the use of telescopes. The use of flexible scopes complements the other diagnostic means.

In histopathology, the use of whole organ sectioning for the study of laryngeal anatomy and surgical pathology has given us a possibility to better evaluate the advantages and shortcomings in the use of CT and MRI. The growth and spread of laryngeal cancer arising in different regions have been documented and has provided the surgeon with a better knowledge of laryngeal pathology and thereby enhanced the chances for a more safe selection of patients for partial, voice conservation surgery. On the other hand the importance of a wide field total laryngectomy has been stressed, when there is a risk for extralaryngeal tumour spread.

The role of malignancy grading and smear cytology in laryngeal diagnosis is well discussed. The more sophisticated methods in the cytological and histological assessment of premalignant lesions and carcinoma, as histochemistry, immunohistochemistry, electron microscopy and cytophotometry are reviewed and this provides a fascinating and comprehensive reading of areas, which will have increasing applications and importance in the future.

Premalignant lesions and carcinogenesis are other areas of great interest and both are very well covered and with a lot of references.

Surgical techniques as well as radiotherapy and combined therapy are more briefly discussed.

The authors have succeeded to produce a book with very interesting chapters on premalignant and malignant squamous cell lesions and carcinogenesis. Other tumours are well covered too and there is an up-to-date reference list. The book is certainly recommended for all oncologically interested otolaryngologists.

Jan Olofsson
(Head of the Department of Otolaryngology
University of Bergen, Norway)

Foreword

In the last two decades clinicians and pathologists have witnessed the discovery of a bewildering amount of new information in the field of oncology. New techniques of tissue and cell examination have been introduced, and some of these methods require specialized knowledge that is not part of general medical training. As a consequence, classifications of neoplastic disorders undergo repeated reappraisals and changes which are not readily intelligible to every physician and, therefore, run the risk of creating more confusion than clarity. There is an urgent need for a common oncological language, particularly in view of clinical trials aimed at studying therapeutic effects in relation to type, grade and stage of neoplastic disorders.

Monographs such as this excellent and beautifully illustrated text by Meyer-Breiting and Burkhardt on tumours of the larynx will thus be welcomed with enthusiasm by all those intimately involved in this subject. Reasons for gratitude on our part are plenty, since this book does not restrict itself to the description and modern classification of laryngeal neoplasms or other lesions, but also provides a comprehensive overview on diverse topics related to the central theme. In particular, the reader will find up-to-date summaries of structural details of the laryngeal region, problems associated with advanced methods of tissue processing, general conditions and risk factors in laryngeal carcinogenesis, recognition and evaluation of precancerous lesions and therapeutic management of laryngeal tumours.

The reader is thus left with the impression that a gap in the field of oncological information has been filled with great care and skill. In addition to pathologists and clinical laryngologists, this book is certain to be of great value to all members of the health professions who are interested in laryngeal disease.

Hans Cottier
(Head of the Institute of Pathology
University of Berne, Switzerland)

Preface

Head and neck surgery, like other kinds of surgery, calls for close cooperation between clinicians and pathologists, who must speak the same language. The degree of cooperation depends on the surgeon's knowledge of the potential and the limitations of morphological methods and on the pathologist's familiarity with tumours of the head and neck and their surgical management. Only in this way can we work together effectively for the good of the patients entrusted to our care.

In the past 15 years there has been a rapid increase in our knowledge concerning the nature and the treatment of tumours of the larynx and a parallel improvement in the technical potential of histopathology. The authors would thus like to bring the whole field of laryngeal tumours – pathology and clinical management – up to date.

The first chapter provides the necessary anatomical basis. Chapter 2 then discusses histological examination procedures. The simple diagnosis of malignancy in laryngectomy specimens and resected portions of the larynx is no longer sufficient: the clinician expects not only information on type of growth and on grading, but also precise details on tumour spread in the various intralaryngeal and perilaryngeal spaces. The conventional small samples taken from the operative specimen are hardly adequate for this task. Differentiated evaluation is possible only with multiple, systematic sections from the whole specimen. In their discussion of the various techniques, the authors were concerned not so much with propagating a personal concept as with presenting as full a description as possible of the methods in use today, so that the reader can then develop his own concepts. Since advanced methods, particularly immunohistology, are gaining everincreasing importance in diagnosis, they are discussed critically and in more detail. The attention is focused on methods for better identification of premalignant changes.

The following chapters deal with the pathology and clinical management of the individual laryngeal tumours. The basis for the sequence and the nomenclature used here is provided by the WHO tumour classification.

Three chapters are devoted to squamous cell carcinoma, the laryngeal tumour with the greatest clinical significance.

Chapter 4 covers carcinogenesis in the area of the larynx, with detailed discussion of the forerunners of the carcinoma, the precancerous lesions. Against the background of experience gained in this and other areas of the mucosa, the clinical-macroscopic aspects of early diagnosis and the histopathological potential for the detection of precancerous and early cancerous lesions are discussed. A uniform, readily understood nomenclature is put forward.

Chapter 5 deals with the histological behaviour of squamous cell carcinoma – grading, spread and metastasis – on the basis of the authors' own comprehensive investigations, while Chapter 6 examines, on the basis of postoperative investigations, the potentialities and the possible sources of error of various surgical techniques. These techniques are briefly described for the sake of clarity. The same chapter goes into the histological findings after irradiation and chemotherapy and their significance for the planning of combination therapy. The discussion of combination therapy is of necessity limited to the experience gained at the Ear, Nose and Throat Hospital in Frankfurt, FRG.

The findings and conclusions reported for squamous cell carcinoma in Chapters 5 and 6 largely apply also to the unusual malignant neoplasms dealt with in Chapter 7, where the patho-histology is given more weight. The therapeutic aspects of management are also examined if it seems demanded by the special nature of the tumour. Pseudotumours are described in Chapter 8 to provide information on which to base differential diagnostic decisions.

The authors fervently hope that this volume will prove a useful tool in the hands of all those involved in the diagnosis and treatment of tumours of the larynx.

Frankfurt/Bern, March 1988

E. Meyer-Breiting
A. Burkhardt

Acknowledgements

The authors are indebted to many people for their support and cooperation. We are grateful in particular to:

Mr. Alfred Müller, photograph and scientific designer of the ENT Department of Frankfurt University, created most of the drawings with great accuracy and assiduity. We appreciate his invaluable cooperation.
Mr. David Roseveare, Heidelberg, has revised our English text and offered valuable advice.
Springer Verlag showed a great readiness to publish this book, and its staff was very helpful and encouraging in all stages of preparation of the manuscript.

The following gifts of pictures and specific advice deserve special mention:

Professor Dr. W. Arnold (ENT Clinic Lucerne/Switzerland) for the picture of ultrastructure of a papilloma cell with virus particles (Fig. 3.3),
Professor Dr. J. Caselitz (Institute of Pathology, University of Hamburg) for electron microscopic pictures of oncocytoma (Fig. 3.6 c, d),
Priv. Doz. Dr. med. J. Lindenberger (Frankfurt/Germany) for light microscopic pictures of a Warthin's tumour of the larynx (Fig. 3.6 a, b),
Professor Dr. W. Schwab, Head of the ENT Department of the University Hospital of the TH Munich, for his kind advice in the actual TNM classification.

Last but not least, we are grateful to all of the collaborators who have helped us in any way in the preparation of this work.

Table of Contents

1 Development, Anatomy, Spatial Compartments and Regions

1.1 Development

Our knowledge of the embryonal development of the larynx has been supplemented by recent studies using the Carnegie system of staging (TUCKER and O'RAHILLY 1972, O'RAHILLY 1973, O'RAHILLY and BOYDEN 1973, O'RAHILLY and TUCKER 1973); this system divides the development of the human embryo into 23 stages which correlate with the appearance of certain morphological structures.

In the human embryo, the first indications of the development of the future larynx are seen in the 3rd week. During this period, a depression forms on the ventral wall of the foregut, a phylogenetic organ of the trunk (stage 9-10: approximate age 18-22 days). From this depression an epithelial sprout develops in a caudal direction and branches to form as the primary anlage of the lung. Cranially this site is severed relatively rapidly to form the laryngo-tracheal groove. From the lateral walls of the foregut, entodermal ridges are formed which join to form the tracheo-oesophageal septum (stage 11-12: approximate age 24-26 days). With further development, this completes the separation of the respiratory and digestive tracts, while caudally the bronchial branches are established. Into the foregut lumen develop two paired hemispherical, mucosal outgrowths, namely the arytenoid swellings (Fig. 1.1 d). In front of them forms the narrow, transversely oriented epiglottic torus (Fig. 1.1 b), which is closely associated with the lingual anlage (stage 13-14: approximate age 28-32 days). Whereas the tongue develops more in a cranial direction, the epiglottis is pushed in a dorsal direction, whereby the valleculae and the associated glossoepiglottic folds arise. The ventricles develop from solid epithelial sprouts by formation of lacunae deep in the laryngeal anlage. When these join the laryngeal lumen, this leads to the formation of the vestibular and vocal folds (stage 15-18: approximate age 33-36 days). Only in the 10th-11th week does the laryngeal lumen proper open. The cartilaginous elements forming principally the mucosal relief, namely, the epiglottis, the vocal processes, the arytenoid cartilages and the cuneiform and corniculate cartilages, are secondary structures of the mucosal mesenchyme. Whilst the mucosa develops from the rump organ foregut, essential parts of the laryngeal framework are derived from the branchial mesenchym and thus from the cephalic anlage. In particular, the lesser horns of the hyoid bone develop from the second and the greater horns from the third branchial arches. The thyroid cartilage is formed from the fourth and fifth branchial arch. First the anlage of the epiglottic cartilage and the hyoid bone develops, shortly thereafter that of the arytenoid and thyroid cartilages as mesenchymal condensations (stage 19-20: crown-rump length 18-20 mm). In the 4th week, the cricoid cartilage develops in the form of a ventral brace (Stage 21-22: crown-rump length 22.5-29 mm). WUSTROW (1963) considers this to be a modified upper tracheal ring.

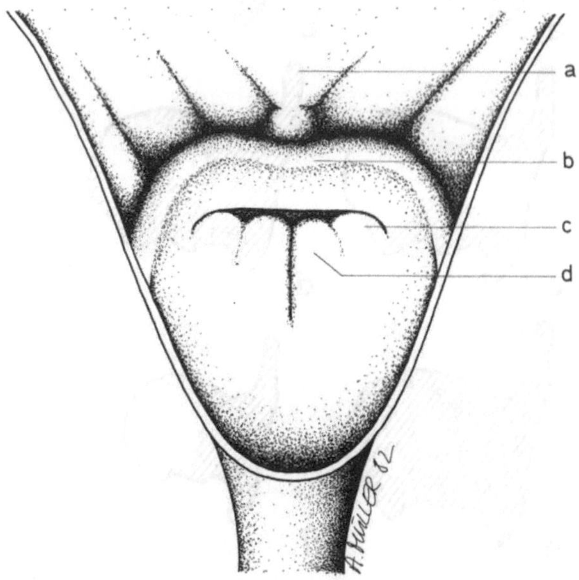

Fig. 1.1 Laryngeal anlage at stage 13-14 (28-32 days). ***a*** Base of the tongue; ***b*** epiglottic torus; ***c*** cuneiform tubercle; ***d*** arytenoid torus. (According to Kallius 1897)

During the 2nd month, the hyoid bone and the components of the thyroid cartilage laminae develop (fourth and fifth branchial arches); these fuse to form the thyroid cartilage proper between the 10th and the 13th week. In the 6th week, the second branchial arch is still an immense connecting structure which reaches from the small hyoid bone horns to the styloid process at the base of the skull. Between the large horns there is a transient cartilaginous connection with the thyroid cartilage laminae, which is later maintained only in the form of the lateral thyrohyoid ligament. Up to stage 23 (age 8 weeks: crown-rump length 30 mm) further mesenchymal condensation takes place, forming the anlage of the most important internal (intrinsic) laryngeal muscles: by this time all essential structures of the future larynx are discernible. Somewhat later, around the 15th week, the cricothyroid joint finally develops with the inferior horn of the thyroid cartilage (KALLIUS 1897, BRAUS and ELZE 1956, WUSTROW 1963, AREY 1965, HAST 1972, O'RAHILLY 1973, STARCK 1975, TILLMANN and WUSTROW 1982). Structures indicating a glottic-supraglottic boundary (Ogura 1955) deriving from the development of the larynx do not exist (HAST 1974).

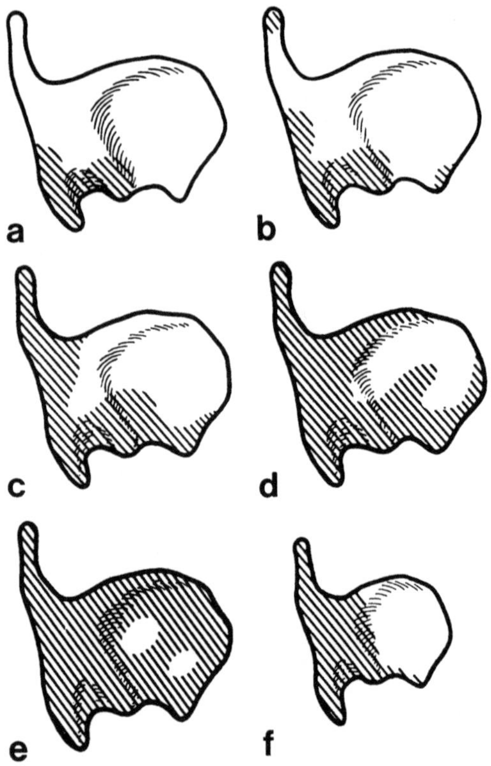

Fig. 1.2a–f Stages of ossification of thyroid cartilage. ***a*** male, puberty: 5% ossified; ***b*** male, ca. 22 years old: 12% ossified; ***c*** male, ca. 25 years old: 25% ossified; ***d*** male, ca. 32 years old: 75% ossified; ***e*** male, over 50 years old: 95% ossified; ***f*** female, menopause: 12% ossified. (According to Lanz and Wachsmuth 1955, Chievitz 1882)

1.2 Postnatal Changes

In the embryonal phase the larynx and the trachea are at the level of C2 but there ensues a slow **descensus** so that in the newborn the larynx comes to lie at the level of C4 and in adults at the level of C6-C7. From puberty on, the thyroid cartilage develops differently in the two sexes: in men the thyroid cartilage laminae lie virtually at right angles to one another, whereas in women they are somewhat more rounded and meet at an angle of not less than 120°.

The age- and sex-dependent **ossification** of the laryngeal cartilaginous structures plays a particular role in the spreading of tumours (KIRCHNER 1969, OLOFSSON and van NOSTRAND 1973, KIRCHNER 1977, MEYER-BREITING and SCHNEIDER 1981). Ossification takes place preferentially in regions of increased tensile stress (Pauwels 1965, Pesch et al. 1980, 1981). It commences in the posterior part of the **thyroid cartilage** (Fig. 1.2a) and in males occasionally in the inferior horn, during puberty. Ossification then extends on the posterior and lower edge of the thyroid cartilage lamina in a cranial and ventral direction. In males a second ossification centre arises in the ventral part of the lower edge of the thyroid cartilage (Fig. 1.2b) and forms a conflux with the first-mentioned zone of ossification, as a rule, at the age of 25 (Fig. 1.2c). Between 30 and 40 year of age, cartilaginous parts are found only on the anterior upper edge and in the centre of the thyroid cartilage laminae (Fig. 1.2d). In women, ossification proceeds somewhat differently, in that the formation of a second ossification centre on the anterior lower edge of the thyroid cartilage is observed only seldom (Fig. 1.2f). Ossification of the **cricoid cartilage** starts with the development of two ossification centres above and below the cricothyroid joint; in men this occurs at the age of 20, and in women at the age of 22. The osseous tissue extends ventrocaudally and dorsomedially from this nucleus into the cricoid cartilage plate. The sex-dependent difference lies in the rate of ossification, which is complete in men, at the earliest, by the middle of the fifth decade (Fig. 1.2e) and in women by the middle of the eighth decade. The ossification of the arytenoid cartilage generally begins 3-5 years later than that of the cricoid and thyroid cartilages. Here too the first ossification centre develops caudally, at the base, in the region of the muscular process. A second ossification zone appears in the region of the apex after ossification of the base is complete. In women it begins somewhat more ventrally and progresses decidedly more slowly than in men. Since the elastic parts of the cartilages, such as the vocal processes, virtually never ossify, there is no complete ossification of the arytenoid cartilage. The same is true of the epiglottis: only in old people is there ossification of isolated areas which are subjected to increased tensile stress (Chievitz 1882, Scheier 1902, Lanz and Wachsmuth 1955, Krmpotic-Nemanic et al. 1985).

In the region of the mucosa, too, age-dependent changes occur which are primarily manifested as the spreading of squamous epithelium at the expense of respiratory epithelium (Sect. 4.4). This expansion is accompanied by fibrous conversion of the supraglottic and subglottic submucosa with atrophy of the elastica and loss of serous glands.

1.3 Anatomy

The larynx is the first portion of the lower respiratory tract. It is a tubular organ with its upper part obliquely pushed into the pharynx at the transition from the middle section (oropharynx) to the lower section (hypopharynx). This results in an especially close relationship between the larynx and both of these pharyngeal regions, particularly the hypopharynx. The entire anterior wall of the latter forms the posterior wall of the larynx. The lateral parts of the upper hypopharyngeal region, the piriform sinuses, extend far ventrally into the lateral wall of the laryngeal framework and here come to lie between the thyroid cartilage and the hyoid bone on the one side, and the posterior part of the cricoid cartilage and the arytenoid cartilage on the other. In turn, the pharyngoepiglottic folds and the epiglottis itself form, with their free part, a common wall which separates the oropharynx on the one side from the larynx and the hypopharynx on the other. The close relationship between these three regions can sometimes lead to difficulties in assigning the origin of advanced tumours to one particular region.

1.3.1 Laryngeal Framework

The base of the laryngeal framework is formed by the **cricoid cartilage** (Fig. 1.3). This cartilage virtually surrounds the laryngeal lumen from below and supports it decisively. The anterior and both lateral parts form an arch, while the posterior part extends,

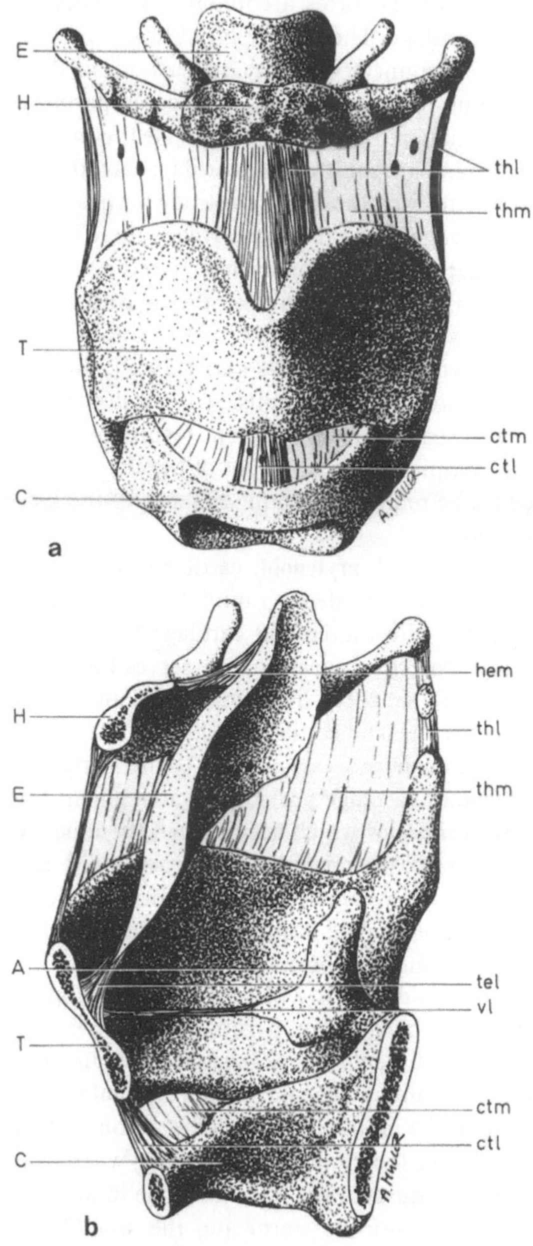

Fig. 1.3 a, b. Laryngeal skeleton and ligaments (**a** frontal and **b** endolaryngeal view) **E,** Epiglottic cartilage; **H,** hyoid bone; **A,** arytenoid cartilage; **T,** thyroid cartilage; **C,** cricoid cartilage; **hem,** hyoepiglottic membrane; **thl,** thyrohyoid ligaments; **thm,** thyrohyoid membrane; **tel,** thyroepiglottic ligament; **vl,** vocal ligament (cord); **ctm,** cricothyroid membrane; **ctl,** cricothyroid ligament

in a laminar form, up to the level of the glottis. The surfaces of the cricoarytenoid joints are situated laterally at this location.

The largest skeletal part of the larynx is the **thyroid cartilage**, which consists of two strong lateral laminae whose free posterior edges come to lie next to the spinal column and which extend upwards and downwards in two pairs of horns, the lower pair of which forms a common joint with the cricoid cartilage. The upper pair of horns, on the other hand, is connected to the greater horn of the hyoid bone on both sides by a very strong, partially ossified ligament of varying length. At the midline, the two parts of the thyroid cartilage are firmly connected to each other and protrude vertically. On the upper edge of the thyroid cartilage there is the more or less pronounced superior thyreoid notch. In contrast to the cricoid cartilage, the thyroid cartilage is involved only to a small extent in the formation of the laryngeal lumen (PERNKOPF 1952); this has also been shown by the results of vertical partial laryngeal resection using different techniques, in which the complete vertical extent of the thyroid cartilage could be removed without collapse of the laryngeal lumen.

The paired **arytenoid cartilages** correspond in form to a three-sided pyramid. Whereas the base articulates with the cricoid cartilage lamina, the ventrally projecting vocal process serves for the attachment of the vocal ligament. The latter is formed largely of elastic cartilage. Both the laterally directed muscular process and the lateral surface of the arytenoid cartilage provide the attachment for a series of muscles which act between the inner wall of the thyroid, the cricoid, and the arytenoid cartilage. The cranially directed apex is surmounted by the paired corniculate cartilages, as mentioned above, and prolongs the posterior laryngeal wall.

The **hyoid bone** is – like a yard on a sailing ship – stretched between numerous muscles without any firm attachments to the base of the skull or to the spinal column. The suprahyoid musculature of the floor of the mouth, including the stylohyoid muscle, attaches to the hyoid bone cranially, whereas the infrahyoid musculature fixes the bone in the direction of the manubrium sterni and the shoulder girdle. The larynx above the thyroid cartilage is suspended on the fixed hyoid bone by the above-mentioned thyrohyoid ligaments and membranes. In purely endolaryngeal and hypopharyngeal tumours, the upper edge of the hyoid bone usually constitutes the uppermost resection line in total laryngectomy.

The **epiglottic cartilage** forms the epiglottis and thereby strengthens the anterior wall of the supraglottic space (Fig. 1.3b). By means of the thyroepiglottic ligament it is fixed with its goose-quill-like prolonged caudal end on the median line in the upper part of the inner wall of the thyroid cartilage. It is also loosely suspended in a dorsocranial position in the vestibule of the larynx by several ligaments and membranes, which will be described individually later. During aspiration it assumes a steeper position and during glutition, a flatter position so that it comes to lie on the remaining ligaments of the laryngeal inlet. The epiglottic cartilage is divided into the pars libera, which projects above the plane of the valleculae, the pars fixa, which is studded with numerous sieve-like perforations, and finally the petiole, which is found caudally (LANZ and WACHSMUTH 1955, PAFF 1973, KRMPOTIC-NEMANIC et al. 1985).

1.3.2 Ligaments and Membranes

The **thyrohyoid membrane**, which has already been mentioned and by means of which the larynx is suspended from the hyoid bone, consists of relatively dense fibre masses, which are pierced only at circumscribed places on each side by the superior laryngeal nerve and the superior laryngeal artery (Fig. 1.3). The membrane is strengthened by a more elastic median thyrohyoid ligament and two lateral thyrohyoid ligaments. The cricothyroid ligament is of a similarly strong nature and stretches from the lower edge of the thyroid cartilage to the upper edge of the cricoid cartilage; it allows the passage of the vessels and nerve branches of the same name only at circumscribed sites where the perforations are sometimes paired, sometimes unpaired. Laterodorsally, this ligament extends into the more delicate **cricothyroid membrane** on the framework and towards the inside, in connection with the vocal ligament, into the elastic cone.

The **hyoepiglottic membrane** is a considerably more delicate connective tissue membrane which stretches from the epiglottis to the hyoid bone (LANZ and WACHSMUTH 1955, BRAUS and ELZE 1956, NORRIS et al. 1970, TUCKER 1974). NORRIS et al. (1970) and TUCKER (1974) divide this membrane into an upper medial section with more horizontal fibres and a lateral hypoepiglottic ligament with fibres which run more vertically. The **aryepiglottic ligaments** and muscles are involved directly in the development of the laryngeal mucosal relief in that they shape the aryepiglottic fold. The aryepiglottic ligament extends caudally into the quadrangular membrane; the latter consists of highly tensile collagenous and to some extent elastic fibres, and is not as strong, or as tight, as the membranes of the laryngeal framework proper. Within the area of the vestibular ligaments, the **quadrangular membrane** sends fibres towards the ventricular ligament, which originates from the inner wall of the thyroid cartilage angle above the attachment of the vocal ligament and is connected to the ventrolateral surface of the arytenoid cartilage. Between the area formed by the quadrangular membrane and the vestibular ligament harbouring it on the one side, and the thyroid cartilage on the other, Morgagni's ventricle in the anterior third of the larynx is pushed far forward in a cranial direction. Comparable to the quadrangular membrane, the **elastic cone** extends in a reflected direction to the vocal folds and here connects with the vocal ligaments and the vocal process of the arytenoid cartilage. Well-known textbooks and reference works describe a transition of the elastic cone into the tunica elastica trachealis. According to OLOFSSON and VAN NOSTRAND (1973), LUND (1974) and TUCKER (1974), as well as from our own observations, this applies only to the smaller part of its fibre masses. The main part inserts on the inner surface of the upper edge of the cricoid cartilage, as will be seen in numerous figures later. In the area of the anterior laryngeal wall, the elastic cone merges with the inner surface of the **cricothyroid membrane**; together, they form the **cricothyroid ligament**. Towards the lumen this portion is immediately covered by a relatively thin mucosa so that there is only a very narrow zone between the endolaryngeal mucosal surface and the external part of the larynx.

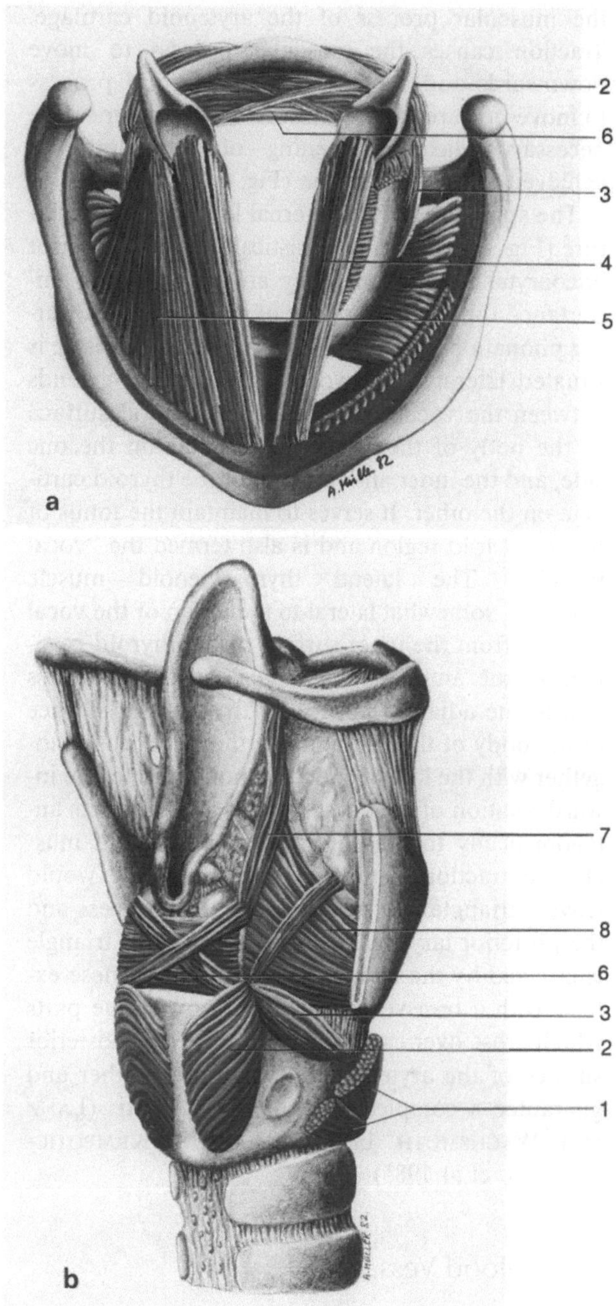

Fig. 1.4 a, b. Laryngeal muscles as seen cranially ***(a)*** and dorsolaterally ***(b)***. **1,** cricothyroid muscles; **2,** posterior cricoarytenoid muscle; **3,** lateral cricoarytenoid muscle; **4,** medial thyroarytenoid muscle (vocal muscle); **5,** lateral thyroarytenoid muscle; **6,** interarytenoid muscles; **7,** aryepiglottic muscle; ***8,*** thyroepiglottic muscle

1.3.3 Muscles

The muscles of the larynx (Fig. 1.4) are divided into the extrinsic and the intrinsic muscles, the latter being subdivided into sphincters and dilatators.

The **extrinsic laryngeal musculature** consists solely of the cricothyroid muscle, which stretches from the outer surface of the lateral cricoid cartilage brace to the lower edge of the thyroid cartilage and here, by a tilting movement of the thyroid cartilage, produces tension in the vocal cord region. The cricothyroid muscle is subdivided into a ventral part (pars recta) and a posterior part (pars obliqua).

Of the **internal laryngeal muscles**, only one brings about an opening of the glottis (dilatator), namely the posterior cricoarytenoid muscle. This muscle originates from virtually the whole surface of the cricoid lamina and extends to the dorsal surface of the muscular process of the arytenoid cartilage. Traction causes the muscular process to move downwards and backwards and the vocal process to move upwards and outwards. In this manner, the necessary maximal opening of the glottis is achieved during inspiration (Fig. 1.4b).

The sphincters of the internal laryngeal musculature (Fig. 1.4a) act antagonistically to the posterior cricoarytenoid muscle. They are of particular importance for the positioning of the vocal cord during phonation. The medial thyroarytenoid muscle is situated lateral to the vocal ligament and extends between the vocal process and the ventral surface of the body of the arytenoid cartilage on the one side, and the inner anterior wall of the thyroid cartilage on the other. It serves to maintain the tonus of the vocal fold region and is also termed the "vocal muscle". The lateral thyroarytenoid muscle stretches, somewhat lateral to the origin of the vocal muscle, from the inner surface of the thyroid cartilage to the anterior wall of the muscular process and to the adjacent portion of the anterior surface of the body of the arytenoid cartilage. It causes, together with the lateral cricoarytenoid muscle, the inward rotation of the vocal process and thus acts antagonistically to the posterior cricoarytenoid muscle. Contraction of these muscles, however, would leave a triangle free between the vocal process and the posterior laryngeal wall; closure of this triangle is effected by the interarytenoid muscles. These extend with a transversal part and two oblique parts which cross over each other from the one posterior surface of the arytenoid cartilage to the other and guarantee a complete closure of the glottis (Lanz and Wachsmuth 1955, Paff 1973, Krmpotic-Nemanic et al. 1985).

1.3.4 Blood Vessels

The larynx is supplied by four major vascular tracts, namely, the paired superior and inferior laryngeal arteries and veins. The **superior laryngeal artery** branches off from the superior thyroid artery only a few millimetres from its exit from the external carotid artery. It runs approximately horizontally as far as to the thyrohyoid membrane, perforates the membrane laterally and stretches ventrally and medially below the mucosa of the piriform sinus. Its end branches, the cricoarytenoid and ventricular rami, anastomose with branches from the inferior laryngeal artery and the cricothyroid ramus respectively. The cricothyroid ramus arises more caudally from the superior thyroid artery, runs in a caudal and ventral direction along the outer wall of the larynx, perforates the cricothyroid ligament and supplies the ventral subglottic area. The **inferior laryngeal artery** branches off the inferior thyroid artery before the latter reaches the capsule of the dorsal parts of the thyroid gland. It stretches, usually paired, cranially along the posterior wall of the trachea, gives off branches in the lateral and dorsal subglottic regions and then communicates, via its end branch on the posterior laryngeal surface, with the superior laryngeal artery. The venous drainage corresponds largely to the arterial supply (Lanz and Wachsmuth 1955, Paff 1973, Krmpotic-Nemanic et al. 1985).

1.3.5 Lymph Drainage

It was at the end of the last and the beginning of this century that much of our knowledge regarding the anatomy of the lymphatic system of the larynx was acquired (Poirier 1887, Most 1899, Poirier and Charpy 1901, Cuneo 1902, Quiret 1906, Bartels 1909). In later decades only isolated additional publications appeared (Rouvière 1932, Pressman et al. 1960, Welsh et al. 1961, Welsh 1964, Beck and Mann 1980).

Since squamous cell carcinomas of the larynx arise from the mucosa, the lymphatic supply (Figs. 1.5–1.7) in this region is of special interest with regard to the tendency to metastasize and the direction of metastasis. The mesh of the lymphatic capillaries in the supraglottic region is particularly dense and their lumina are of noticeably large diameter. This applies especially to the mucosa of Morgagni's ventricle, of the vestibular ligaments and of the free edge of the larynx (Poirier 1887). The region of the vocal folds exhibits a series of remarkable features. It possesses only very sparse, fine lymph capillaries and few drainage facilities. It is just as impossible to fill the vocal cord region of one side from the contralateral side as it is to fill the lymph region below the free edge of the vocal cord from the supraglottic region. The capillary network of the lymphatics is arranged longitudinally in the direction of the vocal cords (Poirier 1887b, Most 1899, Rouvière 1932). In the subglottic space (Fig. 1.5) the capillary network of the lymphatic system is more dispersed, and the vessels themselves are smaller, than in the supraglottic region (Poirier

1887b). According to Most (1899), the lymph drainage from here takes place caudally (Fig. 1.6), whereby the vessels in the region of the posterior wall tend to run more horizontally (Pressman et al. 1960, Beck and Mann 1980).

Lymph drainage from the larynx occurs in three directions (Fig. 1.7). Predominant is the cranial direction, corresponding to the course taken by the laryngeal superior lymphatic vessels (Poirier 1887a). These vessels, together with the lymphatic trunk, course through the thyrohyoid membranes and then in the direction of the carotid triangle, where they join with cranial branches and drain in-

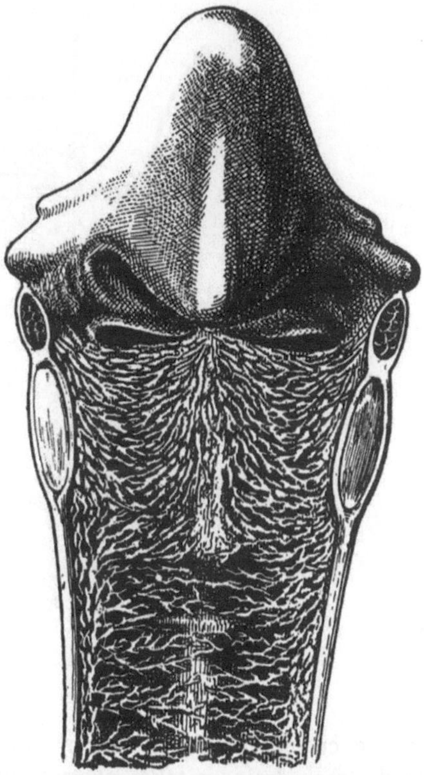

Fig. 1.5 Lymph capillary network in the subglottic mucosa. ▶ (According to Bartels 1909)

Fig. 1.6 a, b. Endolaryngeal spaces and lymph drainage. Drainage ensues in three main directions: **1,** superior; **2,** inferior; **3,** anterior laryngeal lymph vessels. **SPSP,** supraglottic space; **PASP,** paraglottic space; **RSP,** Reinke's space; **SBSP,** subglottic space; **PRSP,** preepiglottic space. **qm,** quadrangular membrane; **vel,** ventricular ligament; **vl,** vocal ligament; **ec,** elastic cone; **hem,** hyoepiglottic membrane; **thm,** thyrohyoid membrane; **tel,** thyrepiglottic ligament ▼

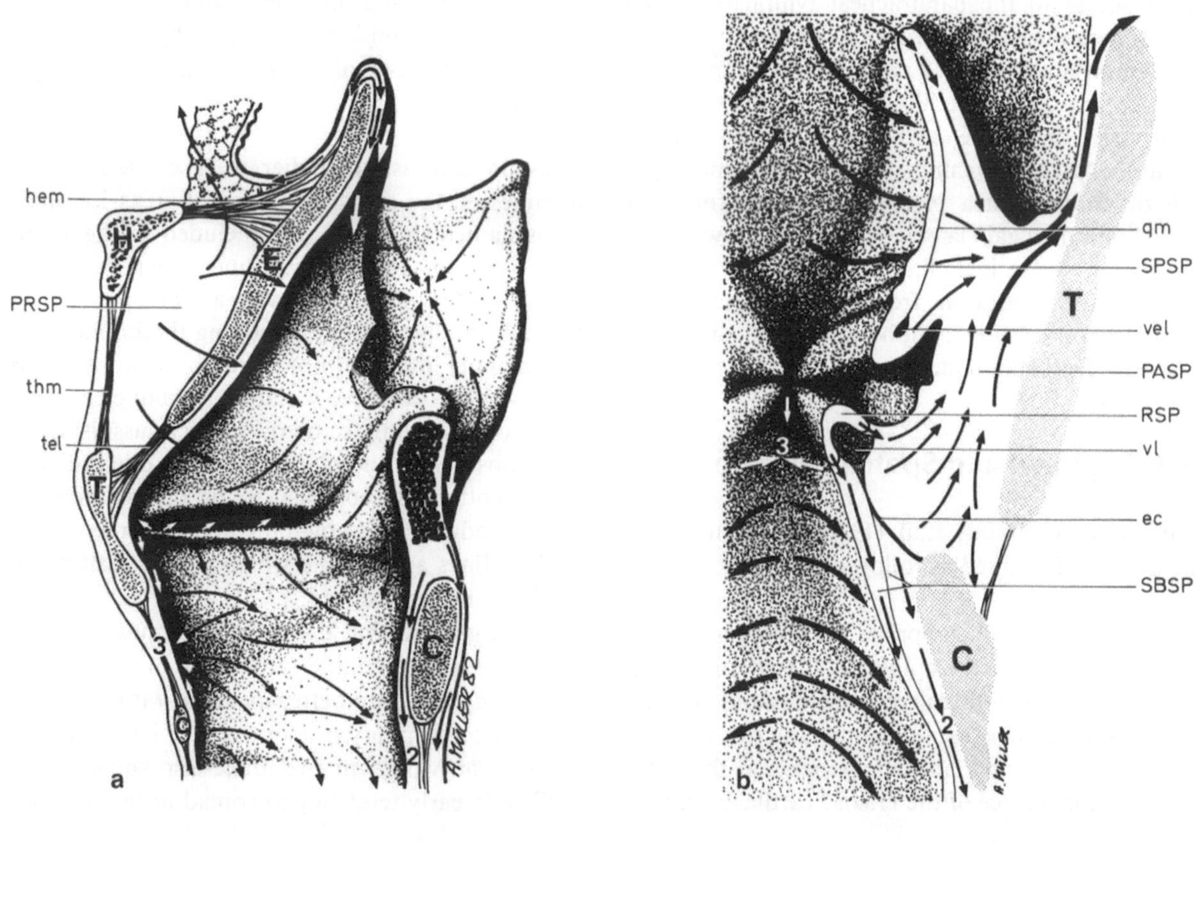

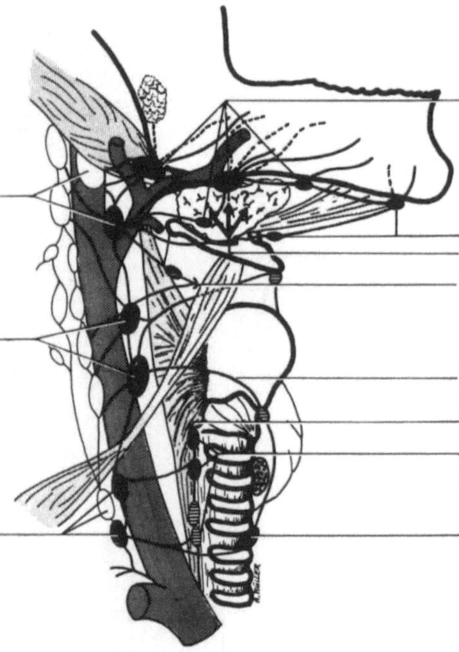

Fig. 1.7 Lymph drainage paths outside the larynx

to the cranial jugular lymph nodes. The second, fairly large drainage takes place dorsally in the region of the subglottic space, where the lymphatics unite laterodorsally on the lower edge of the cricoid cartilage to form the inferior lymphatic vessels and gain access to the paratracheal lymphatic nodes. From here there are connections to the lower jugular lymph nodes and via paratracheal lymph nodes into the mediastinum (Poirier and Charpy 1901, Rouvière 1932). The anterior part of the subglottic space is drained ventrally via several small lymphatic trunks which pierce the cricothyroid ligament, and then gain lateral access to the lower jugular lymph nodes, including the inconstant prelaryngeal lymph nodes in front of the cricothyroid membranes. These lymphatic nodes are often termed "Delphian nodes".

1.4 Regional and Spatial Division

According to Norris et al. (1970), the entire laryngeal region is limited as follows:

1. The anterior wall comprises the laryngeal, suprahyoid surface of the epiglottis, the endolaryngeal surfaces of the thyrohyoid membranes and the thyroid cartilage, as well as the anterior commissure, the cricothyroid membranes and the endolaryngeal surface of the cricoid cartilage ring.
2. The dorsolateral boundaries include the aryepiglottic folds, the arytenoid region, the interarytenoid cleft and the endolaryngeal surface of the cricoid lamina.
3. The upper boundary consists of the free edge of the epiglottis and the aryepiglottic folds.
4. The lower boundary is formed by a horizontal plane at the level of the lower edge of the cricoid cartilage.

Thus, in contrast to earlier ways of defining the boundaries, the so-called marginal areas i.e. those areas named in item 3, are included in the supraglottic region. The dividing line drawn earlier for this so-called epilarynx was a horizontal plane through the hyoid bone. Defining the boundary in this manner proved impracticable, however, since there was considerable variation from one examiner to the other, owing to the difficulty in assessing the exact position of the plane, and from one individual to another. By contrast, fixing the boundary at the free edge of the epiglottis and the aryepiglottic folds defines a clear line which can be readily recognized and reproduced.

The argument that the marginal zones, owing to the more unfavourable prognosis of carcinomas originating here, are better included with the hypopharynx or oropharynx is inadequate insofar as carcinomas of Morgagni's ventricle also show a comparatively early tendency to spread in the direction of the hypopharynx and into the corresponding lymph tracts: accordingly, the prognosis is poor (SHAHEEN 1974). The inclusion of the free epiglottic edge and the aryepiglottic folds in the supraglottic region can be taken as being generally accepted today.

1.4.1 Spatial Subdivision

Pathohistological studies on serial sections of the larynx have shown that in their expansion, a vast majority of squamous cell carcinomas of the larynx respect the skeletal and membranous structures for a long time (TUCKER 1963, OLOFSSON and VAN NOSTRAND 1973, KIRCHNER 1977, MEYER-BREITING and SCHNEIDER 1981). Thus it appears meaningful to subdivide the whole organ "larynx" into individual spaces which are more or less delimited by such structures.

The **supraglottic space** (Fig. 1.6, 5.3, 5.4) is considered as that area which extends from the supraglottic mucosal surface to the lower edge of the vestibular ligaments and the petiole, and is limited in the depth laterally by the quadrangular membrane and the laryngeal surface of the epiglottic cartilage. There is no membranous boundary in the posterior laryngeal wall. The term "supraglottic space" must not be confused with the clinical term of the TNM classification of "supraglottic region" as explained below.

Ventral to the supraglottic space lies the **preepiglottic space** between the thyroid cartilage and hyoid bone, as well as the associated thyrohyoid membrane on the one side and the epiglottis on the other (Fig. 1.6 a). This space is bounded cranially by the delicate hyoepiglottic membrane and caudally by the thin thyroepiglottic ligament.

NORRIS et al. (1970) and TUCKER (1971, 1974) are of the opinion that the lateral parts of the hyoepiglottic membrane, with their more vertical course, delimit the preepiglottic space in a dorsal direction. Since the observations of OLOFSSON and VAN NOSTRAND (1973) and MAGUIRE and DAYAL (1974), in addition to our own, show that there is, rather, a continuous transition of the preepiglottic space, into the so-called paraglottic space which lies behind it. We were not able to confirm a true membranous or ligamentous barrier lateral to the epiglottis. By considering the posterior boundary of the preepiglottic space to be at the lateral side of the quadrangular membrane, CLERF (1944) combined the preepiglottic space of our definition with the supraglottic part of the paraglottic space. MAGUIRE and DAYAL (1974), in an attempt to avoid further misunderstanding, made the proposition that this whole space be termed "periepiglottic space". But since "preepiglottic" space has come to be widely accepted, there appears to be no compelling reason for changing the terminology to "periepiglottic space" with the inclusion of the zone lateral to the quadrangular membrane, especially in view of the fact that the not clearly definable boundary between the preepiglottic space and the paraglottic space involves no more than a relatively narrow zone lateral to the edge of the epiglottis.

There are other grounds on which the inclusion of the space lateral to the quadrangular membrane in the preepiglottic space appears not to be particularly appropriate. This lateral space belongs to the largest connecting spatial structure in the depth of the laryngeal soft parts, the **paraglottic space**, which surrounds the whole of Morgagni's ventricle laterally of the quadrangular membrane without membranous or skeletal barriers and is caudally limited by the elastic cone and the cricothyroid membrane.

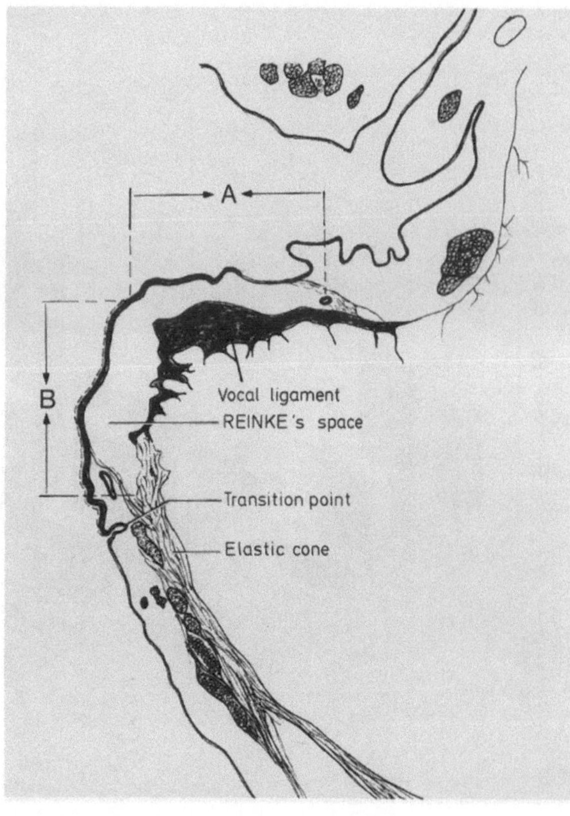

Fig. 1.8 Reinke's space and vocal ligaments in a 52-year-old man; coronal section through the middle third of a vocal cord. A: horizontal extent, B: vertical extent

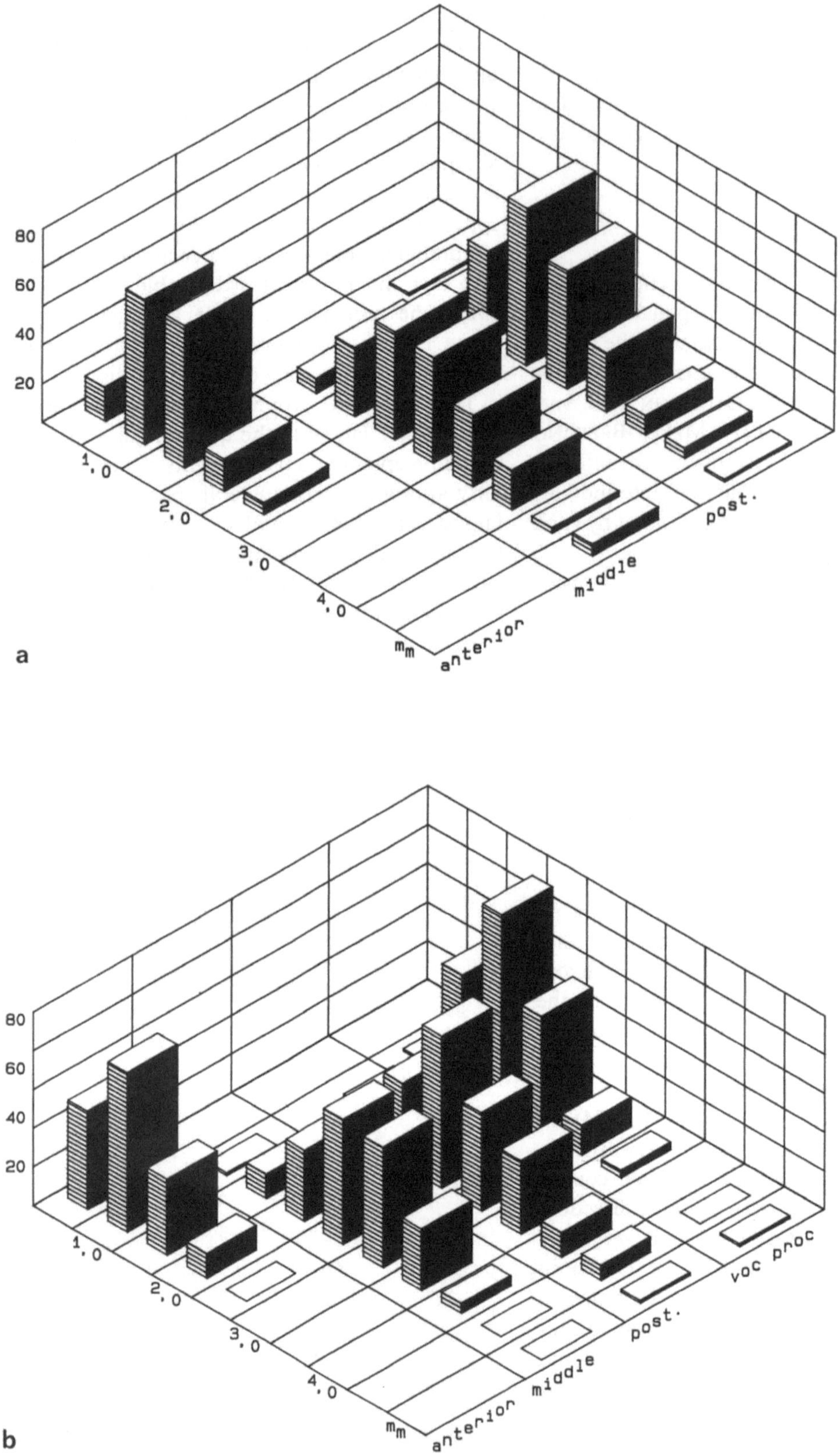

Fig. 1.9 a, b. Extent of Reinke's space in the frontal plane in 225 cases: (**1,** near anterior commissure; **2,** middle third; **3,** posterior third; **4,** vocal process (marked extension in vertical direction only). ***a*** Extent in the ventricular floor; ***b*** vertical extent from the free edge of the vocal cord in the subglottic direction

In the supraglottic direction, the paraglottic space is connected, via the aforementioned communication with the preepiglottic space, to the paraglottic space of the opposite side. Dorsocranially it impinges on the medial mucous membrane of the piriform sinus and on the lapjoint with the lateral mucous membrane. In its dorsal section, the paraglottic space is separated only incompletely from the posterior laryngeal wall and the contralateral side by parts of the laryngeal framework such as the arytenoid, corniculate and cuneiform cartilages and their associated ligaments. Here there are numerous muscular and loose connective tissue structures which favour the penetration of tumour extensions into these zones.

The **subglottic space** lies farthest caudal and has its upper boundary on the vocal ligament and the elastic cone. It reaches to the lower edge of the cricoid cartilage and from here extends continuously into the submucosal region of the trachea. There is thus no right-left barrier.

Of particular importance is the smallest of the spaces to be described here, that between the vocal fold epithelium and the vocal ligament, the abovementioned **Reinke's space**. This is a region with poor lymphatic drainage mediocranial to the vocal ligament. Its maximal extent is in a craniocaudal direction in the middle third of the vocal folds, whereas it narrows markedly towards the anterior commissure and towards the vocal processes (Fig. 1.9).

Corresponding to these spatial divisions, there is no vertical separation of the lymph drainage system of the larynx into a right and a left half, as has often been claimed, most recently by PRESSMAN et al. (1960). Such a division also clearly conflicts with our clinical experience of contralateral metastasis, even in the case of strictly unilateral tumours of the supraglottic and subglottic spaces. Only in the anterior commissure of the vocal cords is there such a separation, as a result of the aforementioned characteristics of Reinke's space. The studies carried out by WELSH et al. (1961) and BECK and MANN (1980) show that there is otherwise no separation of the two sides. In the region of the posterior wall of the larynx, in which the lymph capillaries are predominantly arranged horizontally in all regions. The same is true of the anterior part of the supraglottic and subglottic space where Beck and Mann (1980) again could not establish any vertical separation. The supraglottic part of the paraglottic space is only separated incompletely from the subglottic space by the lymphatically sluggish Reinke's space and the elastic cone, as a result of these communications through the posterior wall.

1.4.2 Regions and Sites

The anatomical regions and areas are defined for oncology according to the International Classification of Diseases (ICD-O, World Health Organization 1976, 1979). Those for laryngeal tumours correspond to the ICD-O topography numbers.

A. The larynx (161) with its supraglottic, glottic and subglottic region (Figs. 5.3, 5.5). These regions are subdivided as follows:

1. Supraglottis (161.1)
   Epilarynx, including marginal zone
   a) upper (suprahyoid) laryngeal epiglottic surface, including free epiglottic edge
   b) aryepiglottic folds
   c) arytenoid region
   Supraglottis, excluding epilarynx
   a) lower (infrahyoid) laryngeal epiglottic surface
   b) vestibular folds
   c) Morgagni's ventricle
2. Glottis (161.0)
   a) vocal cords
   b) anterior commissure
   c) posterior commissure (posterior wall)
3. Subglottis (161.2)

B. The lower, larynx-proximate section of the oropharynx (146). The latter stretches from the boundary between the soft and hard palate to the level of the valleculae. Those larynx-proximate regions of the oropharynx which are relevant as regards tumours of the larynx are:

1. The base of the tongue
2. The valleculae (146.3)
3. The lingual epiglottic surface (146.4)

C. The hypopharynx (148), which reaches from the level of the pharyngoepiglottic fold and the aryepiglottic fold to the plane of the lower edge of the cricoid lamina. It comprises the following regions:

1. The postcricoid region (148.0)
2. The piriform sinus (148.1)
3. The posterior wall of the hypopharynx (148.3)

Unfortunately, within the endolaryngeal regions there are no exactly defined boundaries; these must be constructed as horizontal planes. It is the boundary between the glottic region and the adjacent regions that poses the real problem, however. TUCKER (1974) describes the glottic region as the closable part of the rima glottidis, including the mucosa which covers it, stating that the larger part of the ventricular floor should be considered to belong to the supraglottic space. OLOFSSON and VAN NOSTRAND (1973) tend to classify the ventricular floor with the glottic region, according to the rules laid down by the UICC (1972, 1978, 1986). In so doing, they want to express the fact that in cases of transglottic carcinoma extending cranially via the ventricular floor into the supraglottic region, the primary lesion is nevertheless glottic in origin. The definition of the glottic region suggested by TUCKER (1974) is, per se, more meaningful, since this area largely corresponds to the mucosal area which lies above Reinke's space. If tumours expand to the spaces outside this region, they are subject to other conditions of lymph drainage; this necessarily alters the prognosis. Reinke's space does not have a uniform vertical extension, but is rather more spindle-shaped and thus difficult to assess. According to the international rules of classification (AJC 1972, 1977, 1983, UICC 1972, 1978, 1986), the subglottic region is delimited cranially by a plane which runs horizontally through the mucosal boundary between glottis and subglottis. It should be noted, though, that this boundary is still not exactly defined and may vary, from author to author, between 5 and 10 mm in a caudal direction from the free edge of the vocal cord. If the lymph drainage is taken into account, then this line should be placed where a glottic carcinoma can gain access to the lymph drainage of the subglottic space. This is possible from 5 mm below the free vocal cord edge, at least in the vicinity of the anterior commissure. It must further be taken into account, when using the regional classification of the AJC (1972, 1977, 1983) and the UICC (1972, 1978, 1986) that in terms of lymphatic supply the subglottic space consists of two different spaces. The whole area medial to the elastic cone and within the cricoid cartilage is drained predominantly caudally into the paratracheal lymph nodes and to a lesser extent ventrally via the cricothyroid membrane. In contrast, the soft tissue lateral to the elastic cone belongs to the paraglottic space whose lymph drainage takes place mainly in a cranial direction.

The glottic region is generally defined as the mucosal surface from the ventricular floor to the level of the transition from squamous to respiratory epithelium of the subglottis. This transition takes place, as a rule, maximally 10 mm below the free edge of the vocal cord and varies considerably from individual to individual (MEYER-BREITING and POPESCU 1986). The internationally agreed definition of the laryngeal regions does not correspond at all to the anatomical boundaries and hence to those limits relevant to tumour extension; these boundaries, however, because of their wide interindividual variability, would result in a considerably higher degree of uncertainty in clinical practice than is the case with the international classification.

In our opinion, however, the definition of a region for purposes of classification of malignant tumours should be based on prognostically relevant facts and structures. These are given by Reinke's space and the adjacent ligaments in the anterior commissure and the vocal process, in contrast to the above-mentioned situation in the supraglottic and subglottic region. In the so-called posterior commissure - better posterior wall -, the lymphatic capillary networks of the two regions are confluent; therefore, totally different conditions for the expansion and prognosis of cancer exist here than in the other parts of the glottic region. Figure 1.9 demonstrates the variability of the extent of Reinke's space. However, an analysis of several hundred larynx specimens shows that in the ventricular floor Reinke's space reaches 1-2 mm towards the lateral wall of the ventricle; this is in accordance with the opinion of OLOFSSON and NOSTRAND (1973) and LUND (1974). The vertical limit is nearly identical with the ventricular floor in each coronal section. According to the results of MEYER-BREITING and POPESCU (1986), the glottic region as a rule extends 5 mm caudally from the free edge of the vocal cords. Toward the anterior commissure this extension is reduced to 1-2 mm.

2 Particular Problems of Histological Preparation and Assessment: Advanced Methods

2.1 Whole-Organ Serial Sections

The histological preparation of whole larynges in the form of multiple serial sections is made considerably more difficult by the difference in hardness of the various tissue types in this organ, and in particular by the age-dependent ossification of cartilaginous parts of the skeleton. The detailed knowledge regarding the spread of endolaryngeal tumours that is of invaluable worth for diagnosis and therapy can be most readily gained from whole-organ sections, in which the behaviour of the tumours in relation to the different anatomical structures in the larynx is evident and more exactly discernible.

The first to use whole-organ sections to study the spreading of laryngeal carcinomas was LEROUX-ROBERT (1936). Owing to their thickness, these sections did not lend themselves to the usual methods of staining. Celloidin embedding, first used by KERNAN (1950) and subsequently taken up and improved by TUCKER (1961), is present the technique used most widely in the United States. Its disadvantages lie in the very long time required for preparation (up to 10 months) and in the section thickness of 25 μm, which sets a limit to the histological assessment. Paraffin embedding was introduced for serial section studies of the larynx by FLETCHER et al. (1954). Independently, OLOFSSON and VAN NOSTRAND (1973) employed a technique of paraffin embedding reported to them, but not published, by HYAMS at the Armed Forces Institute of Pathology, Washington DC. HOMMERICH et al. (1971, 1974) similarly preferred paraffin embedding, which offers the possibility of shorter preparation times and thinner sections. Dehydration using different concentrations of tetrahydrofuran solutions in a vacuum, as described by MCCOMB et al. (1967), has not proved of value. We prefer the method of AMTHOR and TOMASKOWITZ (1970). The main problem of paraffin embedding is decalcification. The laryngeal framework is, in the case of total extirpation of the larynx, completely surrounded by soft tissue. When using weak and strong acids, we have found that it takes so long to achieve effective decalcification that a high degree of damage is done to the tissue structure and in particular to the cell nuclei. For this reason, several authors dissect the usually formalin-fixed larynx in order to shorten the decalcification time. KLEINSASSER (1967) and GLANZ (1984) divide the extirpated larynx into vertical sectors (see below). MICHAELS and GREGOR (1980) slice the larynx in an ordinary motorized meat-slicer to horizontal sections of 4 mm thickness before histological preparation. Both methods can be recommended if histological findings of clinical relevance are to be reported as quickly as possible. According to CLAYDEN (1952), BRAIN (1966) and BANCROFT and STEVENS (1977), decalcification accelerators such as electrolysis (RICHMAN et al. 1947) or ultrasonics (THORPE et al. 1963) are encumbered with artefacts which are difficult to estimate, e.g. heat-induced structural changes, and therefore we do not use these techniques. For whole-organ sectioning, the addition of 0.5% chromic acid as recommended by PERENYI (1882) for another purpose, preserves the nuclear structure sufficiently when strong or weak acids are applied for a longer time.

Today we use the following procedure for whole-organ serial sectioning of laryngeal specimens (MEYER-BREITING and WEITH 1982): The specimens submitted are stripped of any surrounding tissue that is not suspected of containing tumour. In cases where the posterior wall has been transsected for clinical diagnostic reasons it is sutured with atraumatic catgut (size 2-0) to avoid distortion of the larynx during fixation and dehydration. During the fixation and decalcification procedure, the solutions are changed daily. For fixation, which takes 4 days, we use 4% formalin solution.

For decalcification, the following solution is used: four parts 5% nitric acid, three parts absolute alcohol, three parts 0.5% chromic acid. Decalcification takes as a rule 12 days in vacuum, but depending on size and age can take as little as 2-3 days. To

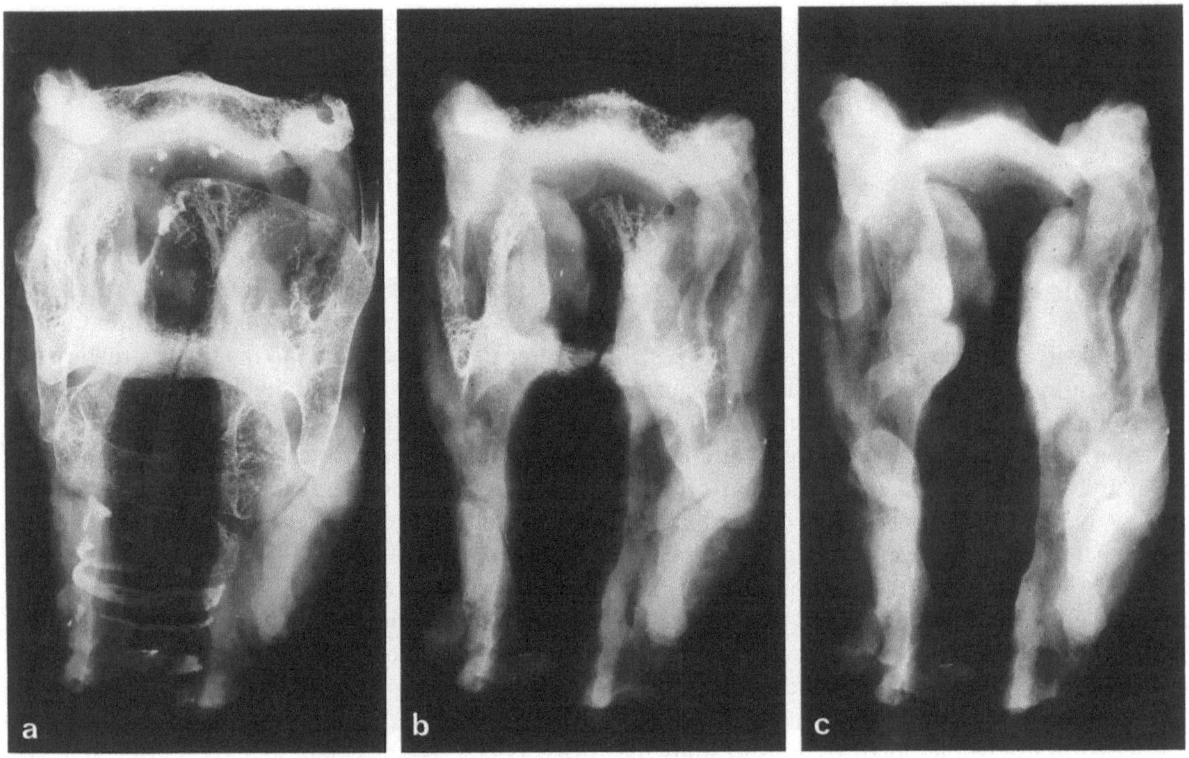

Fig. 2.1 a–c X-ray pictures of different stages of decalcification of whole larynx specimen. **a** before; **b** during (6th day); **c** after the end of decalcification (12th day). Note the main areas of ossification

gain sufficient experience, we recommend X-ray controls (Fig. 2.1). After decalcification has been completed, the specimens are washed for 24 h.

Dehydration is also performed in vacuum. Table 2.1 shows the time-course of dehydration. The specimen must be incubated in methylbenzoate for a minimum of 24 h. After a double floating test, it is transferred into benzene for 2x1 h. Thereafter, the specimen is incubated in liquid Paraplast for the times specified in the table. After this step, the larynx is embedded in Paraplast. The embedding form – a commercial plastic refrigerator container – is filled with Paraplast to twice the height of the specimen since a considerable central retraction of the Paraplast block occurs due to volume reduction. The Paraplast extending over the borders of the specimen is removed with a band saw.

Table 2.1. Timetable of the dehydration procedure in vacuum

Day	Solution	Incubation time (h)
1	Alcohol 70%	2
	Alcohol 95%	7
	Alcohol 95%	7
	Alcohol absolute	8
2	Alcohol absolute	8
	Alcohol absolute	16
3	Methylbenzoate	24
	Benzole	1
	Benzole	1
	Paraplast	8
4	Paraplast	24
	Embedding	

At the bottom of the block a fitting piece for insertion into the microtome is cut. An ordinary hand-operated sliding microtome is, in our experience, better suited for large paraffin sections than a motor-driven microtome, since the "feel" when the knife is drawn across the block is helpful. In general, D-knives should be used, inserted at an angle of 5°–7°. Rolled sections are unfolded in cold water, whereas stretching as such is done in a 50 °C water bath. The sections obtained in this manner are mounted on 10 x 6 cm glass slides which have previously been thinly coated with albumin-glycerin. Subsequently, the slides are put in horizontal position into an incubator, where they are dried at 60 °C.

Histological standards such as haematoxylin-eosin stain (HE), periodic acid-Schiff (PAS), azan and Domagk, as well as silver impregnation, can be applied to these sections in the usual manner. We use special cuvettes for this purpose (size 25 cm x 15 cm x 15 cm) and specially made slide containers. Sections with a thickness of 5 μm can be obtained in the manner described. The total time required is approximately 3½-4 weeks, depending on the size of the specimen processed.

2.2 Histological Evaluation

2.2.1 Plane of Section

Each of the main planes of the body - the horizontal, sagittal and frontal - offers itself as the section plane in laryngeal preparations. Nonetheless, each has the disadvantage that in certain regions, the tumour extensions are cut transversely and thus their relation to the main tumour is difficult to assess, i.e. in such regions the tumour spread can be correctly judged only by evaluation of serial sections. If only the basic principles of tumour spread are under discussion, KLEINSASSER's method (1967) of dividing the larynx into 8-12 vertical sectors of the total circumference of the larynx is convincing. As in the sagittal and frontal section, the plane is always coincident with the respiratory axis and clearly shows the ventral, lateral or dorsal spread of the tumour. Unfortunately, the complete representation of the outer zones of the larynx in relationship to the mucosal surface cannot be completely achieved with this method, and this poses the danger of loss of orientation. If in addition to a general assessment importance is placed on the evaluation of the larynx periphery, for example for the assessment of radiation or chemotherapeutic effects, a technique is necessary which permits the complete preparation of the total tissue section.

Laryngeal tumours spread predominantly in a vertical direction. The region of the vocal fold and vestibular ligaments is arranged in a sagittal direction so that a tumour in this area extends mainly laterally and less often circularly or radially. The sagittal section plane can only depict the tumour spread from the mucosal surface into the depth on the anterior commissure and on the posterior laryngeal wall, whereas the more meaningful, lateral extension and its relationship to the mucosal surface cannot be discerned. A similar situation prevails in the case of the horizontal section technique which in any one section is not capable of showing the relationship to the vertical extent of tumour growth.

As a result of these considerations, we decided upon the frontal plane of section, which is preferably termed the "coronal section" (TUCKER 1971). This plane has the following advantages:

1. The complete larynx can be processed, without loss of material.
2. The plane of section corresponds with the respiratory axis, the direction in which most endolaryngeal tumours spread.
3. This plane of section permits an overview of all parts of the larynx and also a comparison between the affected and the nonaffected side.
4. The results gained can be compared directly with those of numerous international authors.

Figures 2.2-2.5 show the frontal sections in four different regions of a normal larynx. For further detailed studies on the normal larynx we recommend TUCKER's Atlas of Coronal Sections (1971).

Other section planes may prove more useful in answering particular questions, for example in the assessment of the behaviour of carcinomas of the glottic and subglottic anterior wall. For comparative studies of laryngeal sections and computer tomographic pictures we choose horizontal sections conforming to the planes used in the method of X-ray diagnosis (MEYER-BREITING et al. 1982).

2.2.2 Grading

The TNM classification of malignant neoplasms which has come to be in general use today brings with it the danger that no or insufficient importance is ascribed to their histological behaviour (HARRISON 1979). The impression is too readily gained that use of the term "squamous cell carcinoma", by far the most common carcinoma in the laryngeal region, implies uniform behaviour. HANSEMANN, as early as 1890, pointed out that in the cytogenesis of carcinoma cells, anaplastic transformation - characterized by loss of specialized function and of morphological features and increase of uncontrolled proliferation - occurs to different extents.

Accordingly, BRODERS (1920, 1921, 1922) developed a grading of carcinomas which indicates the degree of differentiation, taking into account the

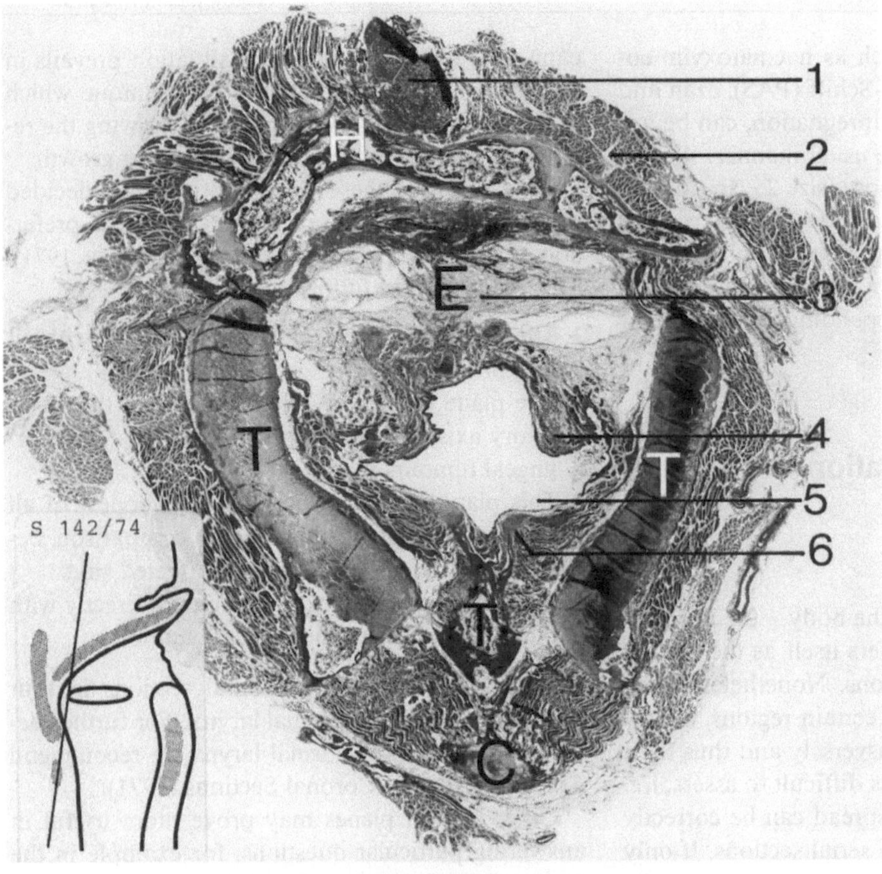

Fig. 2.2 Typical coronal section through a normal larynx immediately behind the anterior commissure. *1*, aberrant goitre; *2*, base of tongue; *3*, preepiglottic space; *4*, ventricular fold; *5*, Morgagni's ventricle; *6*, vocal cord; *H*, hyoid bone; *E*, epiglottis; *T*, thyroid cartilage; *C*, cricoid cartilage

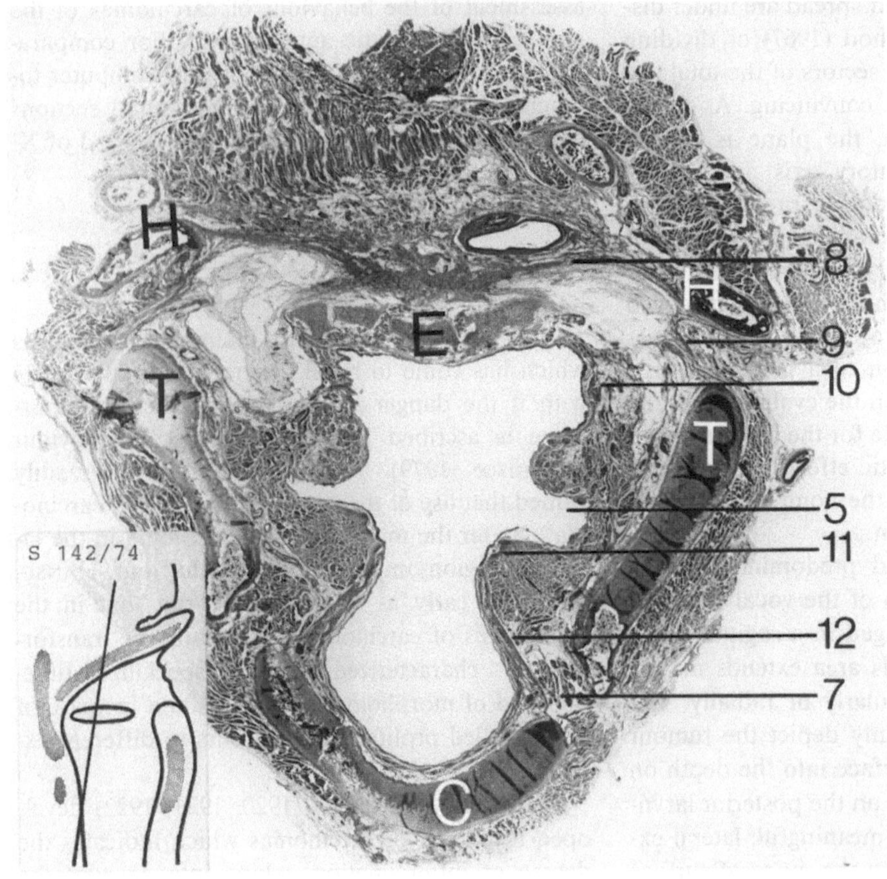

Fig. 2.3 Typical coronal section through the middle part of vocal cords of a normal larynx: *8*, hyoepiglottic ligament; *9*, thyrohyoid membrane; *10*, quadrangular membrane; *5*, Morgagni's ventricle; *11*, vocal ligament; *12*, elastic cone; *7*, cricothyroid membrane; *H*, hyoid bone; *E*, epiglottis; *T*, thyroid cartilage; *C* cricoid cartilage

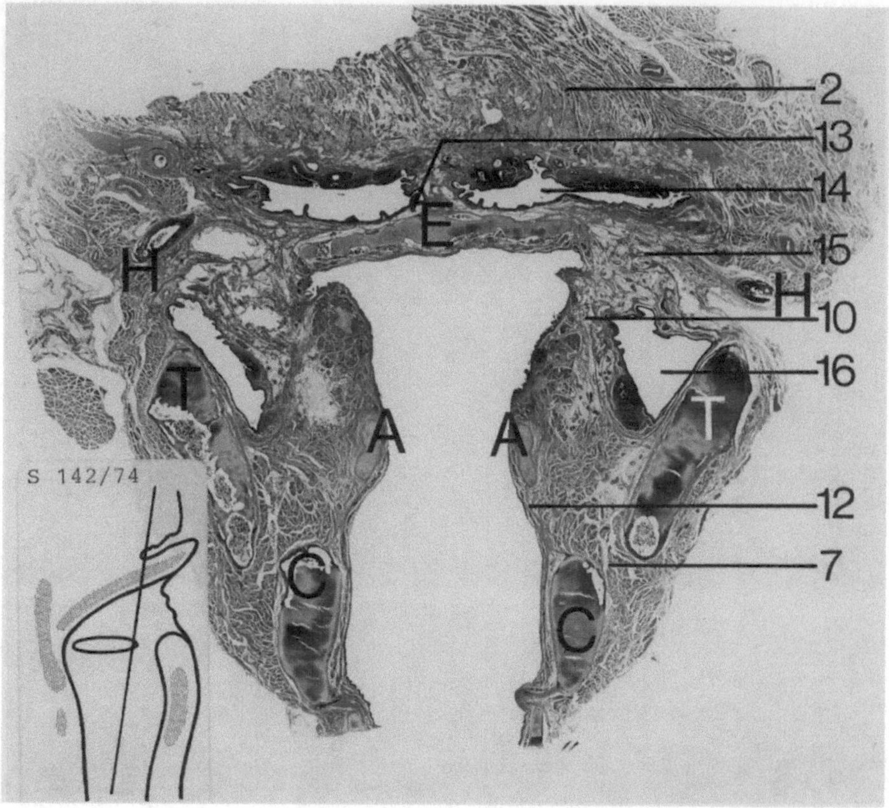

Fig. 2.4 Typical coronal section of a normal larynx through the vocal process of the arytenoid cartilage. *2*, base of tongue; *13*, medial glossoepiglottic fold; *14*, vallecula; *15*, lateral glossoepiglottic fold; *10*, quadrangular membrane; *16*, piriform sinus; *12*, elastic cone; *7*, cricothyroid membrane; *H*, hyoid bone; *E*, epiglottis; *T*, thyroid cartilage; *C*, cricoid cartilage

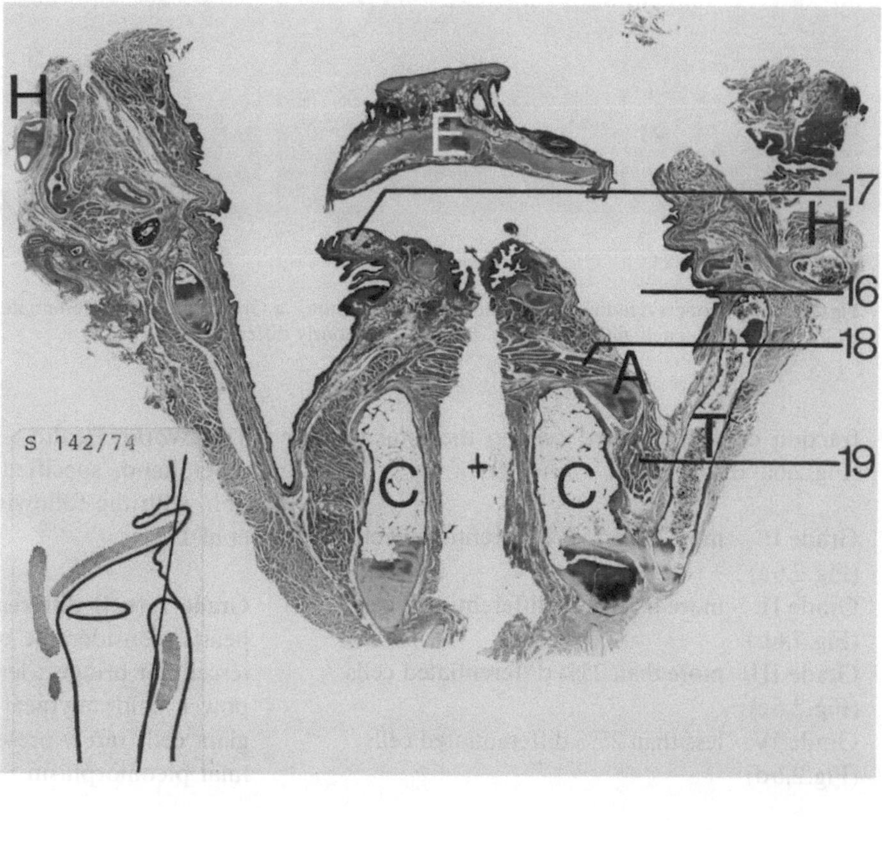

Fig. 2.5 Typical coronal section through the posterior wall of a normal larynx: *17*, aryepiglottic fold; *16*, piriform sinus; *18*, interarytenoid muscles; *19*, lateral cricoarytenoid muscle; *H*, hyoid bone; *E*, epiglottis; *T*, thyroid cartilage; *A*, arytenoid cartilage; *C*, cricoid cartilage

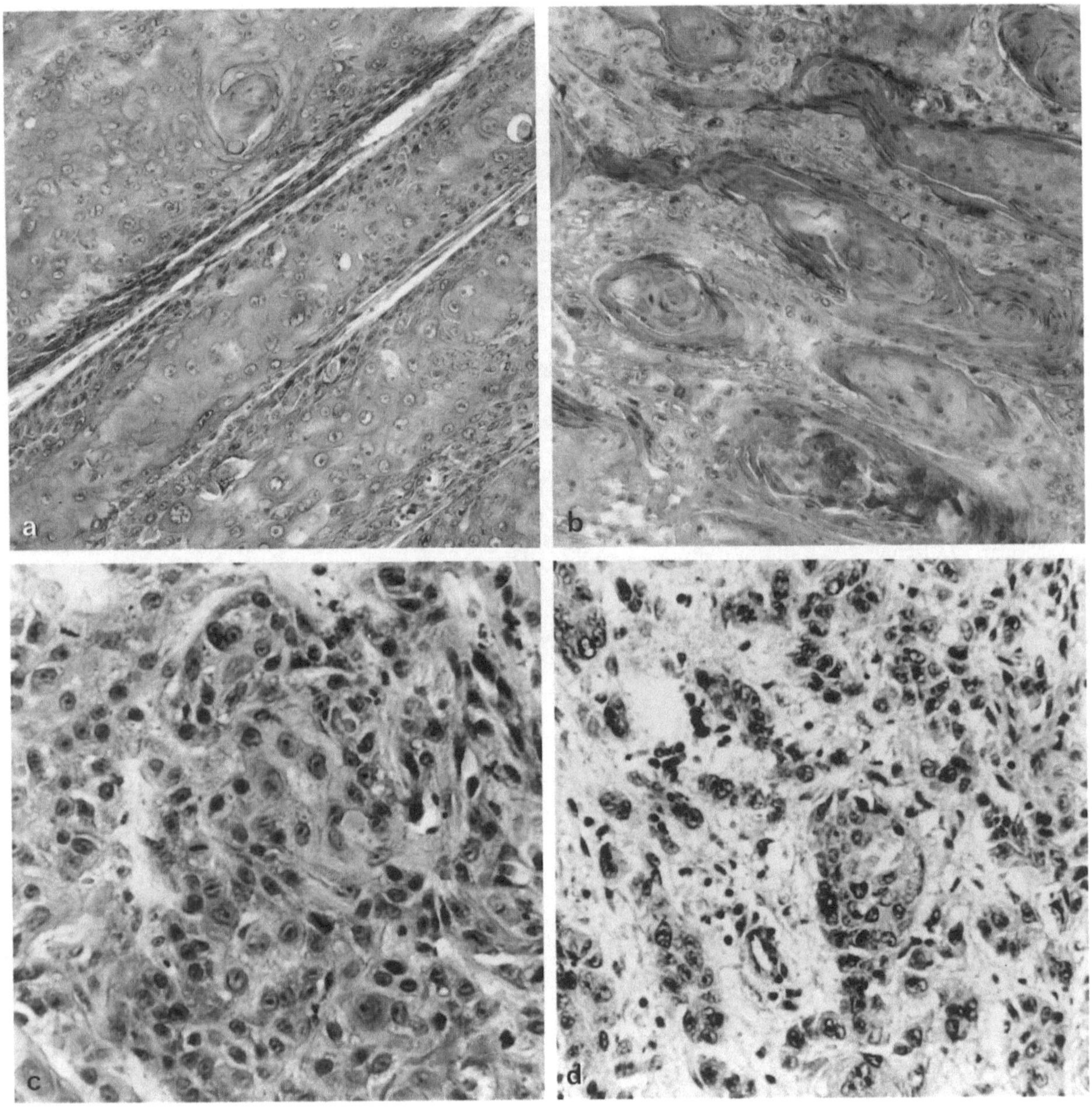

Fig. 2.6a–d. Broders' grading of squamous cell carcinoma. **a** Grade I, highly differentiated; **b** Grade II, well differentiated; **c** Grade III, moderately differentiated; **d** Grade IV, poorly differentiated

fraction of differentiated cells in the total tumour (Fig. 2.6a–d):

Grade I: more than 75% differentiated cells (Fig. 2.6a)
Grade II: more than 50% differentiated cells (Fig. 2.6b)
Grade III: more than 25% differentiated cells (Fig. 2.6c)
Grade IV: less than 25% differentiated cells (Fig. 2.6d)

The World Health Organization (WHO), on the other hand, specified three grades of differentiation, with the following histological criteria (Wahi et al. 1971):

Grade I (well differentiated). Numerous epithelial pearls; considerable cellular keratinization with intercellular bridges; less than two mitoses per high-power field; atypical mitoses and multinucleated giant cells rarely present; minimal nuclear and cellular pleomorphism

Grade II (moderately differentiated). Epithelial pearls infrequent or even absent; neither keratinization of individual cells nor presence of intercellular bridges conspicuous; two to four mitoses per high-power field with occasional atypical mitoses; moderate pleomorphism of cells and nuclei; multinucleated giant cells infrequent

Grade III (poorly differentiated). Epithelial pearls rarely seen; negligible cellular keratinization and no intercellular bridges; more than four mitoses per high-power field with frequent atypical mitoses; marked cellular and nuclear pleomorphism; frequent multinucleated giant cells

The borderlines between the individual categories of this WHO grading system, which has come to be widely accepted in Europe, are not as sharply defined as in Broders' system with its clear quantitative framework. The problems encountered in the determination of tumour differentiation will be discussed in more detail below (Chap. 5).

The grading criteria of Broders and of the WHO rest solely on the cellular differentiation of a carcinoma, and do not take into account the tumour-host relationship, i.e. the growth form of the tumour, its capacity to infiltrate vessels and nerves (Fig. 2.7a-d) and the cellular reaction of the host organism. For this reason there have been repeated attempts to complement or substitute these grading systems by others which include criteria of tumour-host relationship. McGavran et al. (1961) divided squamous cell carcinomas into a more "pushing" type and an "infiltrating" type. Kashima (1976) made further subdivisions of this group into "pushing", "clubbing", "shattering", "splintering" and "infiltrating". These authors observed that carcinomas with disseminated infiltrative and destructive growth had a significantly higher rate of metastatic spread into the regional lymph nodes than carcinomas of the pushing type. For their method of grading, Jakobsson et al. (1973) evaluated, in addition to four characteristics of the tumour cell population, a further four criteria intended to take the tumour-host relationship into consideration:

1. The mode of invasion, similar to the classification by McGavran et al. (1961)
2. The stage of invasion
3. The extent of vascular invasion
4. The cellular response (lymphoplasmocytic), i.e. the capacity of the host organism to react to the tumour

Each of the eight criteria is assigned a score between 1 and 4 according to intensity: by addition a total score is determined (Table 2.2). A score exceeding 20 indicates poor differentiation and high malignancy.

Table 2.2. Jakobsson's histological grading of malignancy (Jakobsson et al. 1973)

	Scoring of features 1	2	3	4
A. Tumor cell population				
Structure	Papillary and solid cords	Strands	Small cords and groups of cells	Marked cellular dissociation
Differentiation	High, well keratinized	Moderate, some keratin	Poor, minimum keratin	Poor, no keratin
Nuclear polymorphism	Few enlarged nuclei	Moderate number of enlarged nuclei	Numerous irregular enlarged nuclei	Anaplastic immature, enlarged nuclei
Mitoses	Single	Moderate number	High number	Numerous
B. Tumor-host relationship				
Mode of invasion	Well-defined border	Cords, less marked border	Groups of cells, no distinct border	Diffuse growth
Stage of invasion	Possible	Microcarcinoma (few cords)	Nodular into connective tissue	Massive
Vascular invasions	None	Possible	Few obvious	Numerous
Cellular response (plasmolymphocytic)	Marked	Moderate	Slight	None

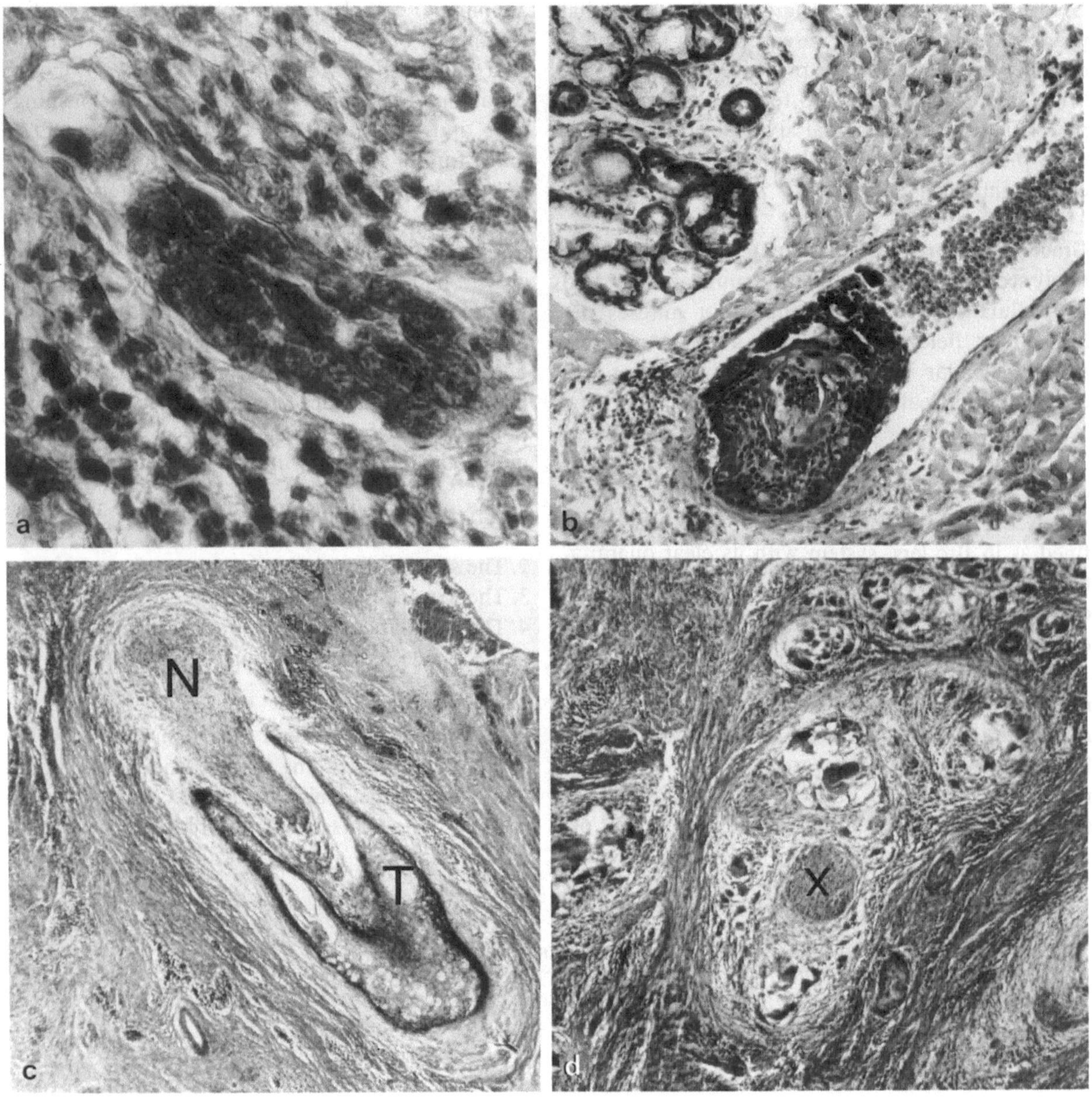

Fig. 2.7a-d. Infiltration of particular forms of connective tissue. **a** Cluster of poorly differentiated tumour cells filling out a capillary. **b** Venous vessel infiltrated by a moderately differentiated squamous cell carcinoma. **c** Nerve *(N)* partially enveloped by tumour tissue *(T)* which has infiltrated the perineurium. **d** Preoperatively irradiated squamous cell carcinoma which has nearly completely destroyed a nerve, with one last fascicle *(x)* remaining. The tumour inside and outside the nerve shows radiation-induced vacuolization and necrosis

LÖBE and QUADE (1982) reduced these criteria to three parameters of the tumour cells (grade of differentiation, nuclear pleomorphism, rate of mitosis) and the stromal reaction. In the same manner as JAKOBSSON et al. (1973) these criteria were assigned to have a score between 1 and 4, and from the total score, the malignancy was established as one of three grades (4-8 = grade I; 9-11 = grade II; 12-16 = grade III). On the basis of statistical evaluation of his material, GLANZ (1984) reduced the number of tumour properties to be assessed to four, weighting the score for the grade of differentiation and the structure of the tumour-host boundary more heavily than the invasion of nerves and vessels and the degree of round cell infiltration at the tumour host boundary (Table 2.3). All the methods of grading described will be discussed in more detail below.

Table 2.3. Histological grading establishing the malignancy index (GLANZ 1984)

Parameter		Score	Grading
I	Differentiation and polymorphism of the tumour	1	Marked keratinization with or without polymorphism
		2	Moderate keratinization with or without polymorphism
		3	Little or no keratinization with or without polymorphism
II	Structure and border of the tumour	1	Solid or compact cell formation with well-defined pushing borders
		2	Small strands and tumour cell cords partially with ill-defined borders
		3	Dissociation of the tumour cells and diffuse infiltration
III	Vascular and perineural invasion	0	Invasion, not proved
		1	Possible invasion
		2	Proved invasion
IV	Cellular response of the host	0	Marked
		1	Moderate
		2	Poor or missing
	Maximal total score	10	

2.3 Advanced Methods in the Evaluation of Precancerous Lesions and Carcinomas

As will be described in Chap. 4, over the past few years there have been considerable advances in the clinical and histological definition of precancerous lesions in the larynx. The term "dysplasia" combines features of deviations from the norm, the extent of which permits a grading (mild, moderate, severe).

Established carcinomas have different biological potentials of aggressiveness. Attempts to define this by histological grading were summarized in Sect. 2.2.2 and will be discussed in Sect. 5.4.

Grading of dysplasia and carcinomas, however, has remained subjective and while statistically clearly related to prognosis its value for the individual patient is controversial.

In recent years many attempts have been made to solve this problem by the application of advanced methods going beyond simple light microscopic histology. Some of these techniques are still largely based on cytological and histological preparations (Table 2.4) while others employ chemical and functional analyses (Table 2.5). BURKHARDT (1985) has recently summarized the results of these studies on oral mucosal lesions. Here an overview with special reference to findings in laryngeal precancerous lesions and carcinomas is given and in addition results from studies on other mucosal lesions will be considered.

Table 2.4. Advanced methods for cytological and histological evaluation of premalignant lesions and carcinomas

Exfoliative and aspiration cytology
Micronucleus test
Quantification of histopathology
Computer-aided studies
Stereological techniques
Histochemistry
Histochemical stains
Enzyme histochemistry
Immunohistochemistry
Surface antigens
Intracellular components/products
Basement membrane zone
Stromal changes (inflammatory reaction)
In situ hybridization (RNA/DNA)
Electron microscopy (transmission, scanning)
Viral/fungal infection
Differentiation

Table 2.5. Advanced methods for functional evaluation of premalignant lesions and carcinomas

Cellular proliferation studies
DNA histograms/cytophotometry
Analysis of immune status
Systemic
Local
Biochemical studies
Tissue homogenates
Body fluids
Analysis of circulating cell products or reaction products
Examination of living tissue
In vivo
In vitro
Experimental models

2.3.1 Predominantly Morphological Methods

2.3.1.1 Exfoliative and Aspiration Cytology

In principle, **cytological smears** can also be obtained from the larynx. Their reliability, however, is limited by pronounced accompanying inflammation and is dependent upon a well-conducted technique (FRANZ and NEUMANN 1978). Cytological smear preparations are divided into five groups:

Group I	No atypia
Group II	Cells deviating from the norm, associated with inflammation
Group III	Dyskaryosis, nuclear atypia and signs of keratinization
Group IV	Atypical cells suggesting malignancy
Group V	Severe cellular atypia

SCHAUER et al. (1973) and HERMANN et al. (1973) were able to document a good correlation between histology and cytology in a parallel study of 300 and 390 cases respectively. LUNDGREN et al. (1981) report, from a prospective study of 350 cases, a positive cytological finding in 157 of 190 lesions involving dysplasia, carcinoma in situ or invasive carcinomas (83%) and a negative finding in 134 of 160 benign changes (84%). Nonetheless, both groups reported one case in which the cytological examination revealed a malignant process which was overlooked histologically. Other authors, too, reported a high proportion of false-negative results (WHITACKER and SIEGLER 1956, FRABLE and FRABLE 1968, THOMSEN et al. 1975, 1976, FRÜHWALD 1979). In addition, the inability to distinguish between severe dysplasia and invasive carcinoma (BICHLER et al. 1985) limits the value of this method. One advantage of the cytological examination is that smears from larger mucosal areas can be taken; it is thus highly suitable for monitoring larger, extensive mucosal lesions in "field cancerization" (BICHLER et al. 1985). No surgical procedure is necessary, and smears can be repeated without limitations; in addition diagnosis of some infectious conditions is possible.

Nevertheless, cytological examination cannot replace a biopsy or, in the case of extensive lesions, "stripping" with subsequent histological examination and thus better assessment and much higher safety.

There have been several attempts to improve the evaluation of exfoliative cytology by additional techniques, like measurement of DNA (Feulgen), assessment of nuclear area, the micronucleus test or immunocytological methods (review: BURKHARDT 1984). No results on laryngeal mucosa have been obtained until now.

In contrast to exfoliative cytology, aspiration cytology has proven valuable in the diagnosis of solid tumours of the laryngeal region.

2.3.1.2 Quantification of Histopathology

KRAMER and coworkers (1969, 1970 a+b, 1980) used a computer-aided discriminant analysis of histological features on different lesions of the oral mucosa. This combines the ability of the pathologist to recognize tissue features with the potential of the computer for pattern recognition (KRAMER 1969). By this method the presence of abnormal mitotic figures, disturbances in the polarity of the basal cells, nuclear hyperchromatism, enlarged nucleoli, cellular pleomorphism, intraepithelial keratinization and the presence of Russell bodies were identified as indicating malignant potential. However, the quality of such evaluations is dependent on the recognition of the features by the pathologist.

Stereological or two-dimensional **morphometry techniques** using light and electron-microscopy have made it possible to measure various parameters in tissues (review: FRANKLIN et al. 1980). In an experimental study on oral carcinogenesis, FRANKLIN and coworkers (1980) found three histological features which were best able to distinguish between benign and premalignant lesions: increases in the nuclear/cytoplasmic ratio, the numerical density of nuclei and the area of the epithelial/mesenchymal interface.

GRÖNTOFT et al. (1978) measured nuclear size in laryngeal lesions. The mean nuclear area for normal, dysplastic and carcinomatous epithelial cells was 48, 41 and 73 μm^2 respectively. The higher the degree of dysplasia displayed by the cells, the greater was the variability of nuclear size. In contrast, no difference between the nuclear areas of normal and keratotic epithelia was found, while two of three epithelia displaying hyperplasia showed slightly elevated values (HELLQUIST and OLOFSSON 1981). The authors concluded that neither hyperplasia nor keratosis alone could be considered premalignant. A differentiated approach was used by OLDE KALTER and coauthors (1985) in measuring the nuclei of 50 cells in the basal, intermediate and superficial cell layers of epithelial hyperplasia with and without dysplasia and carcinoma in situ of the larynx. They determined nuclear area, nuclear contour index, polarity, nuclear crowding and epithelial width. It was easy to separate lesions with and without dysplasia on the basis of mean nuclear area and nuclear polarity, and further classification by discriminant analysis was able to distinguish two grades of dysplasia and carcinoma in situ. The results correlated with conventional histological assessment. A subsequent retrospective study (OLDE KALTER et al. 1986) of 38 untreated patients with dysplastic lesions showed that they could be divided into a group with a favourable course (n=21) and a group with an unfavourable course, i.e. development of carcinoma (n=17). Using five morphometric parameters in linear discriminant analysis, 79% of the cases in the two groups could be correctly classified. In particular, nuclear area in the superficial layer, nuclear crowding in the basal and superficial layers and nuclear pleomorphism (nuclear contour index) in the basal layer were increased in lesions of the patients with an unfavourable outcome. The fifth parameter - nuclear anisokaryosis in the basal layer - was less clearly correlated to poor prognosis. The authors propose additional morphometric study in cases with epithelial dysplasia to separate those at risk.

A number of parameters measured by these methods are estimated quite easily by the human eye during routine diagnostic work. However, it seems possible that quantification will play some part in routine diagnosis in the future.

2.3.1.3 *Histochemistry*

Simple **histochemistry**, i.e. the application of different stain reactions to tissue slides, has become part of routine histology. The PAS stain, for instance, may reveal a loss of glycogen in the epithelium of premalignant lesions, the presence or absence of the basement membrane and the colonization of the epithelium by Candida hyphae. Silver stains also show a thinning or loss of the basement membrane; collagen stains (Masson trichrome, van Gieson), a loss of collagen (due, for example, to high activity of collagenase; see below) in precancerous and cancerous lesions.

Using **enzyme histochemistry**, metabolic activities of malignant and premalignant cells differing from those of the tissue of origin can be demonstrated (Table 2.6). Both qualitative (presence, raised or lowered activity, changes in isoenzyme pattern) and quantitative evaluation are possible. The results of relevant studies of this kind (mainly on oral mucosal lesions) have been summarized by JOHNSON and coworkers (1980).

Table 2.6. Changes in the activity of major enzymes in premalignant lesions and carcinomas

Enzyme	Important for	Epithelial hyperplasia with no dysplasia	Lesions with dysplasia	Carcinoma
Succinate dehydrogenase	Oxidative phosphorylation	↓	↓	↓
Lactate dehydrogenase	Glycolytic pathway	↑	↑	↑↑
Glucose-6-phosphate dehydrogenase	Pentose phosphate shunt	↑↓	↑↑	↑↑/↓
5'-Nucleotidase	Hydrolysis	↑↑	↓	↓↓
Acid phosphatase	Hydrolysis	↑	↑	↑↑
Collagenase (in the stroma)	Collagen degradation			↑↑

One fundamental metabolic change in many premalignant and malignant cells is a shift from predominantly aerobic respiration (oxidative phosphorylation) to predominantly anaerobic glycolysis.

Few studies have been carried out on the changes in enzymatic activities in laryngeal mucosal lesions. The results are consistent with studies on other epithelial premalignant and malignant lesions. GOLABEK and SZYSZKO (1984) demonstrated an increase in total lactate dehydrogenase (LDH) activity and cathodic shift of the isoenzyme pattern in basal and parabasal cells of laryngeal carcinomas, and also considerable changes in the adjacent mucosa.

QUADE and LÖBE (1984) attempted an enzyme-histochemical grading of 146 laryngeal and pharyngeal carcinomas. The activity of the key enzyme of the tricarboxylic acid (Krebs) cycle, succinate dehydrogenase (SDH), was found to be low, but no correlation with survival of the patients could be demonstrated. NADH-cytochrome-c-reductase, also important for oxidative phosphorylation, exhibited nonhomogeneous distribution and no correlation to survival. LDH, which is an important enzyme of glycolysis (the Embden-Meyerhof pathway), showed considerable variation in its activity. Important is the fact that low activity was statistically significantly more often associated with a better 3-year survival than high activity. Glucose-6-phosphate dehydrogenase (G6PD), an enzyme involved in the pentose phosphate pathway of glycolysis, showed considerable variations, but patients with good prognosis were found to have lower activities in tumour tissue than those with a bad prognosis - this was also statistically significant.

As could be expected, both LDH and G6PD exhibited higher activities in poorly differentiated carcinomas (grade 3) than in carcinomas of grades 1 and 2. For patients with low activities of both enzymes 3-year survival was over 90%, for the group with high enzyme activities it was less than 20%. However, in 20% of the group there was no correlation of the activities of these two enzymes.

HEYDEN (1974) claimed that by means of a modified method for demonstrating the activity of G6PD in an atmosphere saturated with oxygen, he was able to selectively identify malignant epithelial cells. He reported that this metabolic "atypia" precedes morphological dysplasia in experimental oral carcinogenesis. However, more recent studies carried out by other investigators have been less conclusive (JOHNSON et al. 1980, EVANS et al. 1983).

Besides enzymes engaged in energy metabolism, activities of hydrolytic (mostly lysosomal) enzymes may also be altered in premalignant and malignant tissues. An increased production of lysosomal enzymes by tumour cells may be related to their invasive capacity.

The activity of **acid phosphatase**, normally found in the keratinizing layers of the epithelium (GARDNER 1965), is often increased in carcinoma cells (QUADE and LÖBE 1984).

Collagenase activity in the stroma of carcinomas is most often very pronounced (ABRAMSON et al. 1975, LIOTTA et al. 1980, 1983). This may correlate with an enhanced loss of collagen. The source of the enzyme (epithelium and/or stromal cells?) is not yet clear. Part of the enzyme activity may be due to tumour cell necrosis; however, collagenolytic activity resulting from lysosomal collagenase has a pH optimum at 6.0-6.5 (see Chap. 5), whereas collagenase activity in the vicinity of vital tumour has a optimum at 7.0-7.8 pH (MEYER-BREITING and WILZ 1988).

Gamma-glutamyl transpeptidase (GGT) is a membrane-associated enzyme normally not present in mature squamous epithelium which can, however, be demonstrated in lesions with dysplasia and in carcinomas of the oral, pharyngeal and laryngeal mucosa (CALDERON-SOLT and SOLT 1985), and also in nondysplastic epithelium of patients at high risk of developing cancer in these regions. The diagnostic value of this test must be further evaluated in controlled studies.

Although the use of enzyme histochemistry for routine purposes has repeatedly been proposed (HEYDEN et al. 1974, MAGNUSSON et al. 1974), these techniques have not been generally accepted as having a place in tumour diagnosis. This is due to the great work load involved in such tests (unfixed tissue and special transport media are necessary), marked regional tissue variations, and the discouraging sensitivity of the reactions to a variety of factors such as duration of transport and unreliability. These difficulties and the success of immunohistochemistry probably account for an apparent loss of interest in enzyme histochemistry. No practical diagnostic test is available.

2.3.1.4 Immunohistochemistry

This technique has become enormously important in recent years. The development was made possible by improvements of methods (immunofluorescence, immunoperoxidase and avidin-biotin complex techniques) which allow for application of certain tests to paraffin sections of fixed tissue. Also the production of highly specific antibodies, especially monoclonals, has contributed to the wide use of these techniques. However, it should be borne in mind that immunohistochemical results have to be regarded with great caution until the reliability of a given test is well established. Control of results is particularly difficult in immunohistochemistry, the

Table 2.7. Antigenic constituents examined by immunohistochemistry in precancerous lesions and carcinomas

Epithelial surface antigens
Blood group antigen A + B + H
Blood group antigen precursors
Lectin binding (nonimmunological)
Ca-antigen
β-2-Microglobulin
Intracellular components/products
Cytokeratin/keratin subunits
Actin microfilaments
Tissue polypeptide antigen
Virus-coded products
Oncofetal antigens/CEA
Constituents of the basement membrane zone
Laminin
Type IV collagen
Fibronectin
Stromal changes
Procollagen
Immunocompetent cells
Immunoglobulins

Table 2.8. Surface antigens of squamous epithelium: reaction patterns and limitations of the methods

"Marker"	Normal mucosa	Dysplasia	Carcinoma	Limitations
Blood group antigens	Cell surface of cells above basal cells	Loss and patchy distribution		Individual variations Loss in wound healing – cellular locomotion – lichen erosivus – irradiation False-negative results False-positive results
Blood group antigen precursors	Cell surface of basal and suprabasal cells	Accumulation in all cell layers	Irregular distribution	Not yet sufficiently studied
Lectin binding	Cell surface of all epithelial layers	Loss of binding with increase in severity of dysplasia	Loss of binding	Partial loss and changes in wound healing and cellular locomotion
Ca-antigen	Negative	Variation	Positive staining in majority of cases	Negative reactions in carcinomas Positive reactions in inflammatory lesions
β-2-Microglobulin	Cell surface of all epithelial layers	Partial loss	Loss	False-negative results False-positive results Not yet sufficiently studied

Table 2.9. Intracellular antigenic constituents and products of squamous epithelium: reaction patterns and limitations of the methods

"Marker"	Normal mucosa	Dysplasia	Carcinoma	Limitations
Keratin (large subunits)	Basal cells negative (thickening of keratin-negative basal cell compartment in hyperplasia)	Positive basal cells	Irregular distribution	Not diagnostic as such
Actin filaments	Basal cell layer positive	Increase in basal cells	Increase in invasive cell groups	Increase in wound healing and cellular locomotion
Virus-coded products (HPV)		Superficial cell layer positive		Questionable significance as of now
Carcinoembryonic antigen	–	–	–	Artefact due to cross-reacting antigens

more so as an increasing number of researchers, inexperienced in the field, make indiscriminate use of the methods without the necessary controls and criticism.

The aim of most immunohistochemical studies has been to determine **tumour-associated antigenic constituents**, in other words, to find a specific "tumour marker". The investigations have been focused on epithelial surface antigens, intracellular products, constituents of the basement membrane zone and changes in the adjacent tissue, including the so-called stromal reaction (Table 2.7). Most work has been done on organs other than the laryngeal mucosa (uterine cervix, urinary bladder, skin lesions, oral mucosa; review and relevant literature: Burkhardt 1985). A summary of the results on premalignant lesions and carcinomas is given in Tables 2.8 to 2.10. The demonstration of viral structural antigens in papillomas and the vicinity of laryngeal carcinomas will be discussed in Chaps. 3 and 4.

For the evaluation of laryngeal dysplasia and

Table 2.10. Antigenic constituents of the basement membrane zone and subepithelial tissue: reaction patterns and limitations of the methods

"Marker"	Normal mucosa	Dysplasia	Carcinoma	Limitations
Laminin	Linear staining of basement membrane zone		Loss of polar deposition Focal accumulation	Not diagnostic as such
Type IV collagen	Linear staining of basement membrane zone		Loss of polar deposition Focal accumulation	Not diagnostic as such
Fibronectin	Network in the basement membrane zone	Breaks and fragmentation	Breaks and fragmentation	Not diagnostic as such
Procollagen	Staining of sub-epithelial tissue	Increase in amount	Increase	Not diagnostic as such

early invasive carcinomas VISSER et al. (1986) used the immunohistological demonstration of intrinsic components of the basement membrane (type IV collagen and laminin). As in other mucosal areas there was a continuous basement membrane containing both elements beneath normal, hyperplastic and dysplastic epithelium, while irregular discontinuities were found in some cases of carcinoma in situ and invasive carcinoma. Such discontinuities were also observed in areas with inflammatory infiltration.

The **local stromal reaction** has been the subject of much speculation, particularly with regard to its role in immunological defence reactions against precancerous and cancerous lesions. Numerous studies have shown a statistical correlation between a marked stromal reaction and a favourable prognosis for patients with malignant tumours of various types, thus forming one of the main bases of the immunosurveillance concept (UNDERWOOD 1974). Immunohistochemical methods combined with electron microscopy have made it possible to study details of changes in cellular infiltrates within the epithelium and the connective tissue of oral lesions (BURKHARDT 1980, 1984). Results obtained mainly on oral mucosal lesions can be briefly summarized as follows:

An overall increase in the number of immunocompetent cells correlating with the degree of dysplasia and differentiation of carcinomas was found. Lymphocytes - predominantly T-cells (OKT8/Leu-2a positive, corresponding to suppressor/cytotoxic cells) - appear in the epithelial/tumoral components and in the adjacent stroma. Plasma cells producing IgG and/or IgA accumulate in the connective tissue. So do - in certain cases - Russell bodies. In the epithelial component typical Langerhans cells are less numerous and exhibit a reduction of their complex dendritic network.

Investigations by MÜNZEL and MEISTER (1976) confirmed that in laryngeal lesions too, epithelial hyperplasia and dysplasia are associated with an increase of inflammatory cells. GRUNDMANN (1973) observed signs of tumour regression and lack of mitotic figures in the vicinity of a dense inflammatory cellular infiltrate. DANIELSON and FRANKLIN (1984) demonstrated plasma cells containing mainly IgG and to a lesser degree IgA and IgM in the stroma of laryngeal carcinomas. RABIN et al. (1984) and HARABUCHI et al. (1985) in series of head and neck carcinomas including five and nine laryngeal carcinomas respectively, were able to show that the majority of lymphocytes present were T-cells (suppressor/killer and helper), with very few B-lymphocytes and natural killer cells.

As this short summary has exemplified, immunohistochemistry is a very promising field of research which has contributed much to our understanding of tissue alterations in relation to malignant tumours. However, as far as the assessment of premalignant lesions and carcinomas is concerned, results so far are disappointing; no test is available for routine use. The fact that most methods necessitate the use of frozen sections of unfixed tissue limits their applicability.

2.3.1.5 In Situ Hybridization

Single-stranded nucleic acids have a tendency to form double-stranded helices (hybrids) with nucleotides in complementary sequence. The use of radioactively labelled nucleic acids makes it possible to demonstrate viral DNA or RNA in situ in tissue sections (see Sect. 4.2). However, due to the occurrence of intervening repetitive sequences in nucleic acids of different species, false-positive results may be obtained, and the in situ hybridization technique should be corroborated by molecular hybridization.

2.3.1.6 Electron Microscopy

Electron microscopy can give insight into the ultrastructural details of cellular differentiation in epithelial tissues, demonstrate viral or fungal infection and reveal immunological phenomena.

The ultrastructure of laryngeal precancerous lesions with and without dysplasia and squamous cell carcinomas has been the subject of a number of studies (SUGAR and FARAGO 1966, SCHENK and KONRAD 1979, SCHENK 1980 a+b, 1981, 1983). The results correlate well with observations on oral leukoplakia without or with dysplasia and on squamous cell carcinomas summarized in monographs by BURKHARDT (1980) and BANOCZY (1982).

Ultrastructurally, epithelial hyperplasia without dysplasia is characterized by a higher degree of differentiation (prosoplasia) or "metaplastic keratosis" imitating epidermal structures (Table 2.11). Typical are also a multilamellar basement membrane, increased numbers of tonofibrils with "premature keratosis", and the formation of "keratin pools" due to a disturbance of the desquamation of the keratin lamellae.

Lesions with dysplasia and carcinomas show common features in different degrees (Table 2.12). Nuclei and nucleoli are enlarged (Fig. 2.8). Anomalies of the cell surface are most conspicuous, and are expressed by a deficient formation of the base-

Table 2.11. Ultrastructural characteristics of hyperplasia of squamous epithelium without dysplasia

Nucleus and nucleolus
No constant alterations
Cellular organelles
Increased in numbers
Signs of activation
Keratinosomes more numerous
Keratohyaline granules more numerous and enlarged
Tonofibrils
Increased numerically
Coarse bundles
Concentric arrangement
Premature keratosis
Keratin lamellae
Uneven keratinization (filamentous/amorphous)
Uncoordinated shedding ("keratin pools")
Desmosomes
Numbers increased or normal
Structure normal
Lack of intercellular contact layer
Basement membrane
Multilamellar
Gaps rarely seen

Table 2.12. Ultrastructural characteristics of dysplastic lesions and carcinomas of squamous epithelium

Alterations of nuclei and nucleoli
Enlargement
Multiple nucleoli
Alterations of cellular organelles
Reduction in numbers of specific and highly organized organelles (mitochondria, keratinosomes)
Numerical reduction of mitochondrial lamellae
Myelin-like figures, multiple membrane complexes and osmiophilic inclusions in mitochondria
Increase in numbers of polyribosomes
Aggregation of cisternae of the endoplasmic reticulum
Increase in numbers of microfilaments
Loss or decrease in numbers of keratohyaline granules
Alterations of tonofibrils
Decrease/increase in numbers
Premature keratosis
Formation of coarse clumps
Perinuclear spirals
Dyskeratotic necrosis
Fibrillar dyskeratosis
Formation of immature keratin with remnants of organelles
Lack of stable membrane formation
Organoid keratosis (keratinous pearls)
Alterations of the cellular membrane
Spongiosis
Formation of cytoplasmatic protrusions (microvilli)
Pinching off of cytoplasmatic processes
Reduction of the number of junctions
Alterations of desmosomes
Reduction in numbers
Reduction of length
Predominance of simple forms
Lack of intercellular contact layers
Reduction of attachment plaque formation
Lack of insertion of tonofilaments
Loss or extraction of desmosomes
Intracytoplasmatic desmosomes
Alterations of the basement membrane
Multilamellar
Presence of atypical material
Incomplete half-desmosomes
Thinning
Gaps
Cytoplasmatic protrusions

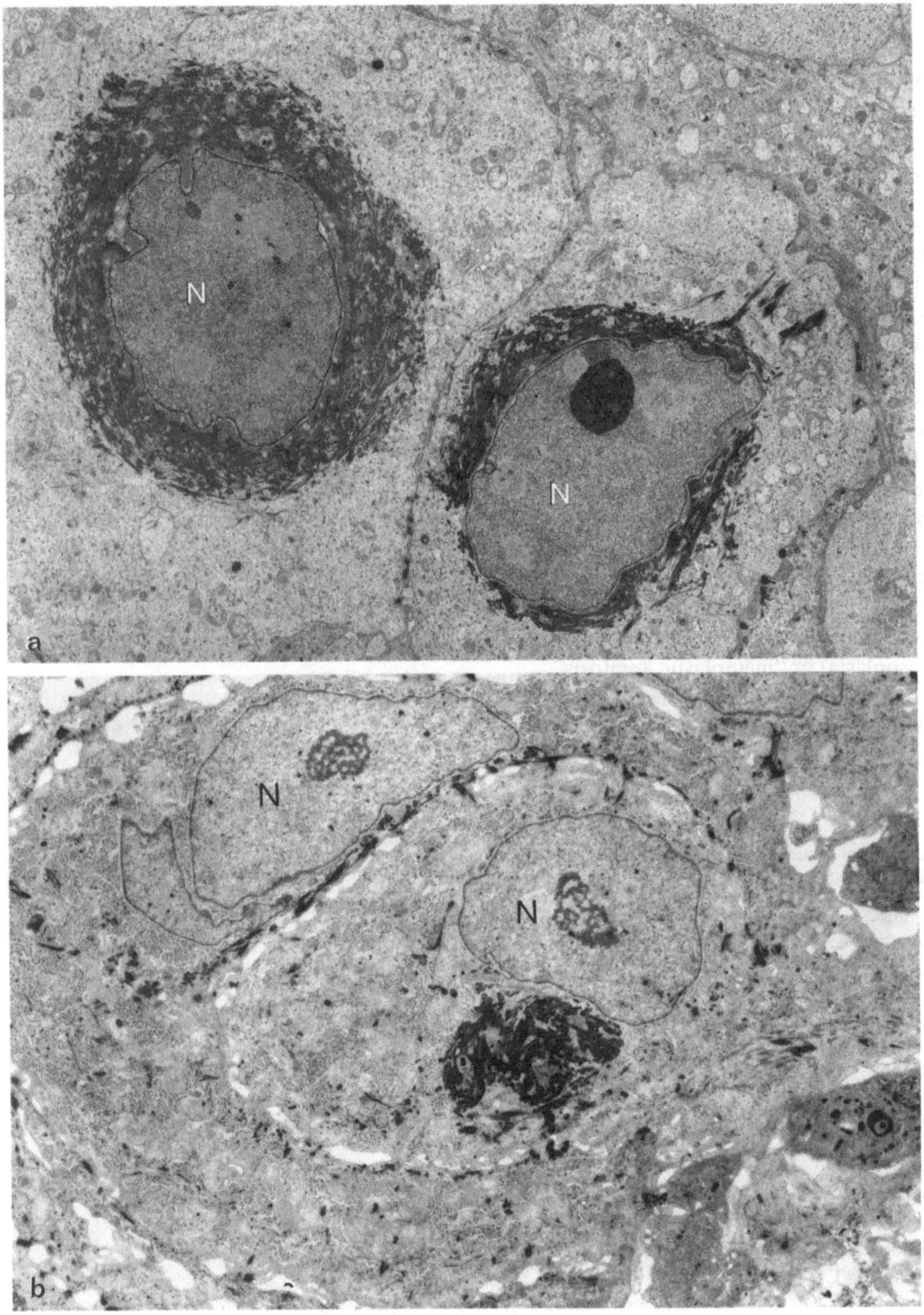

Fig. 2.8 a,b. Electron-microscopic features of squamous cell carcinomas. **a** Tumor cells with large nuclei *(N)*, one containing a dense nucleolus. Conspicuous perinuclear spirals of condensed tonofibrils. The peripheral cytoplasm is free of fibrils and contains only scarce organelles (mitochondria, polyribosomes). The closely apposed cell membranes form only a few short rudimentary junctional complexes without insertion of tonofibrils. × 5400. **b** Tumour cells with large nuclei *(N)* containing loose nucleoli. The tonofibrils do not form spirals but are clumped together near the nucleus as an electron-dense mass. Few, rudimentary desmosomes with occasional short tonofilament bundles inserting. Focal widening of the intercellular space. × 5800.

ment membrane with progressive loss of the lamina densa and hemidesmosomes. At these sites cytoplasmic protrusions and pseudopodia with an increased number of microfilaments (actin) are formed and protrude into the connective tissue (Fig. 2.9). This process has been termed microinvasion. Intercellular junctions are reduced in number, which often leads to a widening of the intercellular space. Deficiency and structural alterations of cell junctions and desmosomes result in reduced intercellular cohesion and/or communication. Insertions of tonofibrils in desmosomes are reduced, leading to a lack of three-dimensional orientation and arrangement. Tonofibrils clump together and form perinuclear agglomerations, often in concentric arrangements, around the nucleus (Fig. 2.8). As a consequence, dyskeratotic necrosis or fibrillar keratosis may occur. Lack or deficiency of the basement membrane barrier, reduced intercellular adherence, pressure exerted by uncontrolled growth and active cellular locomotion play a role in invasive growth.

Scanning electron microscopic studies reveal changes of the cell surface in dysplasia and carcinomas (LUNDGREN et al. 1983, HANSON and BRUCHMÜLLER 1983). Normal squamous cell epithelium and epithelium in simple hyperplasia are uniform with polygonal cells of similar size and shape. The surface is covered by branching microridges. In dysplasia an increasing irregularity appears, giving a cobblestone appearance (LUNDGREN et al. 1983). Carcinoma in situ and invasive carcinoma show a highly disorganized picture, cells are protruding with ill-defined intercellular junctions, microridges are disrupted and irregular microvilli and deep wrinkles appear. The so-called echelon phenomenon is supposed to be typical of carcinomas (HANSON and BRUCHMÜLLER 1983).

Electron microscopy in this context cannot contribute to routine diagnostic procedures, but it certainly can add to the understanding of the biology of disturbances of epithelial differentiation in malignancy.

2.3.2 Additional, more Functional Methods

Besides the predominantly morphological methods described above, more functional approaches to the problem of assessing the biological potential of precancerous lesions and carcinomas have been employed (Table 2.5).

2.3.2.1 Cellular Proliferation Studies

Methods used in proliferation studies and their limitations, the kinetics of epithelium and their changes in hyperplasia and other abnormal states have been extensively reviewed by HUME and POTTEN (1979), SCRAGG and JOHNSON (1980, 1982) and HUME (1981).

Many investigators have demonstrated that cellular kinetics in hyperplasia, dysplasia and carcinoma are altered - as could be expected. Cellular proliferation studies include the counting of mitotic figures in conventional tissue slides (mitotic index) or after mitotic arrest in metaphase, and radioactive labelling, especially with tritiated thymidine (3H-TdR).

In hyperplasia of the oral epithelium an increased mitotic index and labelling index, and linear increase of these parameters with increasing dysplasia, can be observed (review: HILL 1980, SCRAGG and JOHNSON 1982). This is associated with a distribution of mitotic figures and labelled cells also in suprabasal layers, indicating an enlargement of the proliferative pool. In laryngeal carcinomas a correlation of the 3 H-TdR labelling index and the frequency of lymph node metastasis was observed (ELÖ 1983). However, radioactive labelling, the most reliable method, and mitotic arrest are for obvious reasons limited in their application in humans, and in vitro methods are of questionable biological significance.

Evaluation based simply on mitotic indices has very limited value for various reasons. For instance, "normal" control values are difficult to obtain; diurnal variations must be taken into consideration; the progenitor pool is not known and not necessarily identical with the basal cells, the duration of mitosis and the synthetic phase is often not known and mitoses can progress after sampling, resulting in underestimation of the mitotic activity. Consequently, an increase in mitotic index does not necessarily correspond to enhanced cell production, and both hyperplasia and dysplasia are also characterized by altered cell loss. Finally, there is an increase in mitotic figures of the epithelium in regeneration, e.g. as a response to various noxious agents and in wound healing, and also in inflammation and in hyperplasia. In addition, nonepithelial, interepithelial cells may contribute to the total of mitotic figures, although their number may be negligible under most conditions (BOS and BURKHARDT 1981).

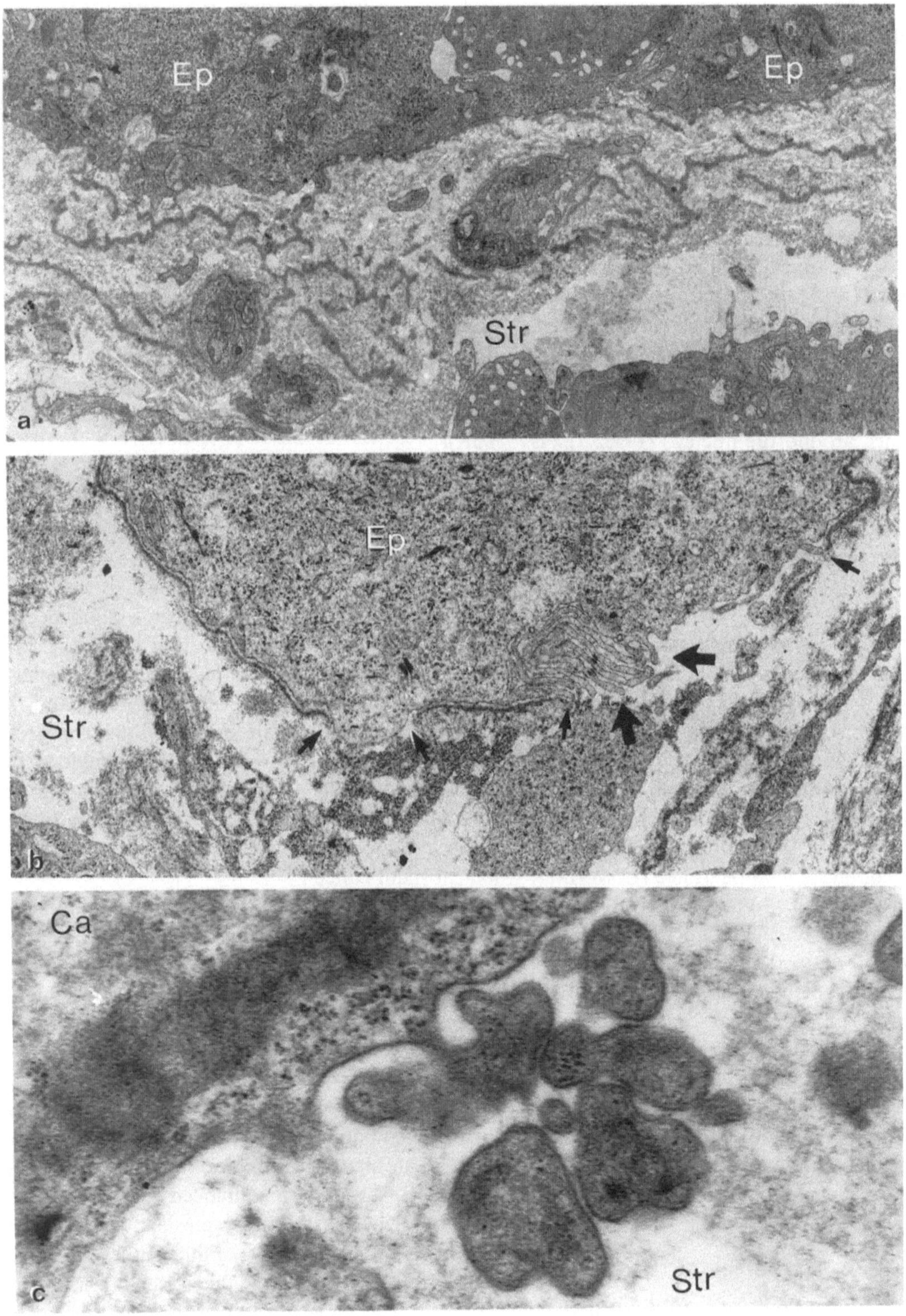

Fig. 2.9a–c. Changes of the basement membrane in epithelial dysplasia and carcinoma. **a** Multilamellar basement membrane in an epithelial hyperplasia with moderate dysplasia. The dark bands of basement membrane material on the epithelium *(Ep)* and in the stroma *(Str)* running irregularly parallel are conspicuous. × 8750. **b** Basal cell *(Ep)* of epithelial hyperplasia with severe dysplasia. There are several gaps in the basement membrane *(between small arrows)*. In these areas there are cytoplasmic protrusions *(large arrows)* and fine tentacle-like projections. × 10900. **c** Microinvasion of a carcinoma cell *(Ca)* without a basement membrane forming cytoplasmic protrusions into the stroma *(Str)*. Some processes apparently have been pinched off and are being conveyed into the stroma. × 56500.

For all these reasons the mitotic index as such gives limited information which can be used only in the context of other criteria of dysplasia and histological features; cell death rate should also be taken into consideration.

Recently the newly developed antinucleoside immunoperoxidase (or immunofluorescence) labelling index (ANIF-LI) has been shown to be equivalent to autoradiography (3H-TdR). By immunohistochemical methods single-stranded nucleic acids can be decorated in the nuclei of tissue sections, making it possible to recognize the cells actively replicating DNA. First evaluations of carcinomas of the head and neck, including six laryngeal carcinomas (CINBERG et al. 1980, 1983) showed that the ANIF-LI could be valuable for the assessment of the growth fraction of laryngeal carcinoma.

2.3.2.2 DNA Histograms, Cytophotometry

DNA histograms obtained by cytophotometric measurements should be based on cell suspensions or cytological smears after staining (Feulgen cyto- or microspectrophotometry) or fluorochromation (cyto- or microfluorometry) of the nuclear DNA. By means of computerized evaluation large numbers of cells may be measured (flow cytofluorometry). DNA histograms obtained from tissue sections, with the cutting of nuclei of different size and on different levels, give no exact values.

These methods have been applied to laryngeal lesions by GIARELLI et al. (1977), GRÖNTOFT et al. (1978), HOLM et al. (1980), HELLQUIST and OLOFSSON (1981), HOLM (1982), BJELKENKRANTZ et al. (1983) and CRISSMAN and FU (1986) and to oral lesions by MITTERMAYER et al. (1981), SAKU and SATO (1983) and other authors (review: BURKHARDT 1985). GRÖNTOFT et al. (1978) in a study of normal, dysplastic and carcinomatous laryngeal tissue, observed a greater variability of the DNA content with higher degrees of dysplasia. The values of their arbitrary units were 69 for normal, 71 for dysplastic and 118 for carcinomatous nuclei. Subsequent studies and investigations by other authors confirmed a correlation of the increase in nuclear DNA content obtained by DNA measurement to the grade of dysplasia (GIARELLI 1977, HELLQUIST et al. 1981). Compared to normal epithelium, epithelial hyperplasia by itself exhibited no marked difference in the nuclear DNA content (HELLQUIST and OLOFSSON 1981), confirming the well-agreed fact that hyperplasia without dysplasia is not a premalignant lesion.

The DNA ploidy pattern has implications for the prognosis of a lesion. A low diploid deviation (2c deviation factor, 2c DI) is characteristic of lesions with a low risk, a high diploid deviation (aneuploid values, dispersion) indicates a high-risk lesion, and the occurrence of hypertetraploid nuclei (4,5c exceeding rate, 4,5c-ER) is considered a "neoplastic marker" by some authors.

In a single-cell DNA fluorometry study on laryngeal hyperplastic, dysplastic and carcinomatous lesions by BJELKENKRANTZ et al. (1983), hypertetraploid nuclei were not found in hyperplastic or mildly dysplastic epithelia, but were present in four of 14 specimens of moderate dysplasia, in five of 19 specimens of severe dysplasia, and in nine of 15 invasive carcinomas. In precancerous lesions the presence of hypertetraploid nuclei was associated with more frequent recurrences and progression, in carcinomas with a worse prognosis.

With such techniques there is, however, a high percentage of false-negative results. In a study by HOLM and colleagues (HOLM et al. 1980, HOLM 1982) 24% of carcinomas showed uncharacteristic changes and predominantly diploid patterns. Of 15 invasive carcinomas measured by BJELKENKRANTZ et al. (1983) the modal DNA value was diploid or nearly diploid in 13 cases. In two cases the tumour was probably polyploid with a diploid basic peak. However, the nondiploid carcinomas and those with more than 50% of cells with DNA values exceeding the modal diploid value + 2 standard deviations showed more advanced stages and had a poorer prognosis than predominantly diploid carcinomas (HOLM et al. 1980, HOLM 1982).

Cytophotometry is at present time-consuming and requires expensive hardware and considerable experience; improvement of technical applications and combination with other techniques, however, could make it a valuable addition to conventional histology.

2.3.2.3 Changes in Immune Status

A number of systemic immunological alterations – enhanced or reduced reactivity and dysfunctions – have been observed in patients with "head and neck" carcinomas and lesions with or without dysplasia (review: CHRETIEN 1975, WANEBO 1979, BURKHARDT 1980, SCULLY 1982 a + c, 1983 b; recent observations on patients with laryngeal cancer:

PAPENHAUSEN et al. 1979, TAYLOR and SAFFORD 1982, MAKIMOTO et al. 1983, WATANABE et al. 1983, MORRA et al. 1984, CORTESINA et al. 1984, DAWSON et al. 1985, GIEREK et al. 1985, WALTER and DANIELSON 1985, WUSTROW and ZENNER 1985). These changes include the humoral and cell-mediated specific immune system as well as the natural killer cells and associated nonspecific defence mechanisms. Most of these changes persist after elimination of the tumour, have been found to be nonspecific and bear no prognostic implications (BIER et al. 1983). Some alterations may be due to associated factors such as alcohol consumption (PALMER 1978, BIER et al. 1983) or smoking (CHRETIEN 1978). Serum levels of circulating immunocomplexes are raised in laryngeal cancer patients, and might be of value for monitoring the efficacy of therapy and detection of recurrences (DENARO et al. 1985). Local immune reactions (stromal reaction) have already been mentioned above (Sect. 2.3.1.4).

So far, no affirmative test indicating the presence of carcinomas or of premalignant lesions has evolved from these investigations.

2.3.2.4 Analysis of Cell Products in Circulating Blood

A number of cell products, especially components of the cell surface of malignant cells and enzymes involved in the metabolism of nucleic acids, may be shed or otherwise freed and thus circulate in the blood. In particular, concentrations of **β2-microglobulin** (SCULLY 1981b) and activities of **alkaline deoxyribonuclease** (SCULLY 1981a) and **thymidine kinase** (SCULLY 1982b) are often raised in the serum of patients with dysplastic lesions and oral cancer.

The levels of **carcinoembryonic antigen** (CEA) may also be raised in the serum of patients with cancer of the head and neck (SILVERMAN et al. 1976). As increased CEA levels are also found in a number of non-neoplastic conditions - notably in heavy smokers - this sign has no real value for the primary diagnosis of laryngeal cancer, which is very often associated with habitual smoking. However, a correlation between CEA titres and the post-therapeutic course of the disease may be of clinical interest.

The suppression of cellular immune reactions mentioned above has tentatively been linked to raised levels of **serum glycoproteins** (haptoglobin, α1-antitrypsin, α1-acid glycoprotein) in patients with head and neck squamous carcinomas. An increase of serum levels of these proteins seems to correlate with tumour extent and clinical stage; levels in cured patients are usually somewhat lower but tend to remain higher than in normal subjects (WOLF et al. 1979).

Serum tests may possibly become useful in the prediction of malignant transformation and control of established carcinomas, especially for the recognition of recurrences. At present too little is known about the reliability of these tests.

2.3.2.5 Examination of Living Tissue

In vivo or in vitro testing of living tissue from premalignant lesions or carcinomas can give important information on the potentials of the respective lesions.

Growth of tissue samples in the athymic nude mouse, which largely lacks a thymus-dependent immune system, is one approach which has been used to examine to what degree oral leukoplakic lesions are reversible (HOLMSTRUP et al. 1981).

The **angiogenic activity** of a tumour, i.e. its capacity to induce capillary proliferation, is clearly related to its ability for invasive growth and metastasis and can be tested by implantation of tumour tissue into the rabbit iris (rabbit iris assay). The angiogenic activity of transitional cell carcinoma of the bladder was tested by CHODAK and coworkers (1980). Over 95% of malignant and premalignant specimens stimulated capillary proliferation, but only 10% of normal mucosa had this effect. To our knowledge this approach has not been applied to lesions of the laryngeal mucosa.

The **invasive capacity** of a tumour can be examined on human amnion membrane in culture. FELIX and coworkers (1982) showed in squamous cell carcinomas of the tongue and larynx that individual tumours behave differently. No correlation between the natural aggressiveness and the course of the disease in patients has yet been established.

The **cloning efficiency** (in vitro stem cell assay) of carcinomas grown in soft agar (or agarose or methyl cellulose) culture (HAMBURGER and SALMON 1977), depends on the presence of vigorous tumour stem cells. This test may become a prognostic indicator in squamous cell carcinomas of the head and neck (MATTOX and VAN HOFF 1980, JOHNS and MILLS 1983, SCHIFF and SHUGAR 1984). Of 73 carcinomas examined, 49% demonstrated clonal growth, with a cloning efficiency ranging from 0.001% to 1.67% (JOHNS and MILLS 1983). There was a correlation of high cloning efficiency with advanced stages of the disease and decreased survival.

Acrylhydrocarbon hydroxylase (AHH) inducibility is genetically determined and can be assessed in cultured lymphocytes. AHH mediates the activation of polycyclic aromatic hydrocarbons to epoxides and is thus an activator of carcinogens. High AHH inducibility is statistically overrepresented in, for example, patients with lung cancer, oral cancer and laryngeal carcinoma (TRELL et al. 1981, ANDREASSON et al. 1982). Testing for AHH inducibility may identify a group of patients at risk.

The testing of living tumour tissue in vitro seems to be a promising method which may be expected to gain more importance in the future. In such systems one can also test the sensitivity of tumour cell lines to cytostatic drugs and radiation. At present, however, standardized methods for routine purposes are still lacking.

2.3.2.6 *Experimental Models*

Experimental models of carcinogenesis - mostly based on the use of hamsters, mice and rats - have contributed considerably to our knowledge of the pathogenesis of squamous cell carcinomas (review: EVESON 1981). Most of these studies have been done on skin and oral mucosa, very few on laryngeal mucosa. A number of enhancing (alcohol, tobacco, trauma, corticosteroids, antimetabolites, irradiation) and suppressing/retarding (retinoids, immunoenhancing agent) influences on carcinogenesis have been identified (review: SHKLAR et al. 1979, SHKLAR 1981). It seems reasonable to assume that the same factors may be acting in carcinogenesis in humans, including the larynx. Recognition of this could contribute to prevention both by elimination of enhancing factors and by treatment (e.g. retinoids in precancerous lesions). No consequences for the assessment of individual lesions have yet emerged from these studies.

2.3.3 Conclusion

There are many promising aspects of the advanced methods presented. Future developments and progress are to be expected, especially from modified cytological examinations, computer-aided quantification, immunohistochemistry, proliferation studies with immunological labelling, cytophotometry, determination of circulating tumour products and testing of living tumour tissue in vivo or in vitro.

At present, there is no all-embracing answer to the many questions related to the diagnosis of precancerous lesions and cancer in the larynx. The assessment of the biological potential of precancerous lesions and established carcinomas still relies on **light-microscopic histological examination.** There is no alternative to this old and well-proven approach.

The grade of dysplasia of presumably premalignant lesions (with all the subjectivity inherent in its evaluation) remains the most important indicator of malignant potential (see Chap. 4). Any advanced method proposed to replace it, must be shown to predict the true biological potential more accurately than conventional histology. The oft-mentioned correlation of the results of an "advanced" method with the grade of dysplasia is not sufficient for acceptance. The aim must be to find a method that unmasks those few cases (about 3% of oral precancerous lesions; BURKHARDT and MAERKER 1981) in which lesions with a seemingly harmless histological picture develop into carcinomas.

2.4 Advanced Methods in the Determination of Tumour Types

Classification of benign and malignant neoplasms is based on the cells or tissue of origin. The latter can be recognized quite easily in the overwhelming number of cases by simple light microscopy and standard stains, as there are enough characteristic features, e.g. architecture, cell shape, cell products. Fortunately the most common neoplasm of the larynx - squamous cell carcinoma - can as a rule be easily diagnosed by these methods. However, there are cases of undifferentiated and uncommon tumours which cannot be classified by conventional light microscopy; sometimes even determination of epithelial or mesenchymal nature is not possible. Rather differentiated tumours of similar histological appearance may also be hard to distinguish, as will be shown for the rhabdomyoma and granular cell tumour (Chap. 3).

As correct histological classification is in many cases the basis for a differentiated therapeutic approach and assessment of prognosis, it is highly desirable to determine the histogenetic origin of every neoplasm. In this endeavour most of the predominantly morphological advanced methods discussed in detail above (Sect. 2.3.1., Table 2.4) have been applied with varying success.

Cytological smears, obtained by exfoliation, aspiration or as imprints from excised tumours, can reveal details not discernible in histological sections. In tumours of uncertain nature, therefore, parallel examination of histological and cytological preparations is valuable.

Morphometric quantification has attracted little attention in this context. Certain cytological features, e.g. characteristics of nuclear shape, can be quantitatively assessed (nuclear contour index measurements) and contribute to discrimination of certain cell types, especially lymphoid cells (rounded nuclear contour) versus histiocytic cells (lobulated nuclear contour).

Histochemical stains are indispensable for routine diagnosis of neoplastic lesions. Important are: Papanicolaou stain for detection of keratinization in undifferentiated squamous cell carcinomas, PAS and alcian blue stain for demonstration of mucus production in adenocarcinomas, Giemsa stain in lesions of haematopoietic origin and the Fontana-Masson stain for neuroendocrine tumours. Silver impregnation reveals the reticulin fibre network. A dense network between tumour cells is often found in mesenchymal neoplasms, while formation of cellular nests free of fibres is typical of epithelial tumours.

Enzyme histochemistry is most frequently employed in differentiation of haematological neoplasms. The demonstration of activities of chloroacetate esterase, which is also possible in fixed paraffin embedded material, is often helpful in recognizing infiltrations of granulocytic elements and their precursors.

Immunohistochemistry has without doubt become the most important tool in tumour differentiation today (see Sect. 2.3.1.4). The cellular differentiation can be deduced from more or less specific products of the tumour cells, which selectively bind specific polyclonal or monoclonal antibodies. Bound antibodies are made visible by secondary antibodies and an enzyme conjugate, e.g. peroxidase-antiperoxidase (PAP) complex, giving a brown reaction product after incubation in hydrogen peroxidase/diaminobenzidine substrate solution. Alternatively, secondary antibodies coupled with fluorescent markers can be employed. Examples of cellular products important for the assessment of tumour differentiation which can be demonstrated by "immunostaining" (TAYLOR and KLEDZIG 1981; incorrectly called "tumour markers" by some authors) are shown in Table 2.13. The importance of such methods is discussed in the relevant sections, e.g. papillomas (Sect. 3.2.1), rhabdomyomas (Sect. 3.3.1.5), granular cell tumours (Sect. 3.3.2.3), malignant melanoma (Sect. 7.2.2.1), spindle cell squamous carcinoma (Sect. 7.1.1.2), and radiogenic tumours (Sect. 7.3).

Special importance for diagnostic purposes is attached to the discovery that the intermediate filaments of the cells - functioning as an inner skeleton - are a constant feature of normal and tumorous cells, giving evidence of their basic origin. The diagnostic implications of the demonstration of intermediate filaments are summarized in Table 2.14. In laryngeal neoplasms the differentiation of spindle cell squamous carcinoma (cytokeratin positive) from malignant mesenchymal tumours (vimentin/desmin positive) is of special importance (see Sect. 7.1.1.2).

Electron microscopy today retains only very limited application in routine diagnostic problems, principally because of the high degree of refinement of the immunohistochemical methods available. The ultrastructure of tumour cells may display tonofilaments and desmosomes (epithelial), cross-striated filaments (myogenic), premelanosomes (malignant melanoma), dense core granules (neuroectodermal), Birbeck granules (histiocytosis X), lysosomes (histiocytic) and other more or less specific organelles or cell products. Electron-microscopic findings are mentioned in the sections dealing with rhabdomyomas (Sect. 3.3.1.5), granular cell tumours (Sect. 3.3.2.3) and spindle cell carcinomas (Sect. 7.1.1.2).

Table 2.13. Cellular constituents important in tumour diagnosis demonstrated by immunohistochemistry (selection)

Cellular product	Diagnostic implications
Intermediate filaments	Basic histogenetic typing
Epithelial membrane antigen (EMA)	Epithelial origin
Cell surface antigens T- and B-cell antigens Membrane immunoglobulins Cytoplasmatic immunoglobulins	Typing of malignant lymphomas/plasmocytomas Demonstration of monoclonality
Enzymes	
Lysozyme	Histiocytic origin
Neurone-specific enolase (NSE)	Neuroendocrine origin
Oncofetal antigens	
Carcinoembryonic antigen (CEA)	Adenocarcinomas of enteric origin
Hormones	
Thyroglobulin	Thyroid carcinomas
Other cellular products	
S-100 protein	Neurogenic tumours, malignant melanoma Langerhans cell tumours (histiocytosis X)
Factor VIII-associated antigen	Tumours of endothelial origin
Myoglobin	Tumours originating from skeletal muscles
Viral structural antigen	
Human papilloma virus	Paillomas, condylomas, Flat warts
Epstein-Barr virus	Nasopharyngeal carcinoma

Table 2.14. Intermediate filaments in tumour diagnosis

Type of filament	Diagnostic implication
(Cyto)keratins	Epithelial tumours
Vimentin	Mesenchymal tumours - sarcomas - malignant lymphomas - malignant melanomas
Desmin	Myogenic tumours - leiomyosarcomas - rhabdomyosarcomas
Neurofilaments	Neural tumours
Glial fibrillary acidic protein	Gliomas

3 Benign Neoplasms

3.1 Definition, Classification, Frequency, General Therapeutic Aspects

VON ALBERTINI (1974) defined true neoplasms as "irreversible autonomic overgrowths of the body's tissue". Autonomic growth excesses are, in part, also represented by those frequent hyperplasias which occur in the larynx, namely, tissue growth as a result of inflammation, polyps and cysts. These so-called pseudotumours must be separated from the irreversible neoplasms. To a large extent, this book follows, as regards content and classification, the International Classification of Tumours of the World Health Organization (WHO) (SHANMUGARATNAM and SOBIN 1978). Pseudotumours (group VIII) and tumour-like malformations and dystopias (group V) will be described in Chap. 8.

Taking the definition given above, and in contrast to MATZKER (1963) we assign the juvenile papillomas to the true neoplasms despite their viral aetiology. As in other organs and systems, a distinction is made in the larynx between benign epithelial tumours, such as papillomas and adenomas; benign mesenchymal tumours, such as fibromas, lipomas, angiomas, rhabdomyomas, chondromas and osteomas; and neurogenic tumours, i.e. neurinomas, neurofibromas, paragangliomas and probably the granular cell tumours. Paragangliomas, haemangiopericytomas and fibrous histiocytomas can behave both benignly and malignantly. The 722 cases of benign laryngeal lesions studied by NEW and ERICH (1938) at the Mayo Clinic included 592 papillomas, 26 haemangiomas, 26 chondromas, one neurofibroma and one adenoma; the remainder were non-neoplastic lesions.

Compiling data from 205 cases of benign neoplasms of the larynx observed over a period of 20 years, FRIEDMANN (1976) found 170 papillomas, 16 adenomas, three chondromas, and 16 other different mesenchymal tumours. JONES et al. (1984) observed, among 269 tumours, 227 papillomas, 15 oncocytic tumours, seven granular cell tumours, five haemangiomas, three lymphangiomas, two cases each of paraganglioma, neurilemmoma and neurofibroma and one case each of chondroma, pleomorphic adenoma, fibrous histiocytoma, fibromatosis and rhabdomyoma.

The symptoms of benign tumours are more or less identical and depend less on the histological type than on the site of origin and size of the lesion. In most cases, conservative excision is adequate treatment. Endolaryngeal ablation via microlaryngoscopy suffices for small superficial tumours, whereas with larger tumours and those lying in the depth of the tissue, it is more advisable to employ pharyngotomy or thyreotomy, depending on the size of the tumour. In some cases, partial or total laryngectomy (Sect. 6.2) may prove necessary. Radiotherapy should be avoided owing to the risk of radiogenic tumours (see Sect. 7.3). Particular therapeutic problems arising with certain tumours will be discussed in detail below.

3.2 Epithelial Tumours

3.2.1 Papilloma and Papillomatosis

Papillomas are benign epithelial tumours with a mulberry- or cauliflower-like surface. They may be broad-based, sessile and wart-like, or polypous and pedunculated, protruding over the surface of the mucosa. The commonest site of occurrence is the vocal cord.

A distinction between juvenile-onset multiple papilloma and adult-onset solitary papilloma must be made according to their clinical behaviour (BJÖRK and WEBER 1956, DEKELBOUM 1965, KLEINSASSER and OLIVERA 1973, PREIBISCH-EFFENBERGER 1970a, WINSTON and EPSTEIN 1958, THOST 1929). The question of malignant transformation of papillomas will be treated separately for both types in more detail in Chap. 4.

3.2.1.1 Juvenile-Onset Papilloma

Juvenile papillomas (Fig. 3.1) appear predominantly in small children and in the second decade of life. Their onset decreases with age and during puberty they may regress spontaneously. They appear to affect both sexes equally (BJÖRK and WEBER 1956). Persistence after 16 years of age is usually associated with a poor prognosis. The true cords, false cords and anterior commissure can be recognized as the sites of origin, but involvement of multiple sites and large areas is the rule. The main symptoms are hoarseness and airway obstruction. There is usually rapid recurrence following removal.

Macroscopically the papillomas appear villous to verrucous and are of a reddish-grey colour. Microscopically there is a typical formation of folds and crypts. The slender fibrous papillae contain a loose, well-vascularized stroma, usually without any dense inflammatory infiltration (Fig. 3.2a). The epithelial lining consists, at the most, of slightly hyperplastic squamous epithelium which as a rule shows no hyperkeratosis and no or mild dysplasia (Fig. 3.2b). Mitotic figures may be found in the basal cell layer. The basal membrane is intact. Often changes in the "prickle" cells can be recognized in the form of so-called koilocytes, i.e. cells with hyperchromatic condensed nuclei and perinuclear vacuoles; these are also characteristic of viral lesions in the uterine cervix.

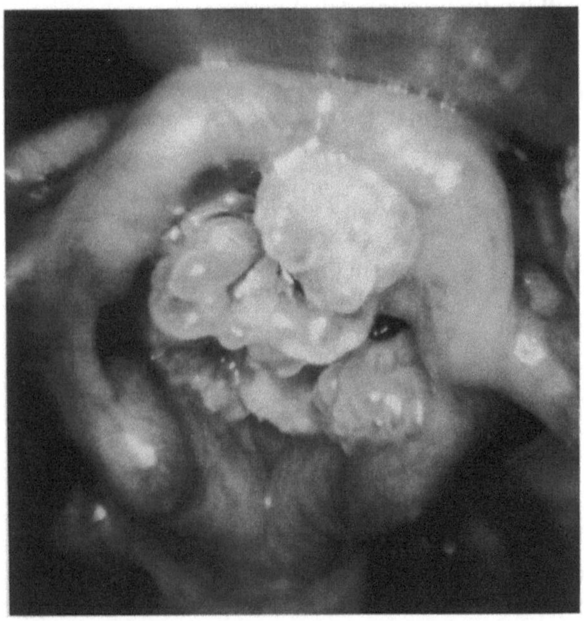

Fig. 3.1. Laryngoscopic picture of a juvenile-onset papilloma in a 2½-year-old boy. Protruding multilocular cauliflower-like tumour in the glottis and supraglottis with almost complete obstruction of the airway

NIKOLAIDIS et al. (1985) distinguished three histological types of papillomas: papillary, acanthomatous and angiokeratotic. The acanthomatous pattern and cellular atypia were associated with an unfavourable prognosis (frequent recurrence), the angiokeratotic type and inflammation with a relatively better prognosis.

Multilocular juvenile papillomas also occur in other regions of the respiratory tract, in particular in the trachea and the bronchi (SHILOVTSEVA 1969, SMITH and GOODING 1974). DWORACEK (1956) reported in his collective study that he observed multilocular papillomas in more than 80% of cases. This multilocular appearance is favoured by the capacity of juvenile papilloma to be transmitted from one site to another (ULLMANN 1923). This transmissibility is a frequent clinical observation, and represents one of the main problems in the treatment of juvenile laryngeal papillomas. Owing to their transmissibility - which includes that from one person to another (DAHMANN 1929, JAKOBI 1955) - an infectious pathogenesis of such tumours was postulated early on. This was confirmed by the detection of the virus, first by MEESEN and SCHULZ (1957), and subsequently by numerous other authors (DMOCHOWSKI et al. 1964, BOYLE et al. 1971, 1973, SOLISCH et al. 1972, LUNDQUIST et al. 1975, ARNOLD 1976, 1977, 1979, SPOENDLIN and KISTLER 1978, QUICK et al. 1978). In contrast to viral warts of the skin, the morphological detection of the virus in juvenile papilloma is seldom successful (SVOBODA et al. 1963, ARNOLD 1976, SPOENDLIN and KISTLER 1978). In only one out of ten cases were SPOENDLIN and KISTLER (1978) able to demonstrate whole virus particles by electron microscopy. Such particles are situated in the cell nucleus (Fig. 3.3), have an icosahedral shape, measure approximately 56 nm in diameter and often exhibit crystalline lattice assemblies (BOYLE et al. 1973). This morphology is identical to that of the papovavirus group (SOLISCH et al. 1972, BOYLE et al. 1973, ARNOLD 1976, 1979, GISSMANN et al. 1977, LIEBERMANN et al. 1978). Members of this group cause verruca vulgaris, condyloma acuminatum and other lesions in man.

An antigenic relationship to condyloma acuminatum (FALSER and SPOENDLIN 1978) and capsid anti-

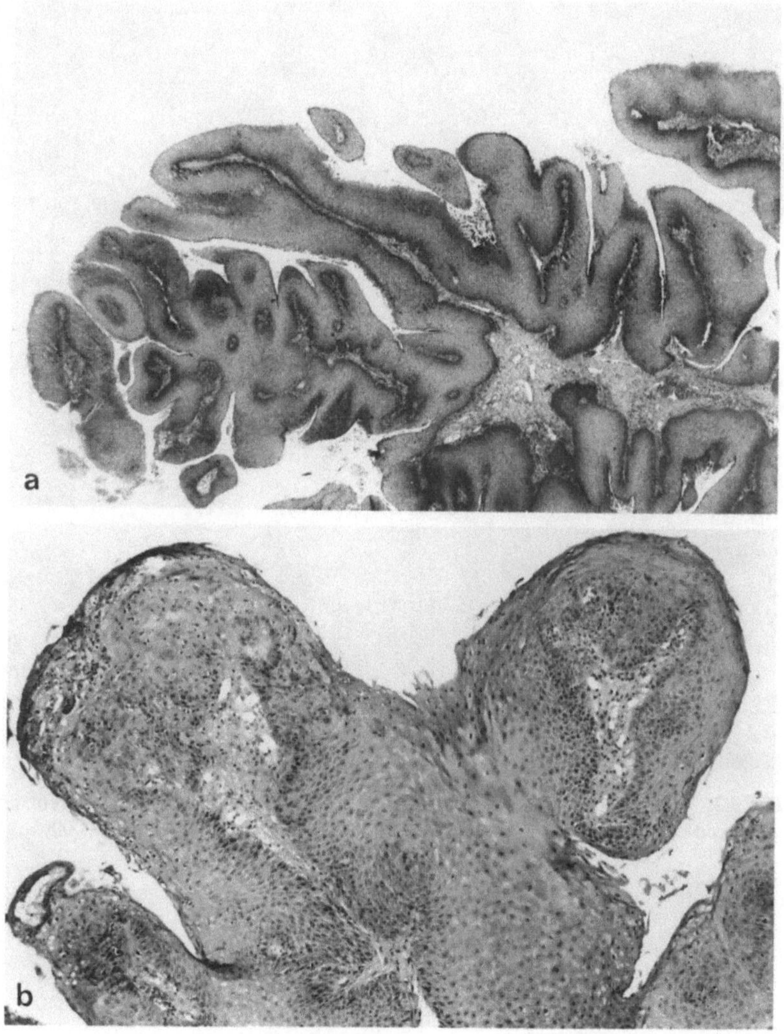

Fig. 3.2 a, b. Juvenile-onset papilloma in a 7-year-old boy with multiple lesions in the glottis and supraglottis. **a** At low magnification multiple, branching, finger-like connective tissue papillae covered by squamous epithelium can be seen. HE, ×20. **b** The regularly stratified squamous epithelium is only moderately thickened, shows slight parakeratosis and only occasional vacuolization ("koilocytosis"). There is no epithelial dysplasia. At the *left*, infiltration of the upper layers by inflammatory cells. HE, ×60

gens common to human papilloma viruses (HPV; BRAUN et al. 1982) could be demonstrated in juvenile-onset laryngeal papillomas using immunohistological techniques (Sect. 2.3). Whilst LACK et al. (1980) observed a positive reaction in more than half of their cases, BRAUN et al. (1982) found a positive reaction in only seven of their 15 cases and MOUNTS et al. (1982) in only two of their 12 cases. In addition to the low frequency of antigen expression, even positive cases only have small numbers of labelled cells in the superficial layers of the epithelium. Using the Southern blot hybridization technique (see Sect. 2.3.1.5) on the other hand, the presence of a papilloma virus genome was confirmed in all cases investigated by MOUNTS et al. (1982) and HEIMBERG et al. (1983), and the virus was identified as four different subtypes of HPV-6. The presence of HPV DNA was demonstrated not only in the tumour itself, but also in the apparently normal mucosa in the vicinity of papillomas and in patients during remission (STEINBERG et al. 1983). These data suggest that a latent, or "silent" infection by HPV viruses possibly with integrated virus DNA is common and accounts for recurrences, whilst capsid formation or production of complete viruses are rare.

Apparently there is a relationship between infections of the mother by condyloma acuminatum and the occurrence of laryngeal juvenile papillomas in children. QUICK et al. (1980) found a history of condylomata in 31 of the mothers of 49 patients with laryngeal papillomas. In 21 cases the condylomatous process was apparent during pregnancy and birth. It is supposed that infection of the children ensues during the perinatal period, especially during birth. In cases of florid condylomata acuminata

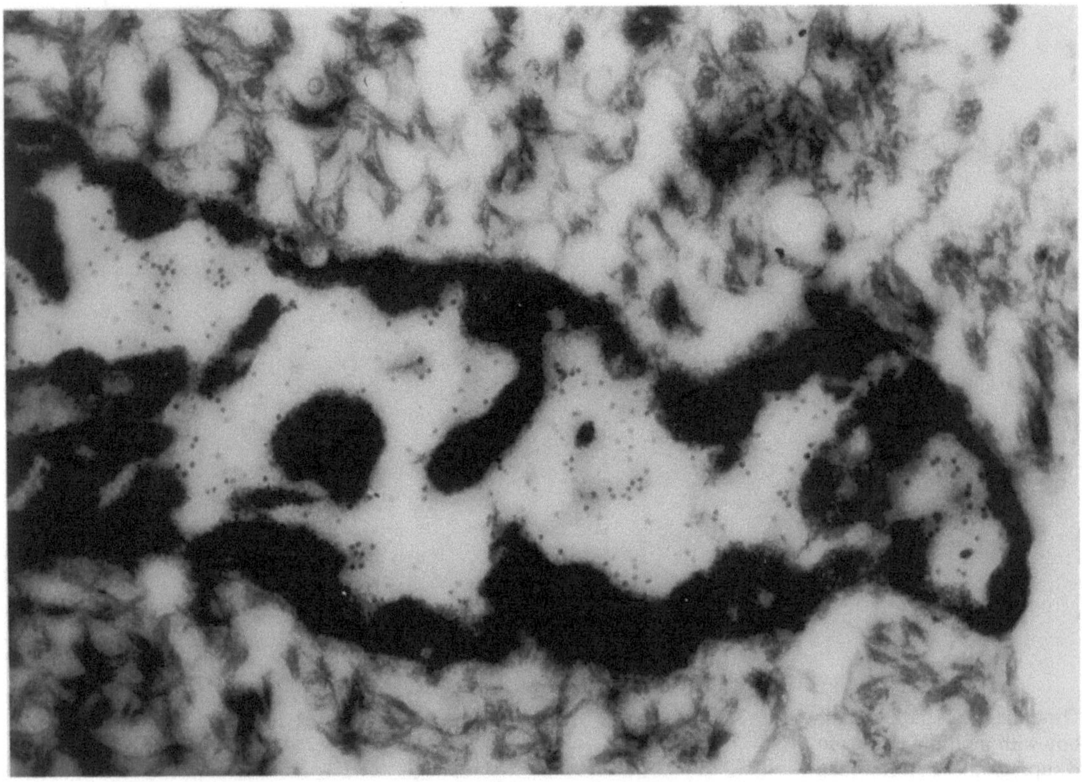

Fig. 3.3. Ultrastructure of a papilloma cell in a 5-year-old boy with recurrent juvenile laryngeal papillomatosis. Marginally displaced chromatin surrounding multiple papilloma virus particles. ×27000

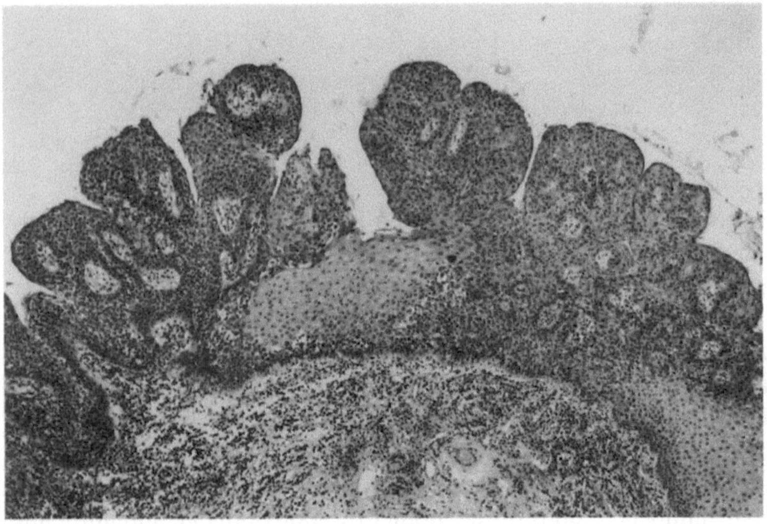

Fig. 3.4. Adult-onset papilloma: 55-year-old man, supraglottis. Irregular papillomatous projection of the epithelium and inflammatory infiltration of the subepithelial tissue. HE, ×45

of the mother caesarean section may be indicated. Another HPV-virus induced lesion - verruca vulgaris of the larynx - has recently been described (FECHNER and MILLS 1982). It must differentiated from verrucous carcinoma (Sect. 7.1.1.1) and will not be discussed in detail here.

The "Story of Warren Bell" (LEJEUNE 1941) is a typical and tragic account of the possible fate of patients affected by juvenile papillomas. This boy suffered from recurrent laryngeal papillomatosis starting when he was 2½ years old, underwent 97 operations and radiation therapy and died at the age of 21 years subsequent to malignant transformation.

Owing to this high rate of recurrence, juvenile papillomas today still present considerable **therapeutic problems**. This is reflected in the large number of trials undertaken to take advantage of new techniques to treat this disease (review: WOLTERS et al. 1984). Nonetheless, only a few methods have proved themselves of worth. The oldest, namely **surgical removal** (HARMER 1903, BLUMENFELD 1927, THOST 1929) has, with the introduction of microsurgery of the larynx, lost virtually none of its importance (BENJAMIN 1973, BOYLE and MCCOY 1970, WOLTERS et al. 1984). A helpful addition provided since the 1920s is **electrocoagulation** which KLEINSASSER (1968) refined in the form of **suction coagulation**. WOLTERS et al. (1984) report intervals without recurrence of 3 years and more in 54.4% of the children and 72.2% of adults treated an average of three times by this method. Since the middle of the 1970s, **laser therapy** has found its way into microsurgery of the larynx. In particular, the CO_2 laser (used in our hospital too), more than the energy-richer neodymium YAG laser, has been used to treat juvenile papillomas (ANDREWS and MOSS 1974, HOLINGER and ANDREWS 1974, LYONS et al. 1978, KARDUK and RICHTER 1979, MIEHLKE et al. 1980, STEINER et al. 1980, review: ROBBINS and WOODSON 1984). It remains to be seen whether the advantages of this expensive technology are really as great as has been anticipated, so that it will be established as a form of treatment. From the chemotherapeutic agents, only the mitosis-inhibiting **podophyllin** has, in our opinion, proved to be effective (HOLLINGSWORTH et al. 1950, DECHER 1961, FABRITIUS 1967, DEDO and JACKLER 1982). Since 1950 application to the surface has been used in the treatment of papillomas (HOLLINGSWORTH et al. 1950).

Cryotherapy does not appear to us to be a suitable means of treating juvenile papillomas, owing to the difficulty in assessing delayed effects on the laryngeal structures which have to be so carefully avoided. Ultrasound, which, after previous removal of the papilloma, was considered to prevent recurrences (BIRCK and MANHART 1963, ARSLAN and RICCI 1966, DOMINOK and KEMMER 1966, JENKINS 1967, PREIBISCH-EFFENBERGER 1970b, RICCI 1974, CANCURA 1977, WHITE et al. 1974, WEHMER 1970) has not been reported on for some considerable time. Radiotherapy of the juvenile papilloma can lead to invasive growth and malignant transformation (WALSH and BEAMER 1950, KLEINSASSER 1958, VLODYKA 1962, MAJOROS et al. 1963, RABBETT 1965, HOLINGER et al. 1968, MAIER 1968, GROSS and CROCKER 1970, DUFF 1971, KLEINSASSER and OLIVERA 1973, FECHNER et al. 1984). It is therefore not only obsolete but even represents malpractice. Local or systemic treatment with antibiotics (HOLINGER et al. 1950, SILVERBLATT 1958, BABLIK 1959), hormones (BROYLES 1940, ZALIN 1948, ARNVIG 1959) and cytotoxic drugs (GAILLARD et al. 1973, SAKURAI et al. 1975, MORGON and GREGOIRE 1976, QUADE and LÖBE 1979, MEHTA and HEROLD 1980) was episodic.

Recently, interferon has been shown to have a beneficial effect (GOEBEL 1981, HAGLUND 1981, GOEPFERT et al. 1982, MCCABE and CLARK 1983, LENARCIC-CEPELJA and KRAJINA 1984) but in our experience with six children treated with interferon between 1982 and 1984, recurrence after cessation of therapy is frequent. This has also been reported by IKENBERG and coworkers (1985).

Malignant transformation of multiple juvenile papillomas without prior radiation is very rare. Among 13 reports, only five withstand critical examination (BARTH 1898, JUSTUS et al. 1970, TOSO 1971, ZEHNDER and LYONS 1975, BRACH et al. 1978, KLEINSASSER and GLANZ 1979a). In addition, we consider the cases described by SHAPIRO et al. (1976), BEWTRA et al. (1982), SOLOMON et al. (1985) and MATSUBA et al. (1985), to be true "spontaneous" malignant transformations of juvenile papilloma. The transformation always appeared after prolonged treatment, at the earliest during the 12th and at the latest during the 64th year of life. Half of these patients were smokers, so that here true spontaneous cancerization is at least questionable. Dysplasias were frequent but were not always indicators of an unfavourable course of the disease.

3.2.1.2 Adult-Onset Papilloma

Papillomas of the adult type, arising after the age of 18 years, represent the most frequent benign laryngeal tumour. Here, in contrast to juvenile onset papillomas, men are more commonly affected than women. Adult papillomas are usually solitary and seldom occur in the form of papillomatosis (STATHEROU 1957). Recurrence following operative removal is rare. The most common symptom is hoarseness; airway obstruction is unusual. The most frequent locations are the vocal folds, the ventricular floor and the supraglottic space.

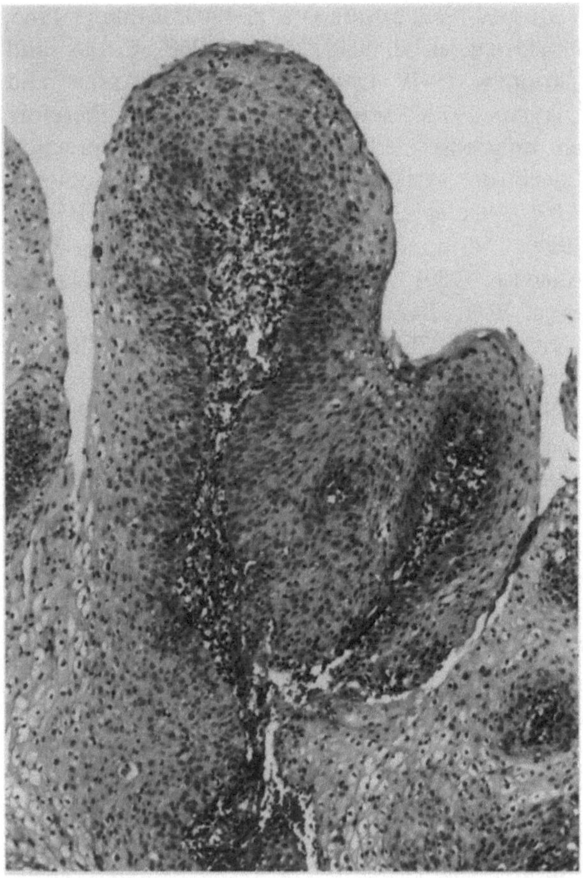

Fig. 3.5. Adult-onset papilloma (same case as Fig. 3.4). High magnification shows disturbance of stratification with increase of cells of the basal-cell type and variations of nuclear size (moderate dysplasia). HE, ×90

Histologically these neoplasms exhibit a coarser surface structure than the juvenile tumours. The stroma is rich in fibres, poorly vascularized, and often chronically inflamed; the squamous epithelium is distinctly more hyperplastic than in juvenile papillomas, with a marked tendency to dysplasia and hyperkeratosis (Fig. 3.5). Even though papillomas belong to the group of benign tumours according to the definition of the WHO (SHANMUGARATNAM 1978), malignant transformation of adult papillomas is not, from the experience of numerous authors, uncommon (SPEISER 1932, COHEN 1933, CUNNING 1950, MATSCHNIG 1954, PUTNEY 1955, DWORACEK 1956, BJÖRK and TEIR 1957, ECKEL 1957, KLEINSASSER 1958, 1963, JACKSON and JACKSON 1959, ABOULKER et al. 1966b, FRIEDBERG et al. 1971, KLEINSASSER and OLIVEIRA E CRUZ 1973, VON ALBERTINI 1974). In our view, based on experience, every papillomatous tumour in adults should be viewed as potentially malignant. Excisions from the surface often give insufficient criteria to classify the tumour as benign or malignant. In nearly all cases of papillary squamous cell carcinoma, only excisions from the depth of the lesion supplied the final diagnosis of malignancy. From this point of view, it can be presumed that in fact some papillomas which undergo so-called malignant transformation were, from the outset, papillary squamous cell carcinomas. This topic will be dealt with in more detail in Chaps. 4 and 7.

In contrast to the juvenile papillomas, no transmissibility of this tumour type has yet been established (BJÖRK and WEBER 1956). For this reason a viral etiology has been rejected. Rather, noxious agents, and in particular smoking or severe mechanical stress, have been considered responsible for the development of adult papillomas. Recent studies by MOUNTS et al. (1982) established, however, that there are in fact indications of a viral etiology also in adult-onset papillomas. In two of eight cases there was a positive reaction with an antiserum to capsid antigens of HPV. The presence of a papilloma virus genome was demonstrated by these authors in all eight cases, suggesting that the etiology of adult-onset papillomas is also viral. In contrast, BRAUN et al. (1982) were not able to detect papilloma capsid antigen in the specimens from six patients with adult-onset papillomas. Possibly there are two types of papillomas in adults: a nonkeratotic type, usually without epithelial dysplasia, as the adult counterpart of juvenile-onset papilloma, and the acanthotic and hyperkeratotic type with dysplasia (KLEINSASSER and OLIVEIRA E CRUZ 1973, JOHNSON et al. 1981).

Fig. 3.6. Oncocytic lesions and oncocytoma. **a** Warthin's tumour (cystadenolymphoma) of the lateral supraglottis. Surrounded by lymphatic tissue, the epithelium shows a tubulopapillary-cystic pattern. HE, ×25. **b** The epithelial cells are finely granular and oxyphilic and this appearance may be mistaken for an oncocytoma. Typically, the cells of Warthin's tumour are arranged in a double layer: the inner cells are round or polygonal, the outer columnar but non-ciliated. HE, ×250. **c** Electron-microscopic picture of an oncocytoma. Three cells in an acinar arrangement. *Left:* a narrow lumen containing proteinaceous substances *(dark)*. The cells form small villous-like projections into the lumen. *Right:* the nucleus (N) of an oncocyte. The cytoplasm contains abundant mitochondria. ×8500. **d** High magnification of the cytoplasm: densely packed mitochondria. The condensation of the cristae is a fixation artefact (human material). ×48000

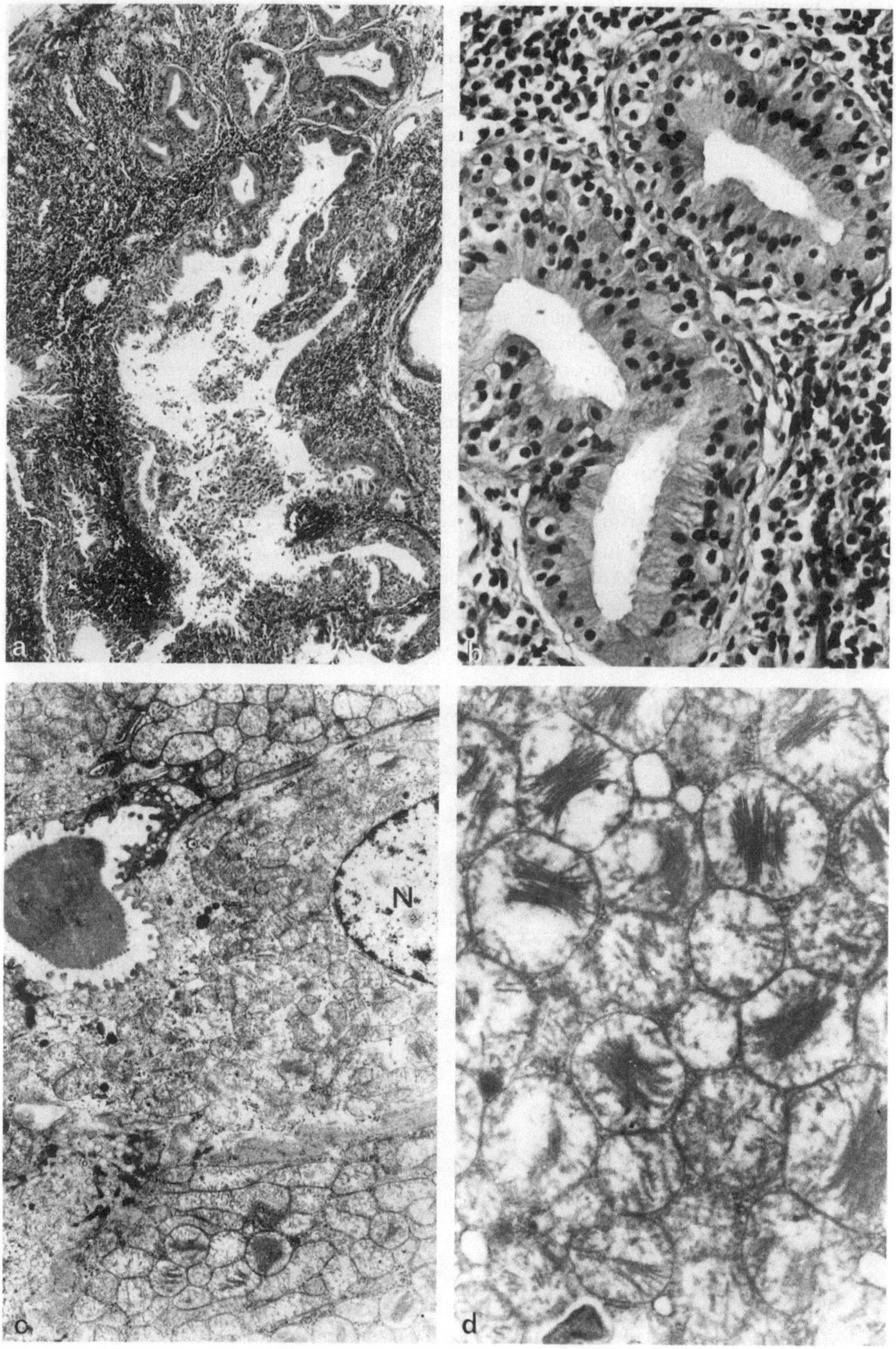
a
b
N
c
d

3.2.2 Oxyphilic Adenoma (Oncocytoma)

The oxyphilic adenoma is composed of so-called oncocytes, cells with abundant eosinophilic cytoplasm interspersed with numerous fine granules which correspond ultrastructurally to mitochondria which are both enlarged and increased in number (Fig. 3.6c, d). The cells arrange themselves in sheets of highly prismatic cylindrical epithelium, and as a rule have small, oval, centrally positioned and somewhat hyperchromatic nuclei. According to NOHERI (1946), oncocytes are probably derived from the excretory duct epithelium of the seromucous glands. They also occur in salivary gland lesions, normal glands and in non-neoplastic changes, e.g. laryngeal cysts; a total of 0.5%-1% of all laryngeal specimens have oncocytic lesions (LUNDGREN et al. 1982).

The oncocytic adenoma or oncocytic cystadenoma, like all other adenomas, can contain cystic formations (HOLM-JENSEN et al. 1977) and follicular lymphatic tissue (FERLITO and RECHER 1981). Focal oncocytic differentiation (Fig. 3.6a, b) can also be seen in papillary cystadenomas (KROE et al. 1967, ECKEDAHL and SCHNÜRER 1969, BARTON 1972, DONALD and KRAUSE 1973). Only rarely do they occur in multiple form as "oncocytic papillary cystadenomatosis" (YAMASE and PUTMAN 1979, LE JENNE et al. 1980, FERLITO and RECHER 1981).

Oncocytic adenomas occur preferentially in elderly patients and are situated more commonly in the supraglottic space and less so in the subglottic. Only NACLERIO (1980) has reported on an adenoma in the glottic region. ARCIDIACONO and MEO (1958) described the malignant transformation of a laryngeal adenoma.

The main symptom of this tumour, as indeed for the majority of laryngeal tumours, is hoarseness.

Oncocytic adenomas were reported by a number of authors: NOHTERI (1946), SOM and PEIMER (1949), HEINZ (1951), VOSTEEN (1954, 1958), COHEN and BATSAKIS (1968), GALLAGHER and PUZON (1969), JOHNS et al. (1973), SASAKI and HOMES (1976), STEINER and PESCH (1976), OLIVEIRA et al. (1977), BELL et al. (1979), FERLITO and RECHER (1981), LINDENBERGER (1982), LUNDGREN et al. (1982), WEIDAUER (1972).

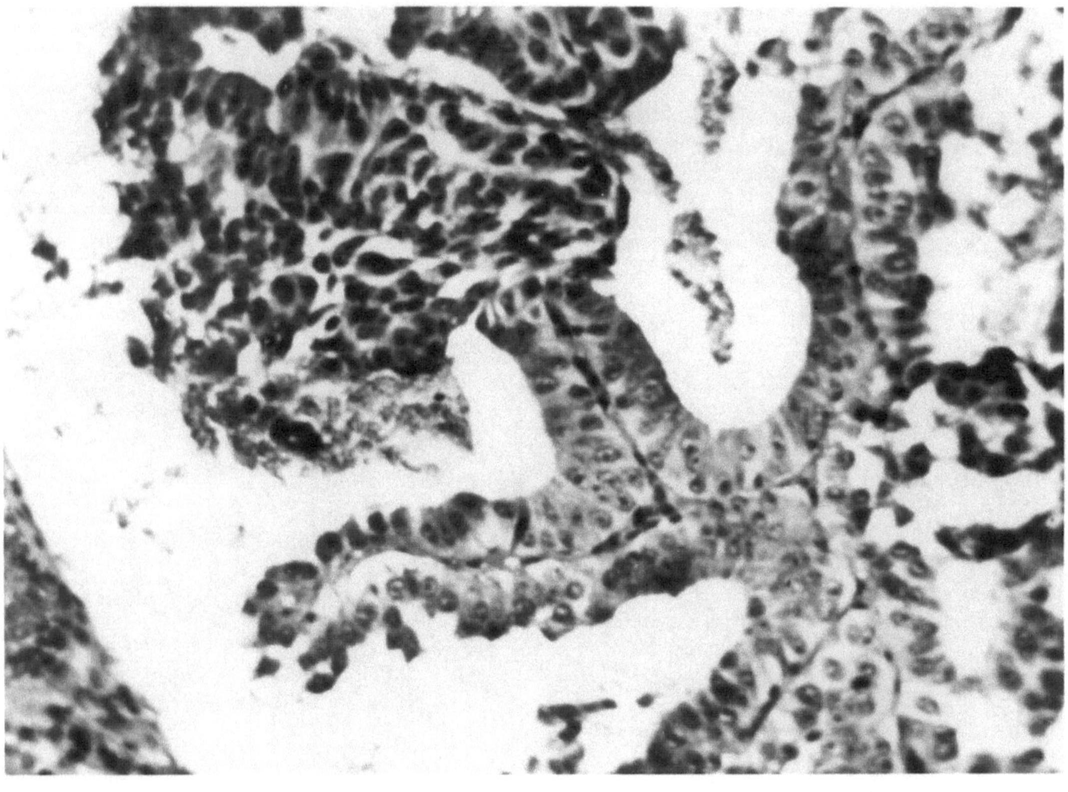

Fig. 3.7. Papillary cystadenoma. 38-year-old man, ventricular fold. HE, ×500

3.2.3 Other Adenomas

Pure adenomas of tubular, acinar or papillary structure occur very rarely in the larynx. BARBACCIA et al. (1956) observed an **adenolymphoma** in the vocal fold region accompanied by follicular lymphatic hyperplasia (Fig. 3.6a, b). Most of the adenomas which do occur in the larynx contain cystic components and are then called **cystadenomas** (WESSELY 1938, FIGI et al. 1944). **Papillary cystadenomas** with formation of folds and villi, usually within the cyst itself, have been observed by RANGER and THACKRAY (1953), ARCIDIACONO and MEO (1958), DONALD and KRAUSE (1973) and by us (Fig. 3.7).

In principle, other benign or malignant tumours (Chap. 7) of salivary gland type can arise from the mucous glands of the larynx. Truly rare examples are **pleomorphic adenomas** in the larynx of which 22 cases have been described in the literature (ZAKZOUK 1985); of these only seven reports are considered convincing benign pleomorphic adenomas by MCMILLAN and FECHNER (1986). The age of the patients ranged from 15 to 70 years, and all tumours were located in the supraglottic region. MCMILLAN and FECHNER (1986) point to the hazard of misinterpreting overlying pseudoepitheliomatous hyperplasia or squamous metaplasia in pleomorphic adenomas as squamous cell carcinomas.

Observations have been reported by FLEISCHER (1956), GIGNOUX et al. (1963), BEHRENDT (1965), TERRACOL (1965), ABOULKER and DEMALDENT (1966), JOKINEN et al. (1974), BETKOWSKI et al. (1978), GAILLARD et al. (1978), SKABANIA and SZLEZAK (1978), SOM et al. (1979), ROZHINSKAIA and CHARTORIZHSKAIA (1980) and YOSHIDA et al. (1983).

3.3 Tumours of Soft Tissue

3.3.1 Mesenchymal Tumours

3.3.1.1 Fibroma, Histiocytoma, Myxoma and Mesenchymoma

Simple **fibromas** are not included in the WHO classification of laryngeal tumours (SHANMUGARATNAM and SOBIN 1978). According to KÖHN (1969), however, fibromas represent the most common benign mesenchymal tumour of the larynx. Older bibliographical references must be reviewed with caution, since pseudotumorous changes in the larynx were previously often classified as fibromas. Further, it cannot be ruled out that many benign tumours of the larynx declared to be fibromas are in fact neurogenic tumours, in particular neurofibromas (FEYRTER 1948, OFFENHAMMER 1954, 1955). The number of true fibromas which have been observed in the larynx should correspondingly be lower than it appears, especially from the older literature. The tendency today to label fibroblastic lesions as histiocytomas is responsible for the fact that MICHAELS (1984) regards fibroblastic tumours in the larynx as uncommon. Traditionally, distinction is made between the more frequent fibroma molle (soft fibroma) and fibroma durum (hard fibroma). Fibroma molle is relatively rich in cells and exhibits loose fibrous connective tissue. Normally submucous, and arising in the supraglottic space, it can occasionally form pedunculate polyps. It occurs at any age but is more prevalent in childhood. TSUI and LORE (1976) reported a case of a congenital, subglottic fibroma molle. The poorly cellular and fibre-rich fibroma durum usually develops in the depth, in the vicinity of the laryngeal framework. Particular variants of this tumour are telangiectatic fibroma (GILBERT et al. 1953, MERZ and GRAF 1958) and giant cell fibroma. Diffuse proliferations of fibrous tissue are rare in the larynx, as are fibromatoses or desmoid tumours (aggressive fibromas) and nodular fasciitis, which is probably reactive in nature (JONES et al. 1984). MCINTOSH et al. (1985) reported a case of a 14-month-old infant in whom congenital solitary fibromatosis of the larynx with fibrosarcomatous changes necessitated total laryngectomy.

In this context we must point out the relationship between histiocytes and fibrocytes. Tumours containing these two kinds of cells have recently often been referred to as **histiocytomas** (JONES et al. 1984). Distinction between benign and malignant forms of fibrous histiocytoma may sometimes be difficult (FERLITO 1978, BIRD and BRYCE 1980).

The so-called **myxoma**, which was observed in the larynx by URFER (1947), ROMUALDI and CORTESI (1947), MATZKER (1963) and CHEN and BALLECER (1986), exhibits, histologically, an abundant gelatinous intercellular substance rich in mucopolysaccharides with few fibres. The stellate, narrow processes of the myxoma cells form a loose reticulate structure. MATZKER (1963) points to the danger of mistaking this for an oedematous pseudomyxomatous polyp. A myxoid liposarcoma, other soft tissue tumours with myxoid degeneration or an oedematous fibroma molle can also, in some circumstances, imitate a myxoma.

Mesenchymomas are mixed lesions consisting of two or more distinct mesenchymal elements in addition to fibrous tissue, e.g. fibrolipoangioma. They are rare in the larynx.

3.3.1.2 Lipoma

Description of laryngeal lipoma date back to that by MEYJERS (1905) who observed a large tumour of this type in the larynx of an 8-year-old boy. There are numerous further references in the literature to the occurrence of laryngeal lipomas. They are most frequent on the epiglottis or the aryepiglottic folds, usually have a lobulated structure, and either project into the laryngeal lumen like polyps or cause a tumorous swelling of the mucosa. Histologically, mature adipose tissue with delicate vessels and narrow connective tissue septae can be seen. Laryngeal lipomas have also been described in connection with diffuse lipomatosis (LAFAYE et al. 1978, MOULONGUET and HAMEL 1976). HUIZINGA (1962), KAPUR (1968) and CHIZH et al. (1980) described malignant transformation of recurrent fibrolipoma into a liposarcoma.

Reports of lipomas have been given by BRUCH (1931), DAVIS (1933), FLYNN (1933), BIRKETT (1934), HEIBERG (1935), DOOTERMANN (1937/38), SCHWARZBART (1937), KLOSE (1938), HARBERT (1951), MACONI (1951), SOM and WOLFF (1952), RICCABONA (1956), GRANT (1961), EAGE (1965), ZAKRZEWSKI (1965), CANNAV (1970), RUDERT (1971a), DI BARTOLOMEO and OLSEN (1973), KONOVALOV (1977), MAREEV and SHKABROV (1980), O'CALLAGHAN et al. (1981) and JONES et al. (1984).

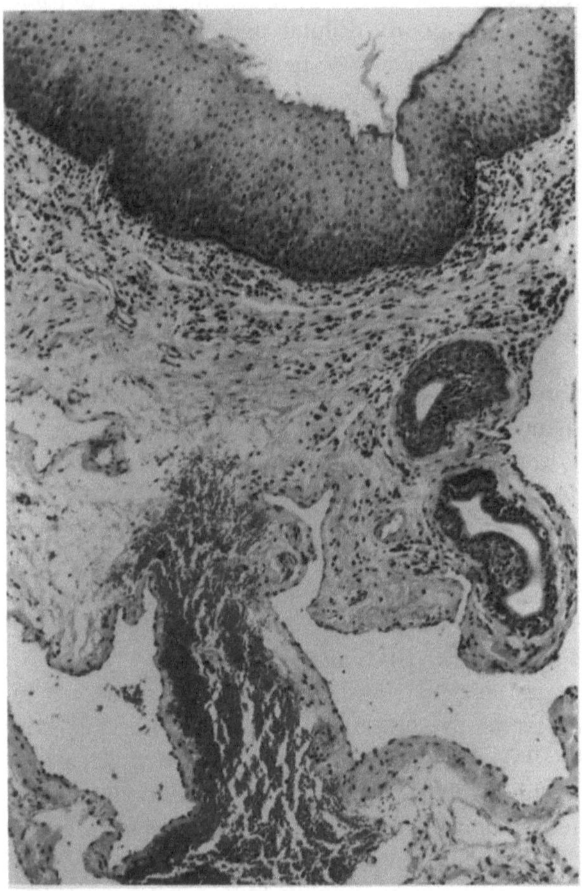

Fig. 3.8. Cavernous haemangioma: 18-year-old woman, supraglottis. Top: the surface epithelium and an excretory glandular duct. Below: cavernous empty spaces lined by a flat endothelium; fresh haemorrhage in the surrounding connective tissue. HE, ×90

3.3.1.3 Angioma

Haemangiomas occur in cavernous and capillary form. In adults, as a rule, the cavernous form (Fig. 3.8) is observed, whereas in newborns and children, haemangiomas of the capillary type are more frequent. The latter must be distinguished from the teleangiectatic granuloma (pyogenic granuloma; see Chap. 8). Haemangiomas of the larynx appear to occur more frequently than was assumed in the past, as reports have increased, especially in the past few years.

According to the numerous reports now available concerning **infantile haemangiomas**, the subglottis is by far the most frequent site of occurrence. Girls appear to be affected more often than boys.

Observations have been reported by SHORP (1939), LAZAR and LEROY (1950), BAKER and PENNINGTON (1956), CAMPBELL (1958), FERGUSON and FLAKE (1961), ZAKRZEWSKI et al. (1963), LEMAIREY et al. (1964), CHRISTAENS et al. (1965), BRIDGER et al. (1970), MINNIGERODE (1970), TOMAS (1971), YEE and HELPER (1973), FEUERSTEIN (1973), JAFFE (1973), HOLBOROW and MOTT (1973), JARVEY and LEVINE (1974), LEIKENSOHN et al. (1976), CHARACHON et al. (1978), BENJAMIN (1978), DILLARD (1979), BEK et al. (1980), HEALY et al. (1980), NARZY et al. (1980), EVANS (1981), JOKINEN et al. (1981), CREPEAU and POLIQUIN (1981), KVETON and PILLSBURY (1982), YOSHIDA et al. (1983) and JONES et al. (1984). A comprehensive survey of older literature can be found in FERGUSON (1944) and KÖHN (1969).

Haemangiomas in adults are less frequent and occur more in the laryngeal inlet and the piriform sinuses (Mounier-Kuhn et al. (1964), Simon (1968), Bridger et al. (1970), Nardi and Rosignoli (1973) and Mirajavsky and Konecny (1974). Among 19 publications by different authors in the period 1978 to 1982, only five reported haemangiomas in adults (Muelfay et al. 1978, Gordon 1979, Kimmelmann et al. 1979, Vlasiuk 1979, Raiz and Kravets 1980).

Macroscopically, haemangiomas are broad-based, sessile, blue-red nodules or elevations covered with mucosa; rarely they present as pedunculate polyps, with smooth or finely bosselated surfaces. The diagnosis can be made macroscopically from the typical picture and biopsies are not indicated. Describing one of his own patients, Simon (1968) pointed out the danger of fatal haemorrhage as a sequel of biopsy.

Similar to papillomas, haemangiomas provide therapeutic problems. Complete excision should be the target. With small haemangiomas this can be achieved by an endolaryngeal approach. Apart from the customary surgical removal (Zöllner 1963), ablation by means of a laser (Simpson et al. 1979, Miehlke et al. 1980, Garfinkle and Handler 1980, Healy et al. 1980, Steiner 1984) and cryotherapy (Schlechter and Biller 1972, Feblot and Dalgroff 1976, Kärjä et al. 1979, Jokinen et al. 1981) have been recommended. We were not able to establish that the risk of haemorrhage with laser ablation is lessened, as is partially conceded by Miehlke et al. (1979). The advantage of almost complete lack of haemorrhage during cryotherapy is counteracted, in our, albeit limited, experience (only a few cases), by the disadvantage that the more sparing the surgery, the more frequently repeat operations are necessary. On the other hand, the more successful the surgical intervention in terms of tumour excision, the more serious are the delayed effects on the laryngeal structure. Large and subglottic haemangiomas are better excised via laryngeal fissure or pharyngotomy following preliminary tracheotomy. Owing to the risk of uncontrollable haemorrhage the removal should be performed under insufflation anaesthesia. Further modes of therapy reported, such as steroids (Cohen and Wang 1972, Schlechter and Biller 1972, Overcash and Putney 1973) and radiotherapy (Tefft 1966, Bourne and Taylor 1972, Feuerstein 1973) appear to us, bearing in mind the consequences, to be especially dubious.

A combination of angiomatous change and proliferation of smooth musculature - the **angioleiomyoma** - has also been observed in the larynx. Six such cases have been described (Neivert and Royer 1946, Quesada et al. 1978, Kleinsasser and Glanz 1979b, Shibata and Komune 1980, Nuutinen and Syrjänen 1983). The tumours are well delimited, usually raised and have been observed on the vestibular and vocal folds. Microscopically they show the typical picture of a vascular tumour with proliferation of smooth muscle fibres, leiomyocytes, in the thickened vessel walls. Fibrosis can be a conspicuous feature.

Hemangioendothelioma - neoplastic proliferation of endothelial cells - is a tumour which can behave benignly or malignantly. Histological distinction is difficult (see Sect. 7.2.1.5). Only two cases of benign haemangioendothelioma seem to have been reported (Nakashima and Watanabe 1985).

Hemangiopericytomas, which are derived from the pericytes of the vessels, have been documented in only six cases (Pesavento and Ferlito 1982). It seems that they can become locally destructive. Since they are difficult to classify as benign or malignant, their radical removal is recommended.

Lymphangiomas occur decidedly more infrequently than haemangiomas. Here too, there are both cavernous and capillary forms. Matzker (1963) reports that he has found a total of seven cases in the world literature. Lymphangiomas have been observed predominantly in the first and second decades of life and at the laryngeal inlet (Kramer and Yankauer 1924, Cordray 1951, Jaffe 1973, Ruben et al. 1975). They are often congenital and form cystic tumours that can lead to progressive dyspnoea (Claros et al. 1985)

3.3.1.4 Leiomyoma

Leiomyomas, which develop from smooth muscles, are, at an early stage, composed of cells which resemble smooth muscle cells with typical cigar-shaped elongated nuclei. Older and usually larger myomas exhibit extensive fibrosis with atrophy of the true myoma cells. Differentiation of such myomas from fibromas can prove difficult. In the larynx, leiomyomas are exceedingly rare. Kleinsasser and Glanz (1979b) found 15 proven case reports of simple leiomyoma of the larynx in the literature, in addition three angioleiomyomas (Sect. 3.3.1.3). We have found only three additional reports (Ebert and Scholz 1979, Matsumoto et al. 1981, Nuutinen and Syrjänen 1983). Those affected are usually middle-aged and there seems to be no sexual predilection. Somewhat older literature can be found in GRACANIN (1947) and GUERRIER (1960).

3.3.1.5 Rhabdomyoma

In the older literature, myoblastic myomas, rhabdomyomas and granular cell tumours were not strictly separated from one another owing to their common large and granular cell character. Tumours of this group were first described by ABRIKOSSOFF (1926, 1931). Observation of cross-striation in the cytoplasm-rich cells is considered to be an indication of an origin from skeletal muscle; but striation is not always detectable. Nowadays a distinction is made between the true rhabdomyomas and those given the noncommital designation "granular cell tumours" whose origin is still unclear but most likely neurogenic (see Sect. 3.3.2.4). With the aid of the electron microscope (BATTIFORA et al. 1969) or, more elegantly, immunohistochemical methods, differential diagnosis can today be accomplished in all cases.

The true **adult rhabdomyomas** occur occasionally in the myocardium, where some are considered, not as neoplasms but as dysontogenetic malformations. In all other organs they form a true rarity, whilst nonetheless showing a predilection for the upper region of the neck, the tongue, pharynx and larynx. In 1964, MORAN and ENTERLINE compiled a survey of 11 reports of proven rhabdomyomas in the literature, adding one of their own cases. Only eight laryngeal rhabdomyomas described in the literature were considered to be of proven origin from skeletal muscle by KLEINSASSER and GLANZ (1979b).

Mainly older people are affected, men more of-

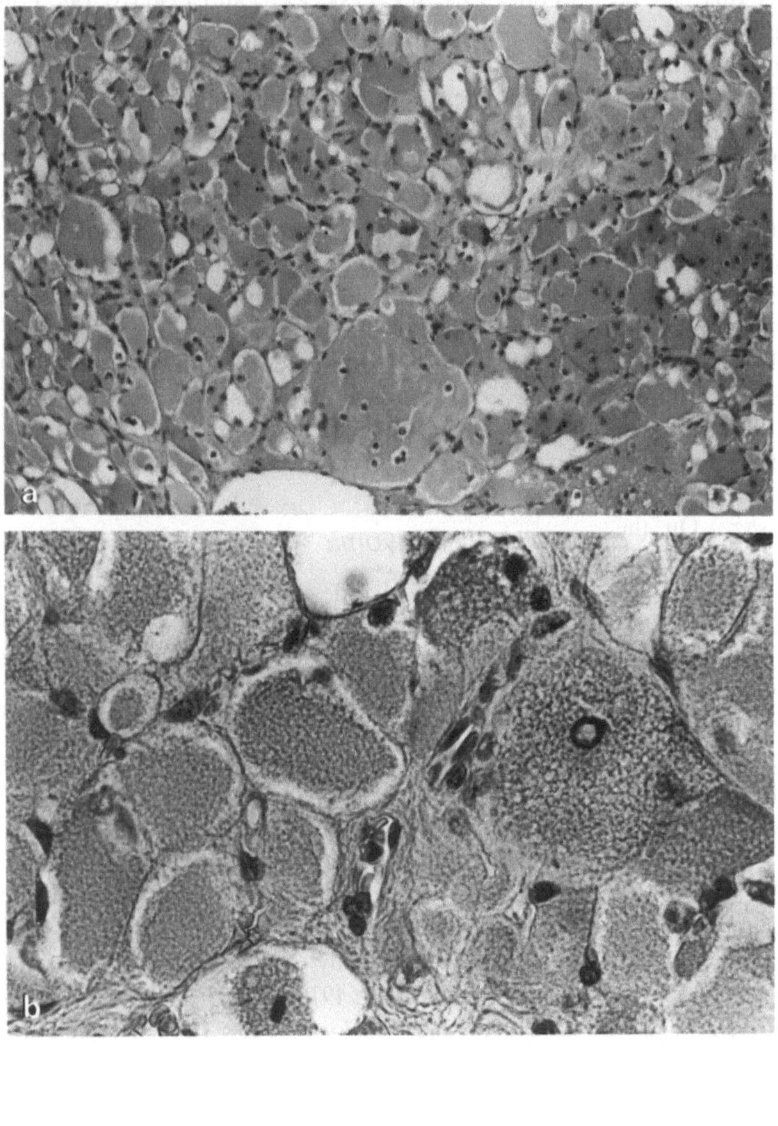

Fig. 3.9a, b. Rhabdomyoma: 64-year-old man with two separate tumorous lesions in the region of the right aryepiglottic fold and in the piriform sinus. **a** At low magnification the large round to polygonal tumour cells with extreme variations of size and mostly multiple nuclei can be seen. HE, ×140. **b** At higher magnification granulation of the vast cytoplasm of the tumour cells is pronounced and occasional faint cross-striation is discernible. HE, ×560

ten than women; multitopical occurrence is not uncommon (GARDNER and CORIO 1983a). The symptoms are hoarseness, stridor, dysphagia and acute respiratory tract obstruction. There is usually no recurrence following local excision.

Macroscopically laryngeal rhabdomyomas are broad-based polypous protrusions which have a smooth surface and a flesh-brown cut surface. Histologically (Fig. 3.9) the tumours are sharply bounded, though they have either no, or only a thin, fibrous capsule. The tumour cells are large (20–30 μm), round to polygonal in shape and contain an abundantly fine to coarse granular, in part fibrillar, marked eosinophilic and PAS-positive cytoplasm with detectable circumscribed cross-striation. Vacuoles containing glycogen and crystalline inclusions are frequent. Usually there are several small nuclei situated eccentrically. Mitotic figures are absent. The interstitial connective tissue is sparse.

On the ultrastructural level (Fig. 3.10a) haphazardly arranged filaments of the myosin and actin type, Z-band material, in part dense bundles of fibrils with incomplete and hypertrophic Z-bands, numerous mitochondria, free ribosomes and rough endoplasmic reticulum can be observed (BATTIFORA et al. 1969, HEIDEN et al. 1978, SCHLOSNAGLE et al. 1983). The cells form, just like normal muscle fibres, a basal lamina on the surface.

Immunohistologically the strongly positive reaction with myoglobin antibodies is proof of the myogenic origin of laryngeal rhabdomyomas (Fig. 3.10b).

Rhabdomyoma must be differentiated from granular cell tumour (Abrikossoff tumour), oncocytoma, mesenchymal hamartoma, mesenchymoma

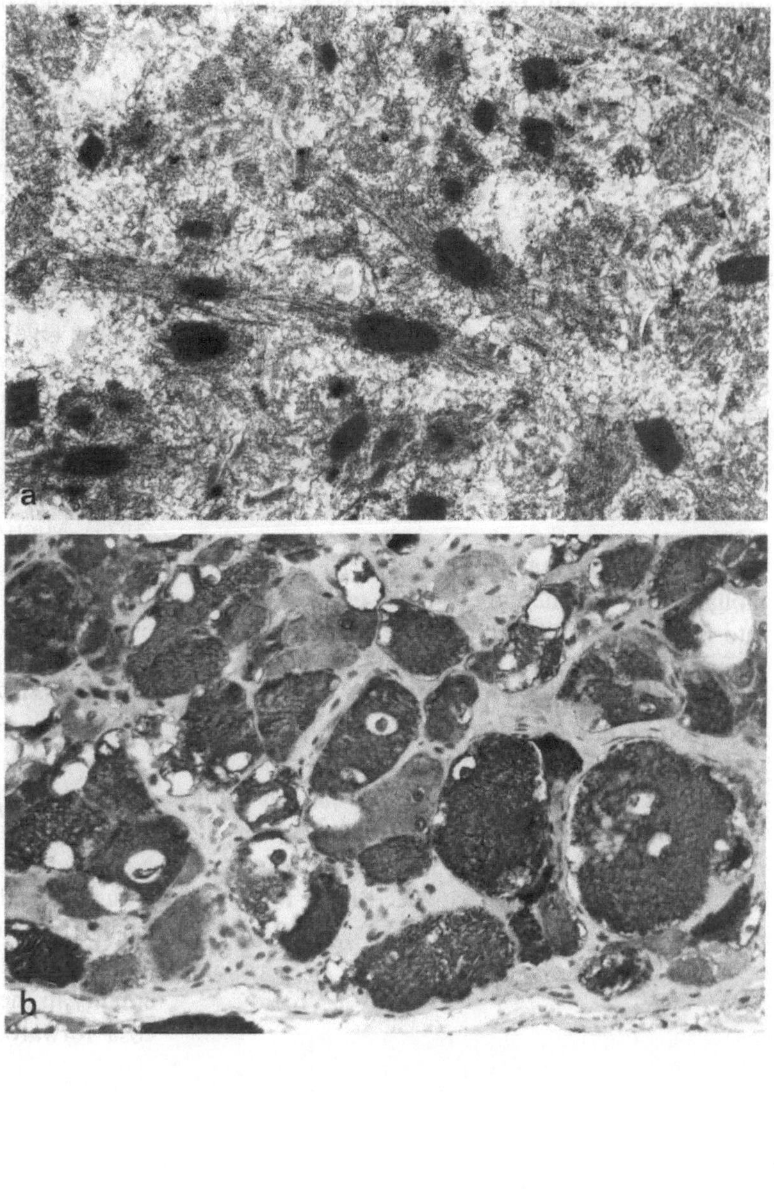

Fig. 3.10a, b. Rhabdomyoma: same case as Figure 3.9. **a** Electron microscopic picture of the cytoplasm with abundant more or less orderly filamentous systems (myosin and actin type) and marked hypertrophic electron dense Z-bands typical for contractile elements. × 25000. **b** Immunohistological demonstration of myoglobin. The cytoplasm of the majority of the tumour cells shows a strongly positive reaction (brown in original slide). PAP, × 220

with myogenic components and rhabdomyosarcoma. Transformation of rhabdomyoma into rhabdomyosarcoma has not yet been observed.

An extremely rare tumour which has been observed mainly in the vulvovaginal region is **fetal rhabdomyoma**, which is subdivided into myxoid and cellular types. There are case descriptions in the oral region (GARDNER and CURIO 1983b) and also in the larynx (GRANICH et al. 1983, ROSENMAN et al. 1986). Both types are much richer in cells than the "adult" rhabdomyoma described above and they contain elongated fusiform cells, usually without cross-striation. In the myxoid type, the tumour has a loose myxoid structure. Especially in the cellular variant there is pleomorphism of cells which can make differentiation from sarcoma difficult. Clinically, fetal rhabdomyomas can present as a polypoid mass. They should not behave differently from the adult form (GRANICH et al. 1983).

More recent reports on rhabdomyomas in the laryngeal region can be found, in addition to those already mentioned, in FERLITO and FRUGONI (1975), BAGBY et al. (1976), WINTHER (1976), BOEDTS and MESTDAGH (1979), MODLIN (1982) and JONES et al. (1984).

3.3.2 Tumours of the Peripheral Nervous System

In the peripheral nervous system predominantly the so-called neurosustentacular tissue (perineural cells or Schwann cells) gives rise to neoplasms. It is of neurocristic origin and can express either fibrogenic, neurosustentacular or melanocytic functions depending on inductive influences from the environment.

According to FEYRTER (1948, 1951), benign tumours of the peripheral nervous system are divided into fusiform, multiform, microcystic, reticular and granular neurinomas. These are rare tumours in the larynx. CUMMINGS et al. (1969) found only 77 cases described in the world literature, up to 1969 without taking into account the individual subdivisions. All age groups are affected, the youngest patient being aged 3 months (CUMMINGS et al. 1969) and the oldest 80 years (MATZKER 1963). No significant sexual predilection can be recognized from the cases described in the literature.

3.3.2.1 Neurilemmoma (Schwannoma, Neurinoma)

The fusiform and multiform neurinomas are the most common type of these tumours and far exceed the other types in number. According to VON ALBERTINI (1974) they originate from the neurilemma, hence the term schwannoma or neurilemmoma. Histologically the whorled and braided arrangement of the fusiform cells and of the accompanying fibres is typical, as is the so-called palisade positioning of the nuclei. Two architectural types can be distinguished: Antoni A (compact with vertical palisades) and Antoni B (loose-textured myxoid). Further classification into cellular, cystic and ancient (hyalinized) types is possible. The tumours are nonencapsulated and may exhibit a certain degree of nuclear pleomorphism. Macroscopically these tumours, which frequently develop from the submucosa, project a usually intact smooth mucosal surface into the laryngeal lumen. The preferred location in the larynx is the supraglottic region, usually on the aryepiglottic fold. NANSON (1978) surveyed 86 cases of laryngeal neurinoma documented in the world literature.

Granular neurinomas are so similar to so-called myoblastic myomas and granular cell tumours that the distinction can be difficult.

References to neurinomas of the larynx can be found, for example, in MARSCHIK (1936), NEW and DEVINE (1947), WALKERS (1947), MCHENRY (1953), RICCABONA (1953), BAUM (1957), GREGG and MYRABO (1959), SZÖNYI and BERENYI (1960), FENDEL (1962), MATZKER 1963, ASH et al. (1964), ABOULKER et al. (1969), THOMAS and REES (1969), WHITTAM and MORRIS (1970), NAEIM and WAISMAN (1973), MICHAELS (1975), PALVA et al. (1975), GAILLARD et al. (1978), NANSON (1978), MÜNZEL and KASTENDIEK (1978), FLEURY et al. (1979), MATIC et al. (1979), MOSTOWSKI (1979), GOODER and FARRINGTON (1980), NATALI et al. (1980) and JONES et al. (1984). ZAKRZEWSKI (1977) reported on a case of malignant transformation.

3.3.2.2 Neurofibroma

Neurogenic tumours with a predominance of loose tissue are called neurofibromas. According to VON ALBERTINI (1974), these tumours originate from the endoneurium. Macroscopically they occur preferentially in the supraglottic region, pushing the mucosa forward. Histologically, simple, cell-rich and plexiform neurofibromas can be distinguished. MATZKER (1963) found neurofibromatosis in association with von Recklinghausen's disease in eight of 17 published cases. Most cases of endolaryngeal neurofibromas described so far have occurred in generalized neurofibromatosis (MORI and TORTORA 1966, SMOLER et al. 1966, JAFEK and STERN 1973, MAISEL and OGURA 1974, PERRIN et al. 1975, CHANG-LO 1977, COHEN et al. 1978, ALTMEYER and MERKEL 1981). YURICH and BEEKHUIS (1960), O'CONNOR and FREELAND (1980) as well as SUPANCE et al. (1980) reported on a regional endolaryngeal neurofibromatosis, which was congenital in one instance. Only BERGER (1967) and TSUKERBERG and ZAKHAROV (1971) described a solitary neurofibroma of the larynx. References to older literature can be found in KÖHN (1969).

3.3.2.3 Paraganglioma, Chemodectoma

Among the paragangliomas, distinction is made between the nonchromaffinic paragangliomas, glomus tumours or chemodectomas and chromaffinic paragangliomas or pheochromocytomas. Their occurrence is exceedingly rare in the larynx and they are derived from the paraganglia of the larynx. In addition to the long-known superior laryngeal glomus situated in the anterior part of the false vocal cord, Kleinsasser described in 1964 a paired inferior laryngeal glomus situated between the cricoid cartilage and the first tracheal ring.

Patients between 14 and 71 years of age were affected by paragangliomas of the larynx, the mean age being 65. According to the literature there is no sexual predilection. The tumors are located, in general, in the supraglottis in the region of the upper laryngeal paraganglia. They are usually still small when diagnosis is established, since they can cause intense pain at an early stage (MICHAELS 1975).

Histologically paragangliomas exhibit a basic alveolar structure, i. e. the tumours are composed of cell clusters (Zellballen) of varying size which are held together by a fine fibre network and lie in a well-vascularized stroma. Occasional acinar structures containing PAS-positive material are formed and may lead to the erroneous diagnosis of adenocarcinoma (SPAGNOLO and PARADINAS 1985). The rate of initial misdiagnosis is high (30%). In general the round to polygonal cells present a relatively monomorphic picture but occasionally considerable variations can be seen in the form and size of the nuclei. The cytoplasm usually contains eosinophilic granules and may be argyrophilic. Using the electron microscope, dense-cored secretory granules can be observed in the cytoplasm. The behaviour of the paragangliomas cannot be deduced from the histological picture; mitotic figures may be the only indicator of malignant potential. As a rule they behave in a benign fashion, although recurrence and metastasis may occur (MICHAELS 1975, HOHBACH and MOOTS 1978, FISHBEIN et al. 1979, WETMORE et al. 1981). Malignant behaviour is reported in about one-third of cases (JONES et al. 1984, SPAGNOLA and PARADINAS 1985).

ZAK and LAWSON (1982) reviewed 33 paragangliomas reported in the literature up to 1979. Further descriptions are given by ANDREWS (1955), BLANCHARD and SAUNDERS (1955), ZEITLHOFER (1955), NEUSS (1956), MATZKER (1963), BAXTER (1965), MARTINSON (1967), VETTERS and TONER (1970), ISHIDA et al. (1971), HOOPER (1972), TOBIN and HARRIS (1972), LAWSPN and ZAK (1974), MICHAELS (1975), HOHBACH and MOOTZ (1978), PERRIN et al. (1978), ANI et al. (1979), GALLIVAN et al. (1979), CLARK-NETO (1980), GEHANNO et al. (1980), JUSTRABO et al. (1980), TRIANTALFILIDI and NASYROV (1980), SCHAEFER et al. (1980), HORDIJK et al. (1981), LEES et al. (1981), LINDELL et al. (1981), THOMAS and BERNARDINO (1981), WETMORE et al. (1981), BASSET et al. (1982) and JONES et al. (1984).

3.3.2.4 Granular Cell Tumour

Granular cell tumours are benign lesions comprising large cells with abundant finely granular cytoplasm. The opinion voiced by FEYRTER (1952) and OFFENHAMMER (1955), namely, that the "myoblastic myoma" of Abrikossoff is, in fact, a granular, neurogenic tumour (granular neurinoma or neuroma), is based on the similarity of the "myoma cells" to the cells in such tumours. For this reason the terms "myoblastic myoma" and "rhabdomyoma" should be reserved for those tumours in which the criteria stated above - cross-striation, myosin and actin filaments, positive myoglobin reaction - are fulfilled (see Sect. 3.3.1.5).

Granular cell tumours appear preferentially subcutaneously and in the oral cavity, with about 10% occurring in the larynx. NOLTE and KLEINSASSER (1982) found 151 cases of granular cell tumours in the laryngeal region documented in the literature and further described four of their own cases. The tumour arises most frequently in the area of the vocal folds, sometimes in the supraglottic region; in children a subglottic origin has also been observed (GARUD et al. 1984, HAR-EL et al. (1985). The patients are mostly young to middle-aged, with the third decade predominating. There is no obvious sexual predilection. Occasionally granular cell tumours are multiple (MOSCOVIC and AZAR 1967). MAJMUDAR et al. (1981) reported on a patient with numerous granular cell tumours in the laryngeal and tracheal region as well as in the tongue, vulva and chest wall.

Macroscopically these tumours appear either as pedunculate polyps or as broad-based sessile growth which push the mucosa forward. The surface shows epithelial hyperplasia in 64% of cases and in 50% a so-called pseudoepitheliomatous hyperplasia (COMPAGNO et al. 1975, AGARWAL et al. 1979; cf. Chap. 4). Occasionally this raises diagnostic problems with regard to distinction from carcinoma.

Histologically the cells are similar to rhabdomyoma cells but somewhat smaller, often elongated and cuspidate; they are weakly eosinophilic (Fig. 3.11 a) but also PAS-positive. As a rule they have only one, slightly eccentrically situated nucleus. Mitotic figures cannot be observed. In making the differential diagnosis, rhabdomyomas, paragangliomas and histiocytic lesions have to be discounted. In the electron microscope no contractile filamentous elements can be seen, but rather abundant osmiophilic membrane-bound granules which are probably derived from lysosomes (BATTIFORA 1969, GARUD et al. 1984). Immunohistochemically, both the neuronespecific enolase and S-100 protein reactions are positive (Fig. 3.11 b).

Although granular cell tumours in general also

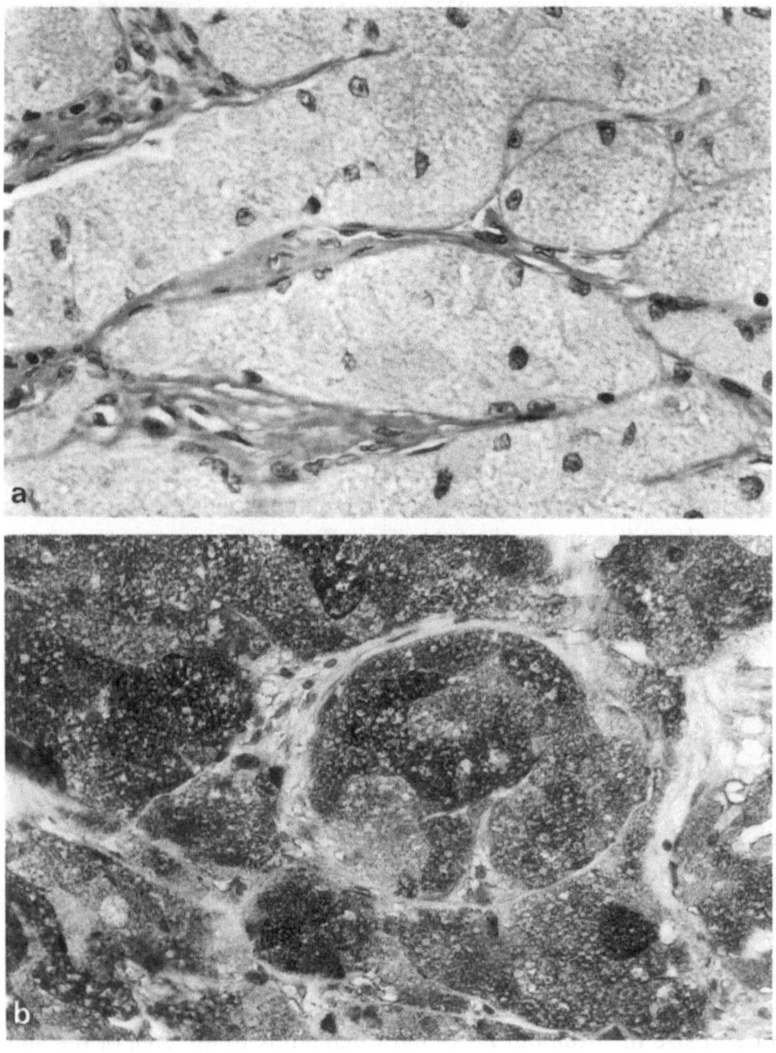

Fig. 3.11 a, b. Granular cell tumour: 23 year-old-woman, supraglottis. **a** Large tumour cells with abundant granular cytoplasm and multiple nuclei reminiscent of the cells of rhabdomyoma. HE ×350. **b** Immunohistological demonstration of S-100 protein. Positive reaction of the cytoplasm (brown in original) PAP, ×350

have no capsule, they are virtually always benign, so that simple surgical removal is adequate. The possibility of malignant transformation was pointed out by BUSANNY-CASPARY and HAMMAR (1958). Owing to the morphological variability of rhabdomyosarcomas, those cases of malignant transformation of granular cell tumours described in the literature (CADOTTE 1974) must be evaluated with caution.

More recent references in the literature to the occurrence of granular cell tumours in the larynx can be found, in addition to those cited above, in HELIDONIS et al. (1978), KENEFICK (1978), FRADIS et al. (1980), GAMMELGARD and JUUL (1980), MCSWAIN et al. (1980) WEISMAN et al. (1980), MROCZKOWSKI (1982), NEVILLE and MCCONNEL (1981), SHEVCHENKO et al. (1981), TOMECKOVA et al. (1981), IVATURY et al. (1982), MODLIN (1982) and EL-GAZALI and EL-GAZALI (1982). KÖHN (1969) provides references to older literature.

3.3.2.5 Ganglioneuroma

Ganglioneuromas (synonyms: gangliocytoma, ganglioglioma) are composed of nerve fibres and mature ganglial cells. They constitute an extreme rarity in the larynx, and as far as we know, have been described only 3 times in the world literature (SPIESS 1930, MATZKER 1963, ZAGARSKIKH 1971). The patients were aged 1, 14 and 31 years. In the first two cases the tumour was situated in the lateral wall of the laryngeal inlet, in the last case in the subglottis.

Macroscopically the intact mucosa was pushed forward. The tumour may consist of multiple nodules. Microscopically it is composed of bands of Schwann cells. The coarse fascicles are similar to those of the neurofibroma. The irregularly distributed ganglion cells are either grouped in clusters or appear singly. They may be multinucleate with prominent nucleoli. The abundant cytoplasm of larger cells often contains Nissl granules. Usually there are no satellite cells, but these may be present and exhibit a typical arrangement. Rather immature ganglion cells indicate ganglioneuroblastoma. Occasionally the fasciculated form is absent in these immature types. The "ganglioma" described by SPIESS (1930) may be such a ganglioneuroblastoma. Since neurogenic tumours may develop in or infiltrate ganglia, there is a danger of mistaking such tumours for ganglioneuromas. Accounts of the occurrence of ganglioneuromas should thus be viewed with appropriate caution (HARKIN and REED 1969).

3.4 Tumours of Cartilaginous and Osseous Tissue

3.4.1 Chondroma

Chondromas are not infrequent in the larynx. SINGH et al. (1980) reviewed 77 cases of chondromatous tumours from the world literature and added two cases of their own.

Chondromas can occur at any age but do tend to occur more in older people (fourth to sixth decade). Men are affected 4 times as often as women. A congenital chondroma was reported by ADLER et al. (1985). Chondromas grow slowly. Dyspnoea, hoarseness and alteration in speech are typical symptoms (NEEL and UNNI 1982). Asthmoid symptoms were described by EPPER and MAURER (1980).

Communications concerning laryngeal chondromas have become so numerous in recent years that we wish to refer only to recent reviews (SINGH et al. 1980, EPPER and MAURER 1980, DAMIANI and TUCKER 1981, ESCHER et al. 1984, WEBBER et al. 1986). Older bibliographic references can be found in KÖHN (1969).

Chondromas take the form of hard, often spherical growths which push the smooth mucosal surface forward and at the same time grow into the deep tissue layers; they originate most commonly in the subglottic region from the cricoid cartilage (70%). The second most common site of origin is the thyroid cartilage (20%) whereas the remaining parts of the laryngeal framework playing only a minor role.

Histologically all cartilaginous tissue types can be imitated, but as a rule the hyaline form dominates (Fig. 3.12). Chondromas may calcify, ossify, exhibit myxoid areas or form lacunae or cavities. MAYOUX et al. (1955), LEROUX-ROBERT (1956), REINHARD (1960), PUTNEY and MORAN (1964), HYAMS and RABUZZI (1970), MITSCHKE (1975), SINGH et al. (1980) and ESCHER et al. (1984), as well as the present authors, have seen chondromas with sarcomatous transformation (Chap. 7). Especially noticeable in the tumours we observed was the interspersion of well-differentiated tissue and areas with undifferentiated tumour growth. The characteristics of chondrosarcomas, as compared to chondromas, are increased cellularity, enlarged nuclei and pleomorphism, mitotic figures and multinuclear tumour cells.

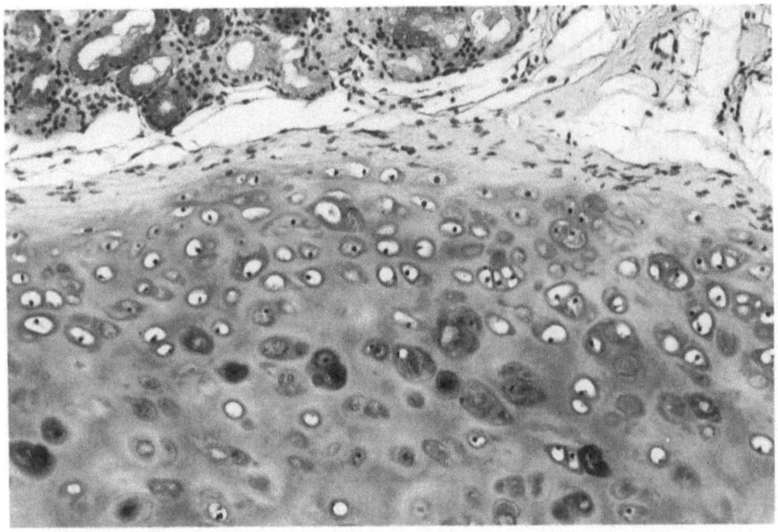

Fig. 3.12. Chondroma: 53 year-old man, cricoid cartilage. The tumour is sharply delineated and composed of hyaline cartilage. The only difference from normal cartilage is slightly higher cellularity and occasionally the presence of two chondrocytes in the chondral cavities. There is no marked nuclear pleomorphism. PAS, ×140

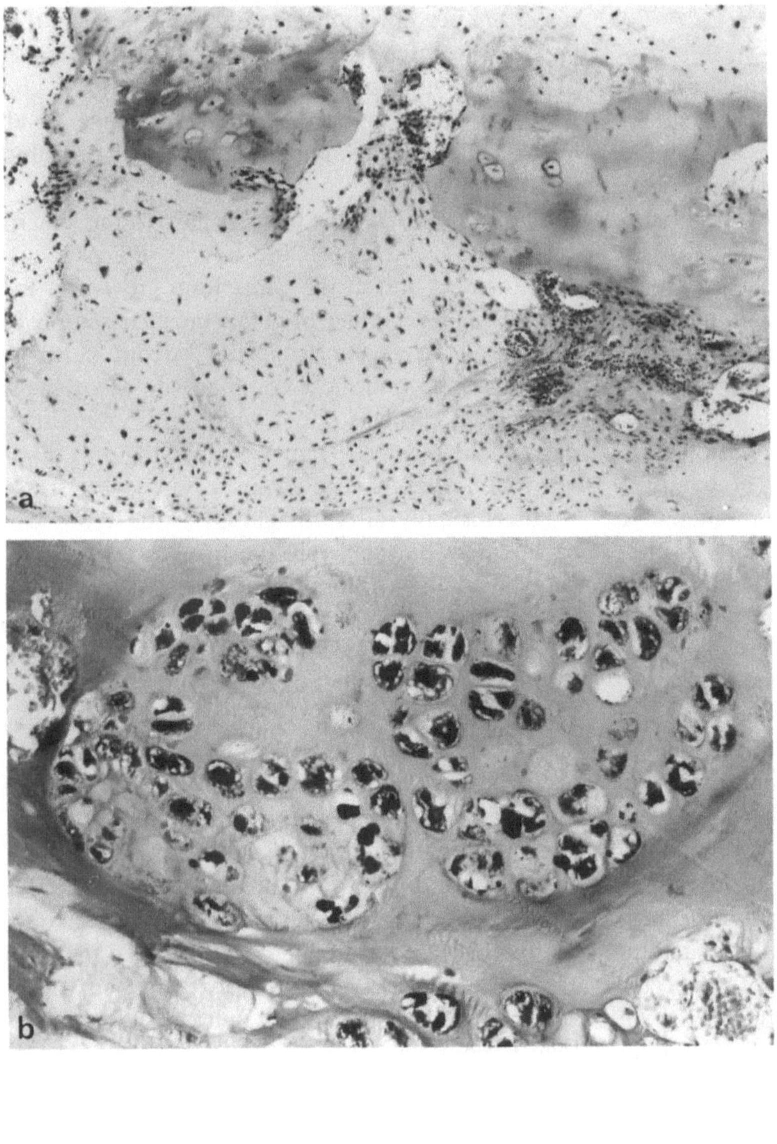

Fig. 3.13a, b. Chondromatous tumour with cellular atypia: 64 year-old man, cricoid cartilage. **a** Irregular composition of the tumour by areas of variable cellularity and vascularity. HE ×90. **b** Higher magnification shows an area with dense cellularity and marked nuclear atypia and hyperchromasia. There are aggregates of more than two cells in the chondral cavities. PAS, ×220

According to ESCHER et al. (1984) a small nodular structure is found mostly in benign tumours, while the presence of spindle cell components and perivascular lymphocytic infiltration is associated with malignancy.

Even relatively benign looking chondromatous tumours may show localized cellular atypia (Fig. 3.13), aggressive behaviour and a tendency to recur. Some can be classified as "low-grade" chondrosarcomas (grade I). Among 33 chondromatous tumours, NEEL and UNNI (1982) diagnosed two benign chondromas, 21 grade I chondrosarcomas and 10 chondrosarcomas. For this reason BATSAKIS (1979) recommends treating chondromatous tumours in general with corresponding respect. MICHAELS (1984) forgoes the division of cartilaginous tumours into benign or malignant.

3.4.2 Osteoma

Corresponding to the different structures of compact and trabecular bone, there are two histoarchitectural forms of osteoma, namely, osteoma eburneum and osteoma spongiosum. In the larynx, osteomas are so exceedingly rare that we could find only two cases registered in the world literature (GERASCHENKO 1957, TSYBYRNE and BOGDANSKAIA 1979). Exostoses occur much more frequently in the larynx; however, they are not to be regarded as tumours, but rather as malformations or overgrowths (VON ALBERTINI 1974). Ossification of other tumours is occasionally observed, such as the fibroma ossificans described by GESCHICKTER and COPELAND (1936). Chondromas may also exhibit ossification (HOPMANN 1935, LESIONE 1965).

3.4.3 Giant Cell Tumour

Although various authors, for example BÜNGELER (1957), have interpreted giant cell lesions in general as reactive tissue proliferations, giant cell tumours originating from osteoclasts are acknowledged as true neoplasms by most authors today (see KÖHN 1969). They have to be differentiated from reactive lesions containing giant cells (giant cell granuloma/fibromas). Their behaviour is generally benign with a tendency to recur; very occasionally an aggressive course can be encountered.

Giant cell tumours of the larynx occur most frequently in the ossified framework and probably originate from the periosteum. They are therefore assigned to the group of cartilaginous and osseous tissue tumours in the WHO classification. They do not show a consistent structure. In particular, the relationship between cell and fibre fraction varies.

Giant cell tumours in the larynx have been described by WESSELY (1939), WAGEMANN (1952), PERRINO (1958), KÖHN (1969), RUDERT (1971b), HALL-JONES (1972), GOTO and NAKASHIMA (1973), KOTARBA and NIEZABITOWSKI (1974), RIBARI et al. (1975), KUBO et al. (1976) and MOUBAYED and WIEBRINGHAUS (1977).

3.5 Tumours of the Lymphatic and Haematopoietic System

3.5.1 Plasmocytoma

Solitary extramedullary plasmocytomas occur fairly frequently in the larynx. In the period from 1962 up to the time of writing we observed five solitary laryngeal plasmocytomas. MANIGLIA and XUE (1983) found 79 cases described in the literature and added three cases of their own. The preferred site was the supraglottic region. Paraproteinaemia is absent in solitary plasmocytoma.

Generalized plasmocytomas appear in older patients as reddish elevations of the mucosa, or in the form of polyps. Histologically there is a dense accumulation of plasma cells, in most cases of an inconspicuous appearance; they are as a rule monoclonal, as can be shown by immunohistology. Amyloid deposition is sometimes seen.

In principle, it has to be established by suitable clinical means of diagnosis to what extent other areas of the body are similarly affected. Surgical removal is the method of choice in cases in which functional disorders are not to be expected. Otherwise radiotherapy and cytostatic treatment should be considered.

3.6 Miscellaneous Tumours, Malformations

Only brief reference will be made here to the very rare **teratomas** (JOHNSON and STRONG 1954, FLEISCHER 1956, FOURNIE et al. 1965, CHUMAKOW and VOINOVA 1973) and **hamartomas** of the laryn-

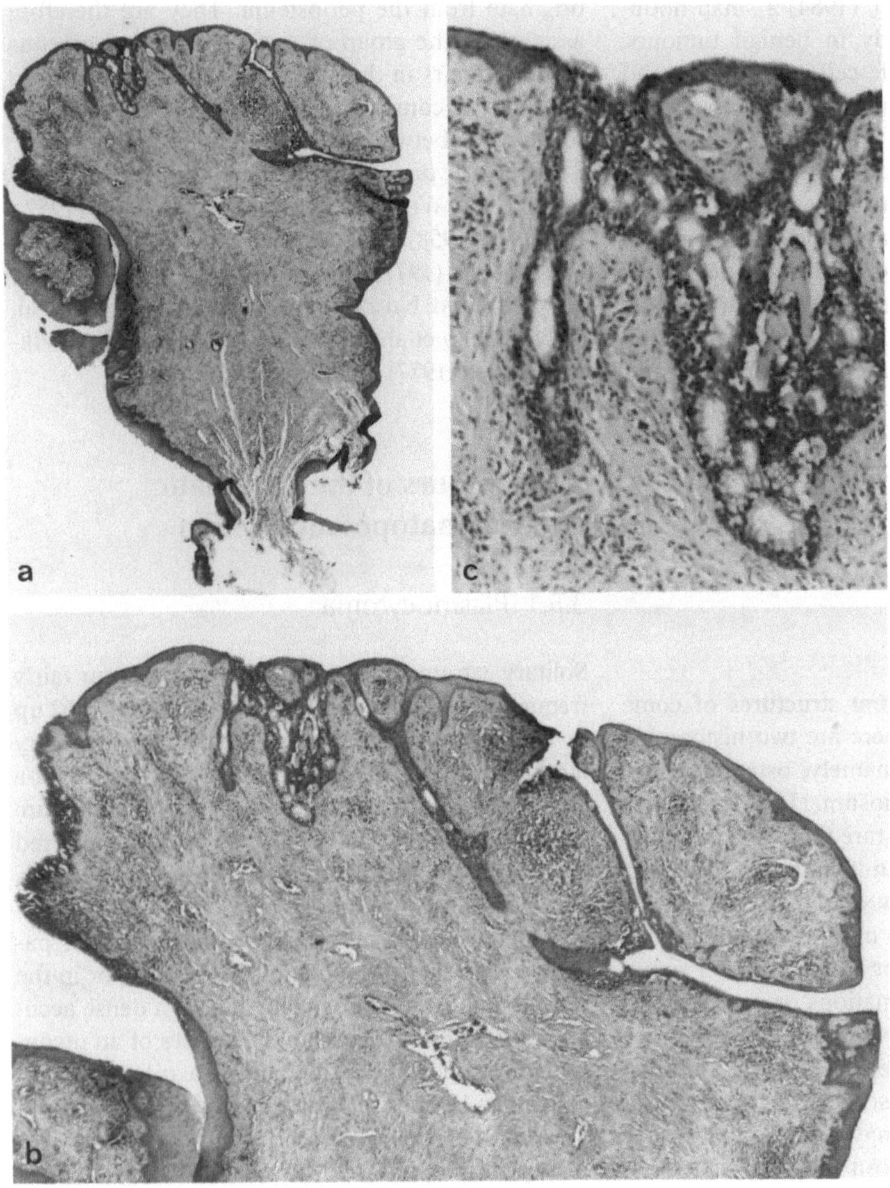

Fig. 3.14a–c. Hamartomatous polyp of the subglottis in a 49-year-old woman with Cowden's syndrome. a Overview of the polyp, which is composed mainly of fibrous tissue covered by epithelium with infoldings into the depth. HE, ×10. b Epithelial infoldings with glandular mucin-producing cells. HE ×90. c The surface of the polyp is covered mainly by squamous epithelium. Below the epithelium, dense fibrous tissue with few ectatic blood vessels. HE, ×35

geal region. Teratomas, i.e. tumorous malformations of different mature tissues, may lead to airway obstruction in newborns. COHEN (1984) described two children with hamartomas of the larynx associated with posterior clefts causing severe episodes of airway obstruction. We observed a hamartomatous laryngeal polyp (Fig. 3.14) in a 49-year-old female patient with **Cowden's disease**. This condition is characterized by fibromatous, in part hamartomatous, overgrowths in various organs (e.g. gingiva and mamma) together with other malformations (LLOYD and DENNIS 1963). A similar isolated polyp was described by ZAPF et al. (1981) in a 6-week-old child with respiratory obstruction. WILHELM et al. (1980) removed a hamartoma in a 42 year-old male patient: the tumour protruded submucosally under the arytenoid region. Such tumours must be distinguished from mesenchymal neoplasms of mixed composition, i.e. mesenchymomas.

Although of malignant nature, **laryngeal blastoma**, recently described in a 65-year-old patient (EBLE et al. 1985), will be mentioned in this context. It corresponds to the rare pulmonary blastoma and is composed of a mixture of immature tissue containing characteristic blastematous components and, in contrast to teratomas, no organoid structures.

Other tumour-like malformations (cysts, laryngoceles) will be described in Chap. 8.

4 General Conditions and Risk Factors of Carcinogenesis, Precancerous Lesions

4.1 Incidence, Age, Sex Distribution and Risk Factors

4.1.1 Incidence

The incidence of malignant neoplasms of the larynx has risen in proportion to the increase in new cases of respiratory tract carcinomas in general (McMichael 1978, Steiner 1984; review Kleinsasser 1983); the overall mortality is 2.5 per 100000 person-years, and in the USA new laryngeal cancers form 1.5% of all new cases of cancer and laryngeal cancer mortality is 0.9% of total cancer mortality.

4.1.2 Age, Sex Distribution and Hormonal Factors

As in malignancies of the respiratory tract generally, elderly individuals, and in particular men, are those most frequently affected by precancerous lesions and carcinomas of the larynx, with a maximum in the seventh decade (Fig. 4.1). This is valid too for malignant diseases in the region of the hypopharynx and the larynx-adjacent oropharynx, i.e. the so-called external laryngeal carcinomas. In the USA only 13% (Devesa and Silverman 1978), in Sweden 9.7% (Olofsson and van Nostrand 1973), in West Germany between 4% and 8% (Schwab and zum Winkel 1975, Bohndorf and Höcker 1976), in the German Democratic Republic 8.1% and in Switzerland 7.6% (in the period 1979–1981; Bundesamt für Statistik 1984) of all laryngeal cancers affected women. However, in the past few years, a backward trend has been noticeable in the predominance of men (Ramadan 1982). Between 1956 and 1976, Wynder et al. (1976) observed a change in the ratio of men to women from 14.9:1 to 4.6:1. They regard this as a reflection of increased cigarette smoking in women. Deitmer (1983) observed two types of women among 71 women with laryngeal cancer: older women who smoked, and younger women showing signs of virilism. Kambic et al. (1984) state, that in Yugoslavia, where there are virtually no differences between men and women in relation to living conditions, work, and smoking habits, there is nonetheless a clear predominance of laryngeal cancer in men. Apparently not only different ways of life of men and women play a role in the development of leukoplakia and carcinoma in the larynx, but also direct hormonal influences. Thus the larynx must be viewed broadly as a secondary sex characteristic, i.e. as a hormone-dependent tissue; the extent of squamous metaplasia correlates with the size of the larynx and the length and thickness of the vocal fold, which are both hormone-dependent and more pronounced in men (Scott 1976). Loewit et al. (1979) were able to demonstrate that testosterone and oestrogen excretion in 15 patients suffering from carcinoma of the larynx was significantly higher than that in a control group. Serum testosterone levels are significantly raised in laryngeal cancer patients – both men and women (Kambic et al. 1984, Haidoutova et al. 1985) but not in patients with epithelial hyperplasia and precancerous lesions (Kambic et al. 1984). Treatment of the latter group of patients with the testosterone antagonist cyproterone acetate, however, produced some cure or improvement in some cases (Hussl et al. 1978).

4.1.3 Endogenous Factors

As with most neoplasms, a genetic (familial) predisposition can be observed for laryngeal cancer. This may be due to metabolic factors. For example, high acrylhydrocarbon hydroxylase (AHH) inducibility is statistically overrepresented in patients with lung cancer, laryngeal cancer and oral carcinomas (cf. Sect. 2.3.2.5).

It is well known that nutritional factors, especially iron deficiency with sideropenic dysphagia (Kelly-

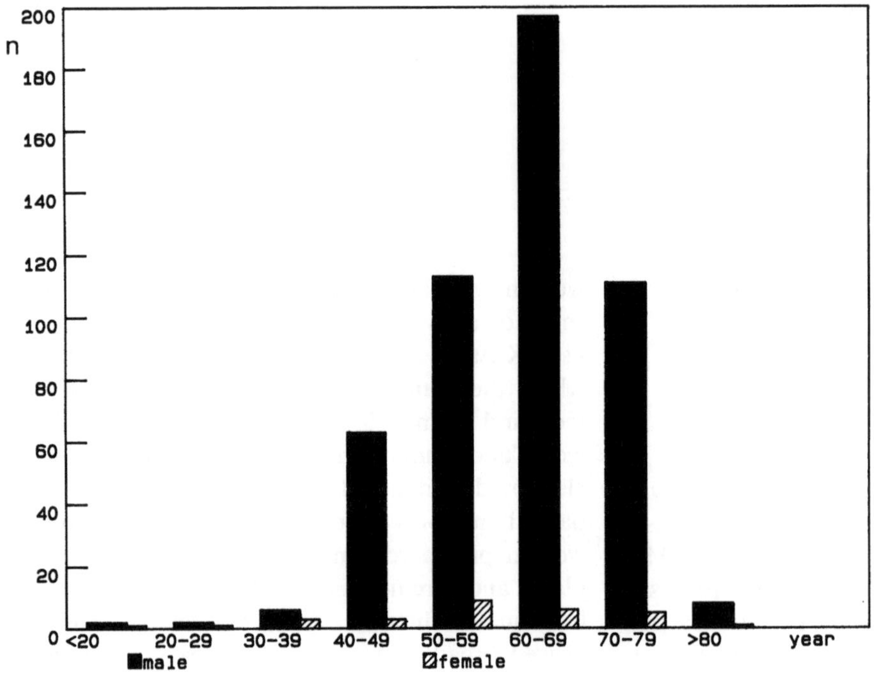

Fig. 4.1. Age and sex distribution of 531 patients with laryngeal carcinomas treated in the ENT Department of Frankfurt University

Patterson syndrome) are associated with carcinomas of the postcricoid region (review: KLEINSASSER 1983). GRAHAM et al. (1981) found that the risk of developing laryngeal carcinoma doubled with a diet low in vitamins A and C. Low magnesium concentrations in erythrocytes and serum were found in patients with laryngeal cancer, while carcinomatous tissue contained higher concentrations of magnesium than normal tissue (SZMEJA and KONCZEWSKA 1986). It is speculated that magnesium deficiency might contribute to carcinogenesis.

Laryngocele may be associated with laryngeal carcinomas (review: KLEINSASSER 1983); however, the nature of the relationship (chronic irritation? disturbance of laryngeal clearance?) is not known.

4.1.4 Exogenous Risk Factors: Tobacco and Alcohol

There is areement among most authors (MCMICHAEL 1978, HERITY et al. 1982, STEINER 1984) with regard to the important role played by tobacco abuse in the development of precancerous lesions and carcinomas of the larynx. STELL (1972) found at a high level of statistical significance, fewer nonsmokers and more heavy smokers amongst 190 laryngeal cancer patients than amongst controls.

Of 50 patients observed by PESCH and STEINER (1979) 96% were men and 94% smokers. BURCH et al. (1981) in a survey of 204 patients and a group of 204 controls, found a marked association between laryngeal cancer, the male sex and the abuse of tobacco and alcohol. The risk of developing laryngeal carcinoma was higher in cigarette smokers than in controls by a factor of 6.1, in cigar and cigarillo smokers by a factor of 2.9, in pipe smokers by 1.6 and in alcoholics by 5.2. ROTHMAN et al. (1980) report that the risk of a heavy smoker is 30 times that of a nonsmoker. Similarly, MÜLLER and KROHN (1980), in a study of 148 autopsies, found severe dysplasia and carcinoma in situ in 47.2% of heavy smokers, in 22.9% of average smokers, in 12.5% of light smokers and in 4.2% of nonsmokers. The occurrence in ex-smokers approached that in light smokers (12.5%). Conversely, they found normal epithelium in only 30.6% of heavy smokers but 83.3% of light smokers. In autopsy material, AUERBACH et al. (1970) established epithelial dysplasia in 99% of 644 cigarette smokers and carcinoma in situ in nearly 16%. In 88 nonsmokers, however, they found epithelial dysplasia in only 4%. Among 116 ex-smokers, 25% showed dysplasia and there was no case of carcinoma in situ. The authors concluded that epithelial dysplasia is dependent to a large extent on the smoking habits of the patient and is in principle reversible. Similarly, DUCHON et al. (1972), after studying 135 patients with vocal cord precancerous lesions for 5 years, reached the conclusion that smoking is liable to influence precancerous lesions of the vocal cords to progress, whereas discontinuation of smoking allows the lesion to recede or reach a standstill.

A prospective study carried out by SCHOTTENFELD et al. (1974) on 733 patients suffering from laryngeal carcinoma showed that the risk of developing a second carcinoma was significantly higher in patients who had been intensively exposed to tobacco and alcohol prior to the development of the first carcinoma. Changing the drinking and smoking habits did not lower this risk during the first 5 years.

An epidemiological study by GRAHAM et al. (1981) on 374 patients with laryngeal cancer and 381 controls similarly showed a high risk to be associated with smoking and alcohol consumption. McCOY et al. (1980) likewise point out the role of smoking and alcohol abuse, and surmise that the latter might lead to a secondary deficiency in various important nutrients and, in addition, exert an influence on detoxifying enzymatic systems. Statistically there is a moderate synergy between alcohol and tobacco in increasing the risk of laryngeal cancer, in that exposure to both factors increased the risk about 50% more than the increase predicted should the effects be simply additive (FLANDERS and ROTHMAN 1982; HERITY et al. 1982).

A study of 466 patients with laryngeal cancer by BRUGERE et al. (1986) showed that alcohol and tobacco consumption of cancer patients varied significantly with cancer location. While only 0.4% of the patients with supraglottic carcinomas were nonsmokers and 4% were nondrinkers, 3.7% of the patients with glottic carcinomas were nonsmokers and 12.8% nondrinkers. This is considered evidence that both risk factors are more involved in supraglottic carcinogenesis.

4.1.5 Inhaled Noxious Agents

Studies by PESCH et al. (1978) and by PESCH and STEINER (1979) showed that the location of laryngeal carcinoma depends, to a certain extent, on the intensity with which the mucosa comes into contact with exogenous noxious agents, in particular smoke, during inspiration and expiration. Owing to the air turbulence during inspiration, contact and deposition of inhaled substances occurs, predominantly in the anterior region of the vocal cords, which forms a bottleneck in the anatomical structure of the larynx and thus constitutes a "smoke trap". Correspondingly, 80% of glottic carcinomas are found in the anterior glottis, whereas carcinomas seldom occur in the region of the anterior commissure (Sect. 5.2.3). The subglottis is protected by the selective deposition described above and only rarely exhibits carcinomatous development. It is thus not surprising that in addition to tobacco smoke, other exogenous inhaled noxious agents play a role in carcinogenesis of the larynx.

4.1.6 Differences in Geographical Distribution – Occupational Risks

Different exposure to exogenous noxious agents probably contributes to the considerable geographical differences seen in the frequency of laryngeal cancer (review: KLEINSASSER 1983). Thus in Switzerland, this form of cancer is found much more often in the west and south and in larger cities (Bundesamt für Statistik 1984).

FLANDERS et al. (1984) report that the 1950-1969 laryngeal cancer mortality for white males in Richmond County, Georgia, was almost double the corresponding rate for the entire USA. In a case control study these authors found that office workers and sales personnel were at a low risk, while farmers, textile processors who separated, filtered or dried textile fibres and all labourers and maintenance personnel exhibited high work-related risk factors for laryngeal cancer.

Similarly in a case-control study in Denmark high risk was found for semiskilled and unskilled workers, workers exposed to dust, outdoors worker, drivers and those working in cement industries and port services (OLSEN and SABROE 1984). Other risk groups are workers in the railroad and lumber industries, sheet metal workers, workers exposed to welding fumes, grinding wheel operators and automobile mechanics (FLANDERS and ROTHMAN 1982, OLSEN et al. 1984). Urbanization is generally associated with a higher risk of death from laryngeal cancer (RAMADAN 1982; review: KLEINSASSER 1983).

Specifically asbestos, nickel, chromium, wood dust and sulphonic acid have been discussed as noxious inhalative agents (review: ROTHMAN et al. 1980, OLSEN and SABROE 1984, SOSKOLONE et al. 1984).

Radiation as a possible cause of laryngeal cancer will be discussed later (Sect. 7.3).

4.2 Papilloma/Papillomatosis and Viral Infection in Laryngeal Carcinogenesis

Papillomas of the laryngeal mucosa (Sect. 3.2.1), which are classified by the WHO as benign tumours, are not regarded as true precancerous lesions. Nevertheless, malignant transformation of papillomas does occur. NEUMANN and KOPP (1980) view every type of papilloma at every age as possessing some risk of malignant transformation.

The **juvenile-onset papillomas**, of viral etiology and usually multiple appearance, tend only very rarely to spontaneous malignant transformation (see Sect. 3.2.1.1). The incidence of malignant change is higher in cases with severe, longstanding, diffuse papillomatous growth also involving the bronchi and bronchioles than in those restricted to the larynx or trachea only. In some patients with a history of many recurrences, a locally "invasive papillomatosis" without marked dysplasia, dissociated infiltrative growth or metastasis has been described (FECHNER et al. 1974) which would be considered malignant by most observers. Frank malignant transformation in juvenile-onset papillomas is found as a rule in lesions which exhibited dysplasia in earlier surgical specimens. Epithelial dysplasia (Sect. 4.6.2) is rare, but tends to increase with the number of recurrences (QUICK et al. 1979, NEUMANN and KOPP 1980, BJELKENKRANTZ et al. 1983). NEUMANN and KOPP (1980) observed severe epithelial dysplasia in one of 19 cases and BJELKENKRANTZ et al. (1983) in one of 23 patients. Epithelial dysplasias, locally destructive growth and malignant transformation are more frequently encountered after previous irradiation (Sect. 7.3).

Adult-onset papillomas, which are usually isolated, can show pronounced keratinization and thereby appears as leukoplakia or verrucous "keratosis" (KLEINSASSER 1963, NEUMANN and KOPP 1980). Malignant transformation is not infrequent, and in addition such changes are often found in the vicinity of established carcinomas. Epithelial dysplasia is much more common here than in juvenile-onset papillomas. The transition to "florid papillomatosis", verrucous acanthosis, verrucous carcinoma and "invasive papilloma" is gradual (FECHNER 1974). JOHNSON et al. (1981) distinguish between papillomas with and without dysplasia, viewing lesions without dysplasia as counterparts of juvenile-onset papillomas and those with dysplasia as premalignant states. PESCH and STEINER (1979) found epithelial dysplasia of varying degree in 87% of papillomas and in 1% of carcinomas in situ. NEUMANN and KOPP (1980) observed severe dysplasia in 9.5% and carcinoma in situ in 4.5% of 22 cases. According to KLEINSASSER (1958), there is a particular risk of transformation in patients over 50 years of age with epithelial dysplasia (in his survey in 50% of cases). Hence it is necessary to determine the grade of dysplasia of all papillomatous lesions. In principle, papillomas, like other types of lesion (leukoplakia/erythroplakia) with severe epithelial dysplasia or carcinoma in situ, have to be regarded as precancerous lesions.

The occasional association between changes caused by viruses, such as juvenile-onset papillomatosis and adult-onset papilloma (see Sect. 3.2.1.2), and the appearance of carcinomas implicates viruses, in particular the human papilloma virus (HPV) in malignant transformation. This is further suggested by histological changes suggestive of HPV lesions, such as acanthotic flat lesions with koilocytosis, endophytic growth or papillomatous patterns in the vicinity of numerous laryngeal carcinomas (SYRJÄNEN and SYRJÄNEN 1981). One-third of the flat and inverted lesions and 42% of the papillomatous lesions contained cells with intranuclear HPV antigens in the cases investigated by SYRJÄNEN et al. (1982). In carcinomatous tissue itself, however, the reaction for HPV antigens is negative. Malignant transformation in experimental papillomatous tumours is also followed by disappearance of viral particles (Shope rabbit papilloma). By means of molecular cloning and DNA hybridization a new HPV type (HPV30) could recently be demonstrated in a laryngeal carcinoma (KAHN et al. 1986).

It is suggested that benign-appearing HPV changes may precede laryngeal carcinomas, and that HPV might be involved in the transformation process (SYRJÄNEN et al. 1982). Also in carcinoma of the uterine cervix (review: ZUR HAUSEN 1978) and in oral white lesions, dysplasia and carcinoma (review: BURKHARDT 1985) such an etiological role of HPV is discussed. However, many questions remain unanswered (BURKHARDT 1985). HPV antigens have also been demonstrated in a number of benign lesions. It should be kept in mind that HPV infection of squamous epithelium might be a frequent transitory phenomenon and is enhanced by differentiation, e.g. keratinization, which is often found in premalignant lesions and in the vicinity of carcinomas. Changes in immunological status in patients with premalignant and malignant lesions could also be of importance. Oral HPV infections are also frequent in patients with immunodeficiency in AIDS-related complex (GREENSPAN et al. 1984). A "passenger status" of viral infections is possible, as has been ascribed to **Candida albicans** in oral leukoplakia and also in hyperkeratotic laryngeal lesions. Although the oncogenic potential of HPV in animals and experimental lesions is unquestionable, an etiological role of HPV in human laryngeal cancer has not yet been proven.

Not only HPV but also herpes viruses have been implicated in laryngeal carcinogenesis. An association of Epstein-Barr virus (EBV) with supraglottic laryngeal cancer could be demonstrated by immunohistochemical reaction for EBV nuclear antigen and by in situ hybridization (see Sect. 2.3.1.5) for EBV DNA in three of five patients by BRICHACEK et al. (1983). Thus at least some cases of laryngeal cancer may be related to nasopharyngeal carcinoma originating from lymphoepithelial tissue associated with EBV infection (see Sect. 7.1.1.4).

4.3 Chronic Laryngitis

A chronic inflammation which may be caused by exogenous noxious agents (see above) and voice abuse as such does not represent a true precancerous lesion. The defect in the epithelial barrier function which arises as a result of such lesions does, however, allows carcinogens (e.g. those present in tobacco smoke) to exert an enhanced effect; increased regeneration, hyperplasia and metaplasia of the epithelium promotes "hyperplasiogenic" carcinogenesis. Possibly, a reduction in the goblet cell density with changes in the clearance of the larynx plays an additional role (NIELSEN and BAK-PEDERSEN 1984a, b). Thus chronic laryngitis must be considered a promoter for the development of precancerous lesions and carcinomas and, in the widest sense, as a disorder which carries a risk of carcinogenesis ("precancerous condition") (GABRIEL and JONES 1960, SUGAR 1970, GLANZ and KLEINSASSER 1976, SHAW 1977).

FURFARO and BARICALLA (1971) found that laryngitis was present prior to carcinomatous disease in between 3.7% and 24% of reported patients. They themselves were able to confirm longstanding inflammation in a high percentage in 115 cancer patients (histology 19.1%, anamnesis 35.7%). SUGAR (1970) presumes a gradual transition between chronic hypertrophic laryngitis and keratosis or leukoplakia.

4.4 Epidermoid Metaplasia

Carcinomas of the larynx are predominantly squamous cell carcinomas and usually keratinizing (SUGAR 1970: 92%, PESCH and STEINER 1979: 98%; in our own patients 97%). These carcinomas generally occur in the skin or in mucosa with a lining of squamous epithelium. It is assumed that squamous cell carcinomas occurring on surfaces not lined by squamous epithelium evolve from undifferentiated basal cells in the course of epithelial hyperplasia or, more often, from squamous metaplasia. In the larynx there is stratified squamous epithelium primarily only in the region of the vocal cords (Fig. 4.2) and the laryngeal inlet; the rest is lined by respiratory epithelium - predominantly columnar pseudostratified ciliated epithelium with mucus-producing goblet cells. With increasing age, the areas of squamous epithelial lining increase; in particular the vestibular ligaments and the supraglottic space are affected (GIARELLI et al. 1977).

SCOTT (1976) histologically examined 111 nonselected larynges in the region of the vestibular ligaments and found no squamous epithelium prior to the 38th year of age, but squamous metaplasia in 57% of older subjects; in men, metaplasia was not only more frequent but also more pronounced. With increasing age, and also depending on exogenous noxious agents and associated inflammation, more extensive squamous metaplasia can be observed in the supraglottic region (GLANZ and KLEINSASSER 1976, PESCH and STEINER 1979). PESCH and STEINER (1979) examined 508 cases and found metaplasia and/or hyperkeratosis in 81% on the glottis and in 19% on the vestibular ligaments, but never in the subglottic region; this distribution corresponds to that observed for carcinomas. STELL et al. (1980), in contrast, were able to demonstrate very small islands of squamous epithelium also in the subglottic region.

A great many reports have shown that laryngeal carcinomas occur most frequently in the region of the vocal folds, i.e. in the region of preexisting squamous epithelium; in the remaining parts of the larynx they are associated with chronic inflamma-

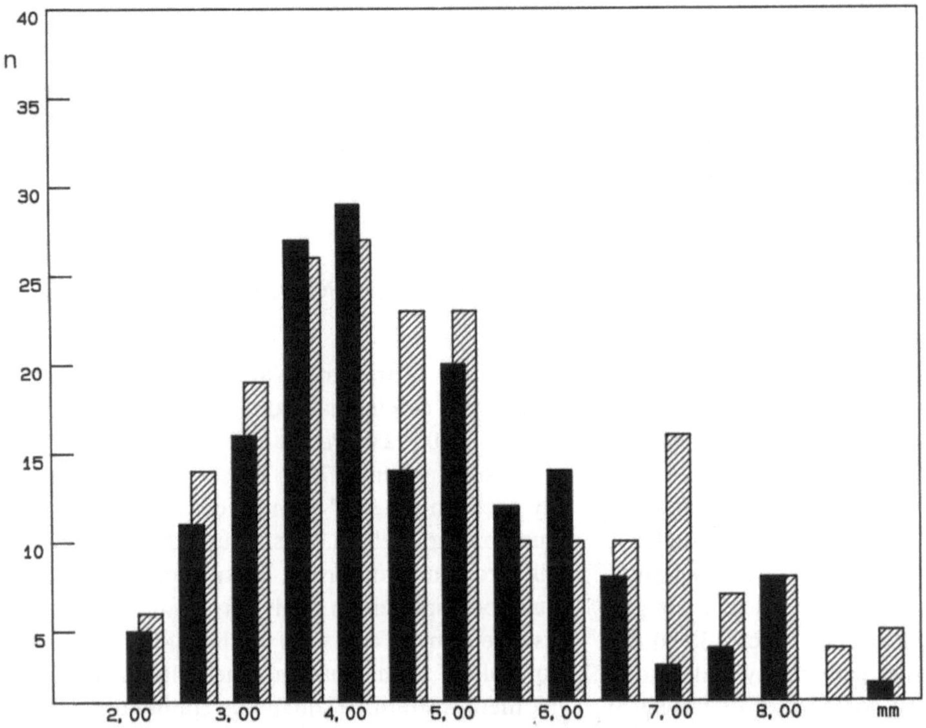

Fig. 4.2. Vertical subglottic extension of squamous epithelium in the middle (black) and the posterior (hatched) third of the vocal cords: morphometric analysis of 225 hemilarynges (age of patients according to Fig. 4.1)

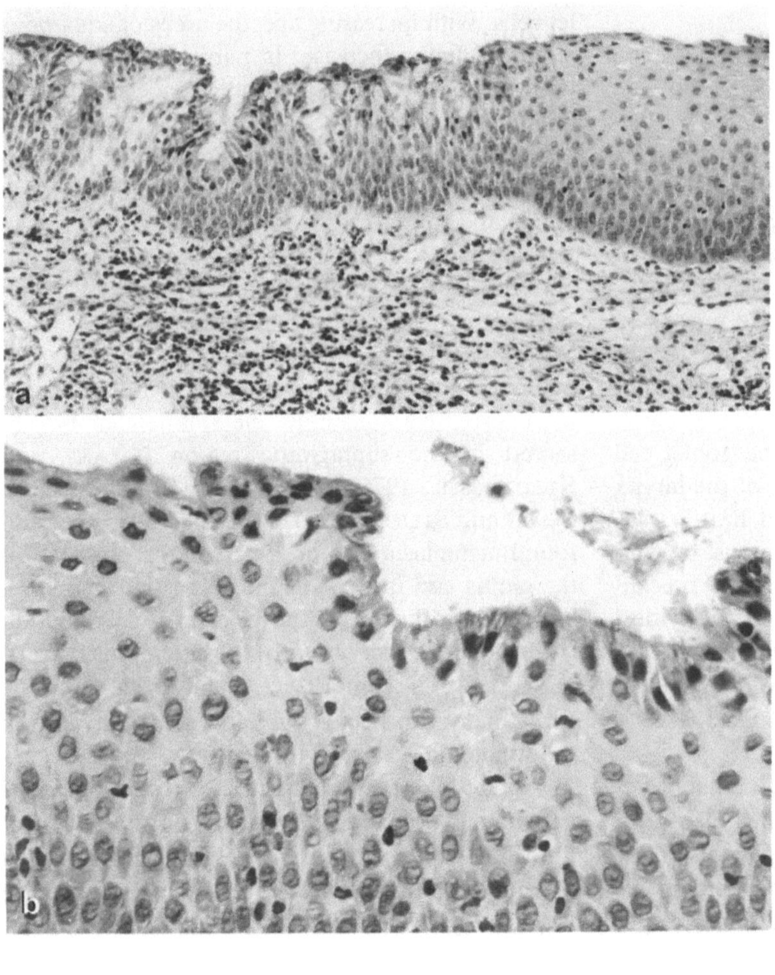

Fig. 4.3 a, b. Squamous metaplasia in the supraglottis: 65-year-old man. **a** The columnar pseudostratified ciliated epithelium on the left is gradually replaced by multilayered squamous epithelium toward the right of the picture. There is marked chronic inflammation. HE, ×140. **b** The squamous epithelium of a recent metaplasia is still covered on top by cylindrical epithelium with mucous production and cilia. HE, ×350

tion, squamous metaplasia (Fig. 4.3) and dysplasia (GLANZ and KLEINSASSER 1976, GIARELLI et al. 1977, PESCH et al. 1978, PESCH and STEINER 1979). In the areas outside the vocal folds, therefore, squamous metaplasia can be regarded as a precondition for the development of a squamous cell carcinoma (KLEINSASSER 1963, GIARELLI et al. 1977).

4.5 Multitopic (Multicentric) Tumour Growth: Field Cancerization

It is an everyday observation when studying carcinomas of different mucosal surfaces that in general, epithelial changes in the vicinity of the tumours are found which, taken alone, would correspond to a precancerous lesion. Indeed, not infrequently further invasive carcinomatous foci can be observed at other sites. This was first demonstrated by PETERSEN (1901) using wax plate models of carcinomas and their surroundings. ZUPPINGER (1938), based on the fact that second tumours are more frequent in patients with oral, pharyngeal and oesophageal carcinomas than would be expected on the basis of pure chance, concluded that there is a "disposition" for cancer in these patients, i.e. an undetected precancerous condition. SLAUGHTER et al. (1953) coined the term "field cancerization" or "condemned mucosa" to describe their findings on examination of carcinomas of the oral mucosa. They detected other, separate carcinomatous foci in 11.2% of cases. These results supported the assumption that in carcinogenesis of squamous epithelium, no strictly localized process (unitopical or unicentric cancerous transformation) is involved, but rather entire mucosal areas may be subject to synchronous or even metachronic cancerization owing to the same endogenous and especially exogenous factors.

Squamous metaplasia in the supraglottic region, squamous hyperplasia with varying grades of epithelial dysplasia, carcinomata in situ and multiple microinvasive carcinomas are virtually always associated with established carcinomas of the larynx (KLEINSASSER and HECK 1959, KLEINSASSER 1963, ROBBETT et al. 1972, GRUNDMANN 1973, BAUER 1974, GLANZ and KLEINSASSER 1976, PESCH et al. 1976, GIARELLI et al. 1977, PESCH and STEINER 1979). Only in the subglottic region are such changes rare.

We know today that some of the cancers in the larynx are primarily multitopical (multicentric; RABBETT 1962). FERLITO (1980) described five cases with two separate primary carcinomas of different histology in the laryngeal and hypopharyngeal regions. KRESPI et al. (1983) reported on a patient with four separate carcinomas in the pharyngolaryngeal area, all of which arose simultaneously.

Not only the mucosa of one organ, but even whole organ systems, like the respiratory tract, and also distant organs, can be affected in the course of multitopical cancerization. The presence of more than one carcinoma is found, according to larger statistical studies, in about 5% of cancer patients (WALLACE 1957, from 3006 cases); the rate seems to be rising in recent years. In two studies on 1231 patients (LAMPRECHT et al. 1983) and 645 patients (BLACK et al. 1983) with tumours of the upper respiratory tract, a second tumor was found in 8.9% of cases. Among 496 patients with laryngeal carcinoma, MARTIN et al. (1979) observed 45 cases (about 10%), who suffered from another malignant tumour in a different site either at the same time or later. This figure is higher than would be expected statistically. WAGENFELD et al. (1980) were able to demonstrate that of 740 victims of glottic carcinoma, 48 (6.5%) presented with a second tumour in the respiratory tract; in an equivalent normal population this would be expected in only 14 subjects. The authors calculate the risk of developing a second tumour in the respiratory tract within 10 years of successful treatment of glottic carcinoma to be 12%. Relevant here are the findings of a study by BROWN (1978), who, among 1600 cases of laryngeal carcinoma treated with radiotherapy, observed a second tumour in 3.8% of cases over a period of 16 years. In two cases the second tumours were located in the area irradiated, but most commonly they were found in the lungs and in the head and neck region. In a series of 1389 patients with laryngeal cancer, MIYAHARA et al. (1985) recorded multiple primary malignancies in 138 cases (9.94%), including triplicate tumours in nine patients and quadriplicate tumours in two patients.

In 600 patients suffering from laryngeal carcinomas observed by the present authors in the period 1966 to 1976 (follow-up to 1982), there were 11 secondary tumours (six bronchial carcinomas, five laryngeal carcinomas). In addition two of the laryngeal carcinomas had been preceded by a hypopharyngeal carcinoma. The development of radiogenic secondary tumours in the marginal area of the field irradiated will be dealt with in Sect. 7.3.

Laryngeal carcinomas are especially frequently associated with bronchial carcinomas (Cahan 1955, Thoma 1974, Sakula 1974, Goldsher et al. 1977, Martin et al. 1979, Lamprecht et al. 1983, Black et al. 1983). The patients affected are usually heavy smokers: thus, probably the same exogenous noxious agents attack the entire respiratory epithelium and, together with endogenous factors, lead to the development of carcinomas.

Apart from second tumours in the respiratory tract, tumours of other organs, especially of the gastrointestinal tract, are also more frequently observed in patients with laryngeal carcinomas. Laryngeal carcinomas are often preceded by premalignant and malignant oral and oropharyngeal lesions (Lipkin et al. 1985). Wenig and Abramson (1983) point out an increased frequency of prostate carcinomas.

These facts are of practical importance in as much as registration of patients with precancerous lesions, as well as carcinoma patients following therapy, allows them to be separated as a risk group. Hereby arises the necessity and possibility of prevention, follow-up and, if necessary, therapy (Steiner 1984, Miyahara et al. 1985). Thus, in every patient in whom the diagnosis of laryngeal carcinoma is established, clinical investigations ("panendoscopy") should be carried out to search for tumours of other organs and check-ups over a period of years are mandatory.

4.6 Precancerous Lesions

A precancerous lesion is defined as morphologically altered tissue in which cancer is more likely to occur than in its apparently normal counterpart (WHO 1972). The definition and nomenclature of clinical appearance and histological changes associated with premalignant lesions nonetheless present considerable difficulties and there is still marked confusion in terminology. This has arisen in particular from the uncritical jumbling of clinical and histological terms, as, for example, in the case of "leukoplakia" and "keratosis" (Miller 1976, Kambic 1978, Crissman 1979, 1982, Goodman 1984).

There is general agreement today that especially in the field of precancerous lesions there should be clear and precise definition of terms and strict separation of clinical, i.e. in general macroscopic, descriptions from histological and cytological diagnostic terms (Kleinsasser 1963b, Miller 1976, Neumann and Franz 1977, Franz and Neumann 1978, Burkhardt 1980, 1985, Axell et al. 1984). Clinical findings and histological cytological assessment should be evaluated critically and used together to contribute to the nosological and diagnostic classification of the individual case; in this manner the basis can be formed for therapeutic considerations.

Since laryngeal carcinoma develops from stratified squamous epithelium (formed primarily or by metaplasia), it is obvious that there are parallels between carcinogenesis of the laryngeal mucosa and carcinogenesis in other organs with squamous epithelial lining. Precancerous lesions of mucosa lined with squamous epithelium have been intensely studied in the region of the portio vaginalis uteri and the oral cavity; investigations have focused on their macroscopic clinical appearance, as well as histological, cytological, immunohistological and ultrastructural changes (Burghardt 1972, Pindborg 1980, Burkhardt 1980, 1985, Burkhardt and Maerker 1981). The results have already led to marked advances in early detection and treatment of precancerous lesions and early stages of carcinoma, especially in the field of gynaecology.

The application of the results gained by these studies on laryngeal mucosal lesions appears desirable. For the sake of better communication it is imperative to have a consistent nomenclature for all mucosal lesions. This of course should not preclude the consideration of local particularities.

4.6.1 Macroscopic Clinical Aspects: Leukoplakia, Erythroplakia

Neither in the laryngeal mucosa nor in any other mucosa, are there absolutely typical macroscopic clinical changes by which precancerous lesions can be recognized (Kleinsasser 1959, Miller 1976). The primary clinical finding should therefore always be formulated only descriptively, being particularly careful to use no histological criteria (see Miller 1976, Bauer 1976). Many terms unfortunately used so often, such as "keratosis", "keratotic lesions", "epithelial hyperplasia", "carcinoma in situ", "dysplasia" and also "pachydermia" are to be dismissed as clinical diagnoses. Some of the terms are a result of the fascination which the often present hyperkeratosis of these lesions exercised on earlier observers. Today we know that this change - which, incidentally, can be recognized only histologically - is of no prognostic significance in itself. Likewise, histological diagnoses which are based on the macroscopic picture, such as "leukoplakia", are not on their own, meaningful (MILLER 1976).

Precancerous lesions of mucosal surfaces lined by stratified squamous epithelium can as a rule be discerned under three different macroscopic aspects: as white mucosal changes, as red mucosal changes and as a mixture between white and red areas. White mucosal changes are designated **leukoplakia** (Fig. 4.4a,b) defined as a white patch or plaque that cannot be rubbed off and cannot be characterized clinically or pathologically as any other disease (WHO 1978). Leukoplakia is further divided into homogeneous and nonhomogeneous (nodular and verrucous) forms (AXELL 1974). Red mucosal changes are termed **erythroplakia**, defined as a bright red patch of mucosa that cannot be characterized clinically or pathologically as any other disease. Mixed forms of white and red mucosal changes are termed **erythroleukoplakia** (Fig. 4c), speckled leukoplakia or speckled erythroplakia. These purely descriptive clinical terms are applied readily to the laryngeal mucosa (LANIADO et al. 1981, HELLQUIST et al. 1982, GILLIS et al. 1983). As a result of the highly refined microlaryngoscopy today not only these basic types of lesions but also more subtle changes can be recognized. They can and must therefore be described further, for example, by attributes such as sharply delimited, diffuse, planar, nodular, granular, villous, wart-like, verrucous, thickened, thinned, smooth, glassy, polypous, papillomatous, disseminated, erosive etc. (KLEINSASSER 1963, MILLER 1976, NEUMANN and FRANZ 1977, HELLQUIST et al. 1981). These are purely descriptive clinical terms which must be supplemented by histology and cytology for the assessment of the biological potential. They always indicate the necessity of excision and mark the area to be removed.

It is true for the laryngeal mucosa, as for other mucosal areas, that nonhomogeneous leukoplakias and the less common red mucosal lesions, i.e. erythroplakias and erythroleukoplakias, in general indicate poor prognosis, i.e. epithelial dysplasia and an increased tendency towards invasive growth (BOSATRA 1977, SHAW 1977, KLEINSASSER 1983). In contrast, HELLQUIST et al. (1981) see no difference in behaviour between leukoplakia and erythro-

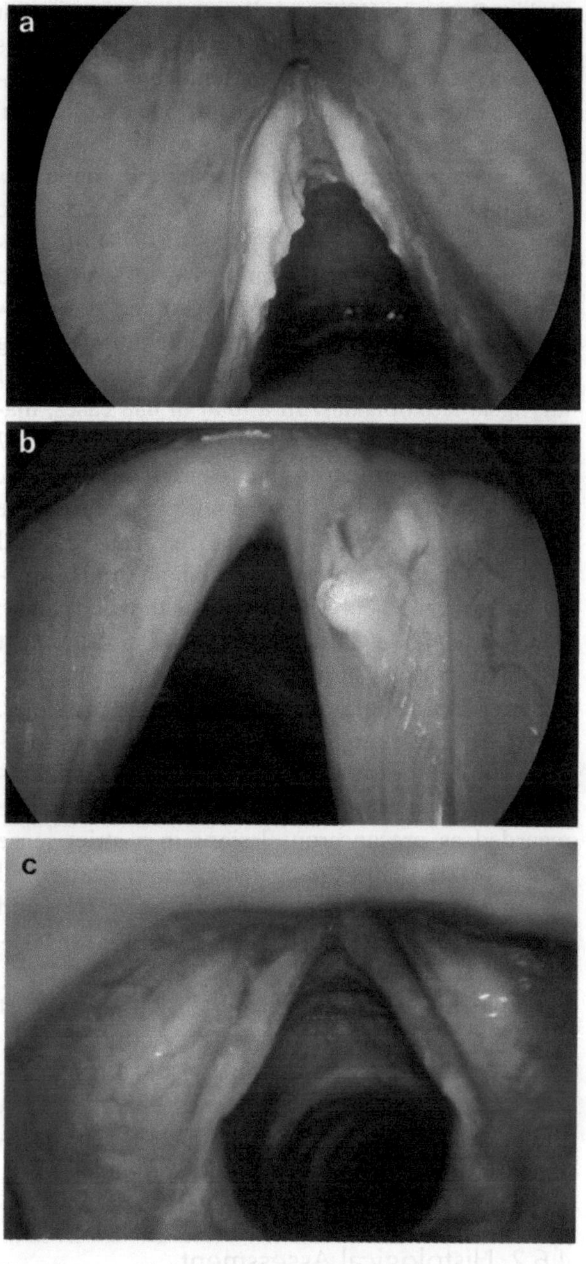

Fig. 4.4a–c: Clinical picture of leukoplakia and erythroplakia in the larynx. **a** Homogeneous leukoplakia of the vocal cords: 59-year-old man. Extensive sharply delineated lesion with only slight wave-like surface protrusions of the thickened epithelium. **b** Nonhomogeneous, verrucous to nodular leukoplakia of the glottic region: 51-year-old man. The lesion is not sharply delineated and protrudes like a wart into the lumen. **c** Erythroleukoplakia in the glottic region: 79-year-old man. Extensive, partly whitish and slightly raised, partly reddish and atrophic mucosal changes

plakia. ROBBETT (1972) ascribes a higher malignant potential to the circumscribed leukoplakial changes - which he considers to be of endogenous nature - than to diffuse forms which he attributes to external noxious agents.

The peak occurence of leukoplakia in the larynx is in the fifth, sixth and seventh decades (LIAPIS and PAPACHARALAMPOUS 1969, HENRY 1979); the lesions develop especially on the vocal cords and usually lead to hoarseness. FURFARO and BARICALA (1971) compiled the data in the literature dealing with the frequency of malignant transformation of laryngeal leukoplakias. In a total of 488 cases, malignant transformation was reported in 3,5% (17 cases), varying in the different reports between 0% and 27,6%. QUANTE (1976) similarly surveyed the literature and found variations between 3% and 40%. He himself observed malignant transformation in at least 3% of 319 patients with leukoplakia; in a further 7% of these patients with development of carcinomas, he suspects an incorrect primary diagnosis. Taking into account histological findings, about 10% of leukoplakias in different organ locations can be shown to exhibit severe epithelial dysplasia or carcinoma in situ and accordingly must be regarded as precancerous lesions in a strict sense (BURKHARDT 1980); the percentage in the laryngeal region is somewhat higher, i.e. between 10% and 20% (GIARELLI et al. 1977, CRISSMAN 1982, HELLQUIST et al. 1982).

Discussing oral precancerous lesions, AXELL et al. (1984) stated that a complete description comprises etiological (see Sects. 4.1.3, 4.1.4, 4.1.5), clinical, topographical and histological characteristics. Without any doubt, excision and subsequent histological examination is the most important step.

4.6.2 Histological Assessment and Classification of Dysplasia

Despite a certain subjectivity, the histological examination of biopsy material still provides the most reliable method of determining malignancy or malignant potential. Most important, histological examination establishes with certainty whether a lesion without infiltrative growth is present, or whether there is already an invasive carcinoma. In addition, over the past few years reliably reproducible criteria have been worked out for assessing the deviation of stratified squamous epithelium from the norm.

Considerable differences exist, however, in the histological nomenclature of these more or less precancerous changes. KLEINSASSER (1963b) divided the changes into three groups:

1. Simple squamous cell hyperplasia
2. Squamous cell hyperplasia with isolated localized cellular atypia (so-called suspect cases)
3. Precancerous epithelium

In group 3 he combines dysplastic epithelium with the so-called carcinoma in situ, since according to his investigations their biological behaviour is similar. In a retrospective study he established that among 70 patients in group 1, six developed a carcinoma during the next 6 years, and of 11 patients in group 2, one developed a carcinoma in this period (KLEINSASSER 1963c). Thus he took groups 1 and 2 to represent facultative precancerous lesions which, from his observations, are in general reversible tissue changes. It is striking that of the 20 patients in group 3 (which would now be termed severe epithelial dysplasia and carcinoma in situ) who were treated either not at all or inadequately as judged by the standards of today, 18 developed a carcinoma.

KAMBIC (1977, 1978), and KAMBIC and LENART (1971) divide mucosal changes, combined under the heading "hyperplastic aberrations", into four groups:

1. Hyperplasia simplex - simple hyperplasia
2. Hyperplasia abnormalis - abnormal hyperplasia
3. Hyperplasia atypia - atypical hyperplasia,
4. Carcinoma with the subgroup carcinoma in situ - preinvasive cancer

Groups 1 and 2 are regarded by the authors as principally reversible and group 3 as precancerous, whereby they state that there is a chance of about 25% of transition to carcinoma.

One endeavours today to supplant the multiform terms which have been used for the histological characterization of the malignant potential of precancerous lesions with a uniform nomenclature applicable to all organ systems (GRUNDMANN 1976). For precancerous changes in other organs - cervix uteri, colon, urinary tract, oesophagus, oral mucosa - the term "dysplasia" coined by KROMPECHER (1924) for "heterotopic differentiation" has come to be widely used as the result of a recommendation by the WHO (1978). It is likewise recommended for, and applied to, the classification of laryngeal mucosal changes (GRUNDMANN 1973, PESCH and

STEINER 1979, MÜLLER and KROHN 1980, LANIADO et al. 1981, HELLQUIST et al. 1982, MICHAELS 1982, 1984, GILLIS et al. 1983).

The use of "dysplasia" has been subjected to criticism inasmuch as (a) it is also used to describe certain malformations, and (b) at least some forms of "precancerous dysplasia" in fact represent true neoplasia (KOSS 1979, RYWLIN 1984). However, other terms like atypia, atypicalities or dyskeratosis, epithelial proliferation and keratosis without or with atypia - (KWOA, KWA) (see HYAMS 1976, CRISSMANN 1982, GOODMAN 1984, BARNES and GNEPP 1985) or proposals such as "intraepithelial neoplasia" or "atypical in situ proliferation" (see RYWLIN 1984) are no more convincing or more logical.

The use of numbers (I-III or I-IV) is also unsatisfactory, as different numbering systems are used in different organs and the system used should be stated in each single case. "Dysplasia", in contrast, is a concise term which in the context of epithelial lesions cannot lead to misunderstandings. So, for semantic reasons, it is suggested that the use of "dysplasia" in its now conventional meaning be continued. Epithelial dysplasia in "tumour-like lesions" is classified under epithelial abnormalities by the WHO (SHANMUGARATNAM and SOBIN 1978).

Dysplasia designates a deviation of the histological structure and the cytological differentiation from normal and is a measure of the malignant potential of a lesion. Although an absolutely definitive assessment of the prognosis of lesions in any individual patient is not possible (FRIEDMANN 1976, KOSS 1978), since inferences regarding a dynamic process are drawn from a static, momentary picture, nonetheless there is at present no other criterion by which the biological behaviour can be prognosticated with more certainty. A summary of other methods employed to determine the malignant potential of mucosal lesions is given in Sect. 2.3.

AUERBACH et al. (1970) were able to show, from histological examination of the laryngeal mucosa of 942 autopsies, that epithelial dysplasia correlates with laryngeal carcinomas with regard to age, sex distribution, risk factors and location. Epithelial dysplasia was most common on the vocal fold (15,6%), less so on the vestibular ligaments (10%) and even more infrequent in the supraglottic space (7,5%) or subglottically (2%).

Clinicopathological studies have clearly shown that moderate and in particular severe epithelial dysplasia and carcinoma in situ are correlated with an increased risk of malignant transformation. Such investigations have been carried out especially on the oral mucosa (MINCER et al. 1972, BANOCZY 1977, PINDBORG et al. 1977, BURKHARDT and MAERKER 1978 and 1981, SILVERMAN et al. 1984), but also on the laryngeal mucosa (KLEINSASSER 1963b, LIAPSIS and PAPACHARALAMPOUS 1969, CRISSMAN 1979, HELLQUIST et al. 1982).

4.6.2.1 Criteria of Epithelial Hyperplasia and Epithelial Dysplasia

Numerous accounts have been given concerning the definition of criteria of dysplasia in various organs with a mucosal lining (review: BURKHARDT 1980) and also in the laryngeal mucosa (KLEINSASSER 1959, 1963b, c, TRENTINI et al. 1973, FECHNER 1974, FRIEDMANN 1976, SCOTT 1976, KAMBIC 1977, 1979, PESCH et al. 1978, PESCH and STEINER 1979, HELLQUIST et al. 1981, 1982, CRISSMAN 1979, 1982, MICHAELS 1984).

First of all it is important to exclude changes that are of no immediate importance as regards the assessment of dysplasia (Table 4.1). These are inflammatory changes, epithelial hyperplasia and epithelial atrophy. Inflammation can lead to spongiosis of the epithelial structure and also to focal destruction of the basal membrane. Epithelial hyperplasia is often found in leukoplakia, atrophy in erythroplakia.

Most frequently epithelial **hyperplasia** (Fig. 4.5; sometimes wrongly termed "keratosis") is present in the lesions under discussion. It can be further characterized by acanthosis (thickening of prickle cell layer), hyperkeratosis (as orthokeratosis or parakeratosis), spongiosis (loosening of prickle cell cohesion) and leukoedema (irregular desquamation of the keratin lamellae with deposition of fluid be-

Table 4.1. Histological and cytological characteristics of epithelial hyperplasia and dysplasia

Characteristics of epithelial hyperplasia	Characteristics of epithelial dysplasia
Hyperkeratosis Orthokeratosis Parakeratosis	Droplet-shaped rete pegs Basal cell hyperplasia Loss of basal cell polarity Cellular pleomorphism
Acanthosis Epithelial edema and spongiosis (leukoedema)	Increase of mitotic figures Dyskeratosis (intraepithelial keratinization) Disturbance or loss of epithelial stratification Reduction of cellular cohesion

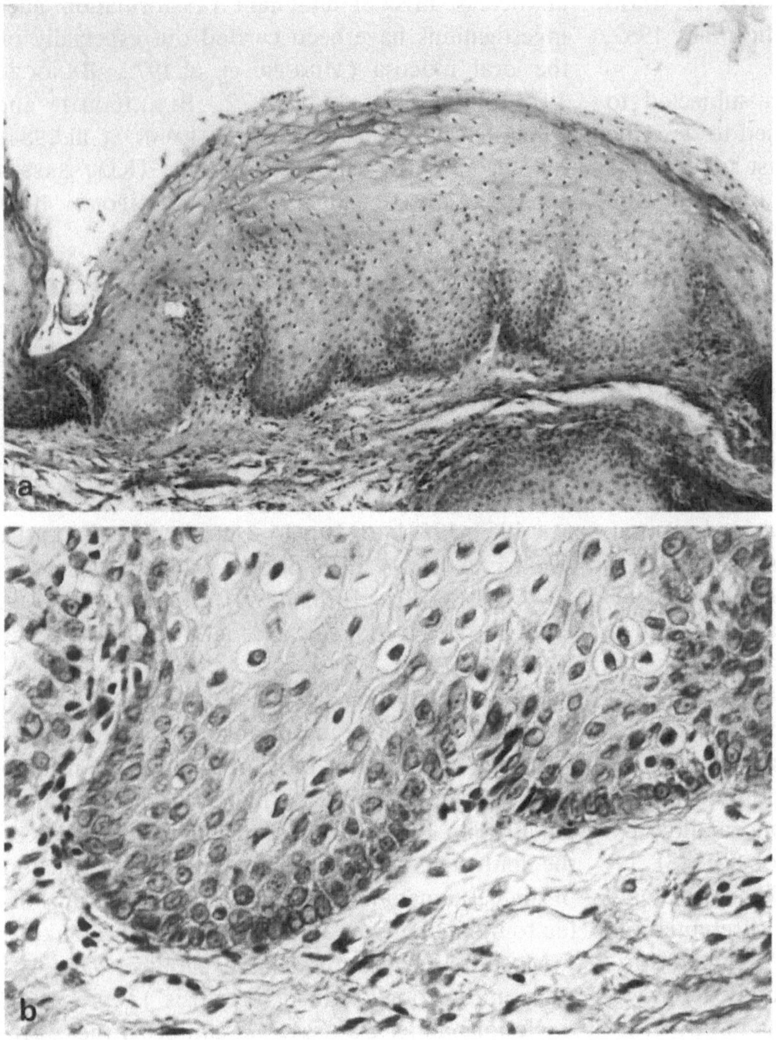

Fig. 4.5a, b. Epithelial hyperplasia with mild dysplasia: 58-year-old man, glottis. **a** The epithelium shows a marked thickening in the centre with hyperparakeratosis. Slight increase of rete ridges at the epithelial mesenchymal interface. The stratification is normal. In the subepithelial tissue there are only few inflammatory cells. HE, ×90. **b** The basal cell layer is well delineated and only slightly widened, there is little variation in nuclear size and staining, and mitotic figures cannot be seen in this field of high magnification. HE, ×350

tween the lamellae; so-called keratin pools). Different authors have discarded the term "hyperkeratosis" in connection with changes in the laryngeal mucosa, since in this region, according to the principles of classical histology, an "unkeratinized" stratified squamous epithelium is normally present. Histochemical, immunohistochemical and ultrastructural studies have shown, however, that in these allegedly nonkeratinizing epithelia there is always keratin formation to some degree (BURKHARDT 1980), although different subtypes of cytokeratins can be demonstrated by immunohistochemistry. If a keratinized layer is clearly recognizable in the laryngeal mucosa by light microscopy, then it is justified to speak of a hyperkeratosis - hyperparakeratosis with preservation of cell nuclei, hyperorthokeratosis with a stratum granulosum and loss of nuclei.

It is important to stress the fact that neither epithelial hyperplasia nor hyperkeratosis, taken on their own, indicate epithelial "degeneration" i.e., possible malignant transformation (KAMBIC 1977, 1978).

The extensive spectrum of cellular and tissular changes indicative of epithelial dysplasia is recognized by the pathologist on the basis of experience, usually without detailed analysis being necessary (MICHAELS 1984).

The numerous characteristics of dysplasia can be reduced to eight essential criteria (Table 4.1): changes in the region of the basal cells (numerical increase of cells of the basal cell type and loss of polarity), cytological changes (cellular, especially nuclear pleomorphism and increase in mitotic figures, often above the basal cell layer) and criteria characteristic of stratified squamous epithelium, namely isolated intraepithelial keratinization of single cells (dyskeratosis) and disturbance of the epithelial architecture, especially loss of cellular cohesion and stratification. In addition, further histological changes are associated, as a rule, with epithelial dysplasia. Whereas the stratified squamous epithelium of the laryngeal mucosa formed primarily or by metaplasia is planar and exhibits a smooth or slightly wavy epithelial mesenchymal interface, in epithelial hyperplasia, and more so in dysplasia, either an increased formation of rete ridges, i. e. endophytic growth, often with drop-shaped rete pegs, is found, or papillomatous exophytic growth which clinically constitutes a verrucous aspect can be observed.

There are no sharp boundaries between papillomatous exophytic epithelial hyperplasia (Fig. 4.6), papillomas of adults (see Sect. 3.2.1.2; KLEINSASSER 1963, GRUNDMANN 1973, NEUMANN and KOPP 1980), verrucous acanthosis or hyperplasia (GLANZ and KLEINSASSER 1978, SHEAR and PINDBORG 1980) and verrucous carcinoma (see Sect. 7.1.1.1). All of these lesions present clinically as verrucous or papillary mucosal thickening.

In addition to epithelial changes, alterations of the subepithelial connective tissue can be observed in dysplasia which are summarized under the term "stromal reaction". This includes alterations of the

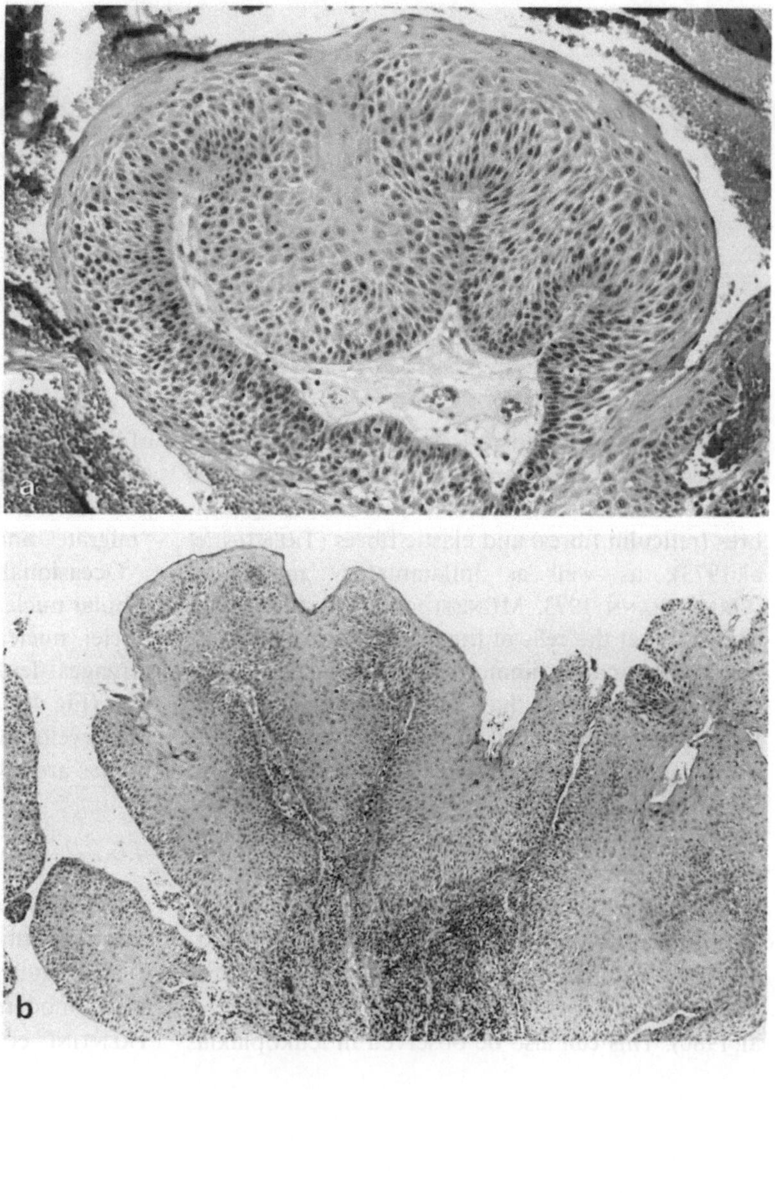

Fig. 4.6 a, b. Papillomatous exophytic epithelial hyperplasia: 90-year-old man, glottis. **a** Blunt protrusion of thickened and parakeratotic epithelium with slight dysplasia. HE, ×140. **b** Papillomatous, markedly thickened epithelium with disturbance of stratification, nuclear pleomorphism, occasional dyskeratosis and marked inflammation (moderate dysplasia). Distinction from adult-onset papilloma with dysplasia is often arbitrary in such cases. HE, ×60

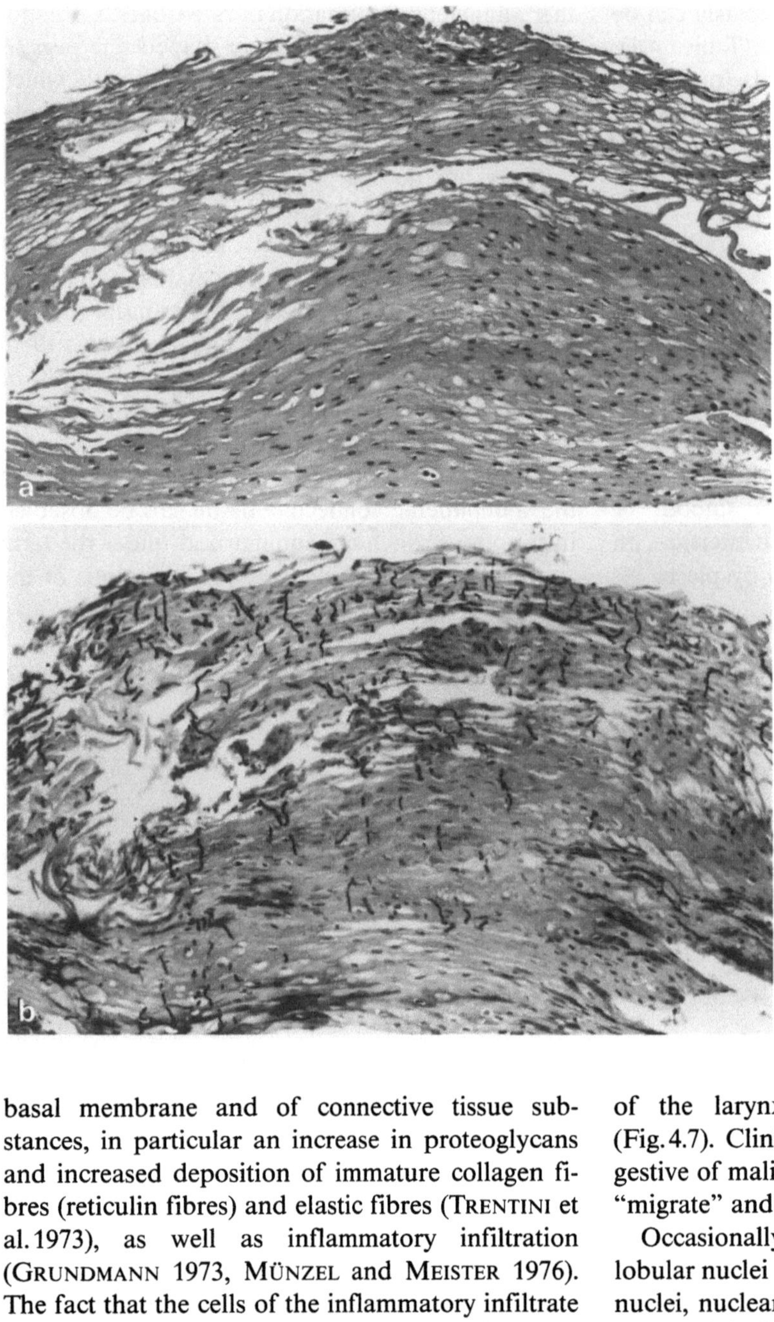

Fig. 4.7 a, b. Hyperplastic epithelium with **Candida** colonization. 64-year-old man, supraglottis. **a** Upper layer of hyperplastic epithelium with considerable hyperparakeratosis (keratin lamellae with nuclear remnants). With haematoxylin-eosin stain there is no indication of fungal growth. HE, ×140. **b** With the periodic acid-Schiff stain many fungal hyphae can be seen growing perpendicularly into the horn lamellae. This is typical of **Candida** species. PAS, ×140

basal membrane and of connective tissue substances, in particular an increase in proteoglycans and increased deposition of immature collagen fibres (reticulin fibres) and elastic fibres (TRENTINI et al. 1973), as well as inflammatory infiltration (GRUNDMANN 1973, MÜNZEL and MEISTER 1976). The fact that the cells of the inflammatory infiltrate are predominantly immunocompetent cells (especially lymphocytes) has led to the now well-founded view that this is the morphological expression of an immunological reaction of the body to the onset of malignant growth (review: BURKHARDT 1980). Such an immunological reaction can be considered to be a basic indicator of the malignant potential of the lesion (GRUNDMANN 1973).

A fungal colonization on the surface of hyperkeratotic lesions is often found in the oral cavity with high degrees of dysplasia (BURKHARDT et al. 1980). This can also be observed in leukoplakias of the larynx, although much less frequently (Fig. 4.7). Clinically, these changes are highly suggestive of malignancy. Typically, the lesions tend to "migrate" and recur following excision.

Occasionally, nuclear alterations - enlarged lobular nuclei with nuclear inclusion bodies, double nuclei, nuclear vacuolization - can be observed in laryngeal leukoplakias which suggest a viral infection (Fig. 4.8). Viral factors that may be involved in the development of precancerous lesions and carcinomas are discussed in Sect. 4.2.

4.6.2.2 Grades of Dysplasia

On the basis of the combination and severity of the criteria mentioned above, it has become customary to distinguish between three grades of dysplasia: mild, moderate and severe (Figs. 4.5, 4.9, 4.10; TRENTINI et al. 1973, FRIEDMANN 1976, MILLER

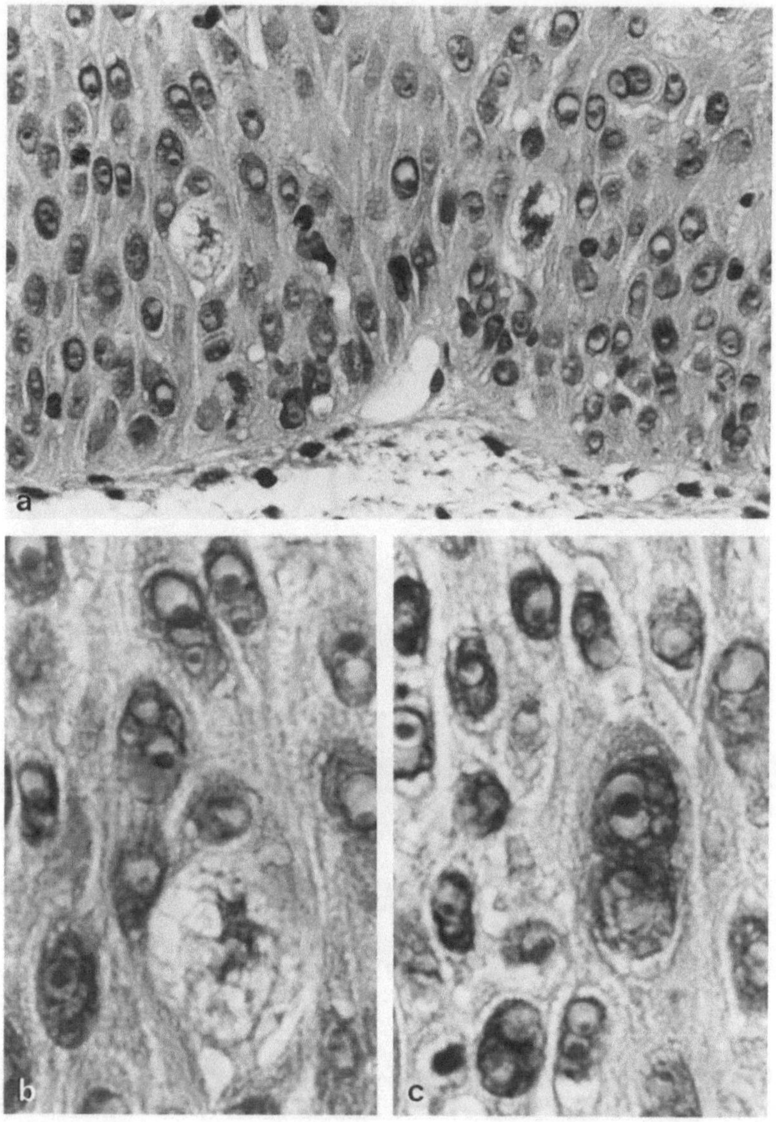

Fig. 4.8a–c. Hyperplastic epithelium with indication of viral infection. 45-year-old woman with chronic laryngitis and white thickening of the left vocal cord. **a** Basal portion of the epithelium with nuclear inclusions in many of the nuclei and two suprabasal atypical mitotic figures ("mitosoid figures"). HE, ×500. **b** Higher magnification of atypical mitotic figure. HE, ×1100. **c** Binuclear "virocyte" with clearly recognizable inclusion body. HE, ×1100

1976, Bauer 1976, WHO 1978, Crissman 1979, 1982, Pesch and Steiner 1979, Burkhardt 1980, Hellquist et al. 1982). In addition, carcinoma in situ can be distinguished by total loss of stratification (Sect. 4.7). Some authors combine severe dysplasia and carcinoma in situ in one group.

Recent morphometric analysis of laryngeal lesions with dysplasia by Olde Kalter et al. (1985) support the distinction of more than two grades of dysplasia, i.e. subdivision of the group 3 of Kleinsasser (1963b); by this method groups 1 and 2 and groups 1 and 3 could be easily distinguished by quantitative parameters, while groups 2 and 3 could be separated into clusters not identical with conventional subdivision. Discriminant analysis of morphometric parameters was able to separate lesions correctly in patients with a favourable and an unfavourable clinical course (Olde Kalter et al. 1986; see Sect. 2.3.1.2).

Table 4.2 sets out proposal for the evaluation of the criteria of dysplasia, employing a classification into three grades and carcinoma in situ. It is taken into account that the individual changes must be weighted differently. Thus basal cell hyperplasia can still be a sign of harmless, increased regeneration of the epithelium, whereas dyskeratosis and impairment in the epithelial stratification indicate higher malignant potential. Since in general the latter alterations are found in combination with the more harmless changes, a temporal sequence – basal cell hyperplasia → loss of polarity of basal cells → cellular pleomorphism, increased mitotic rates

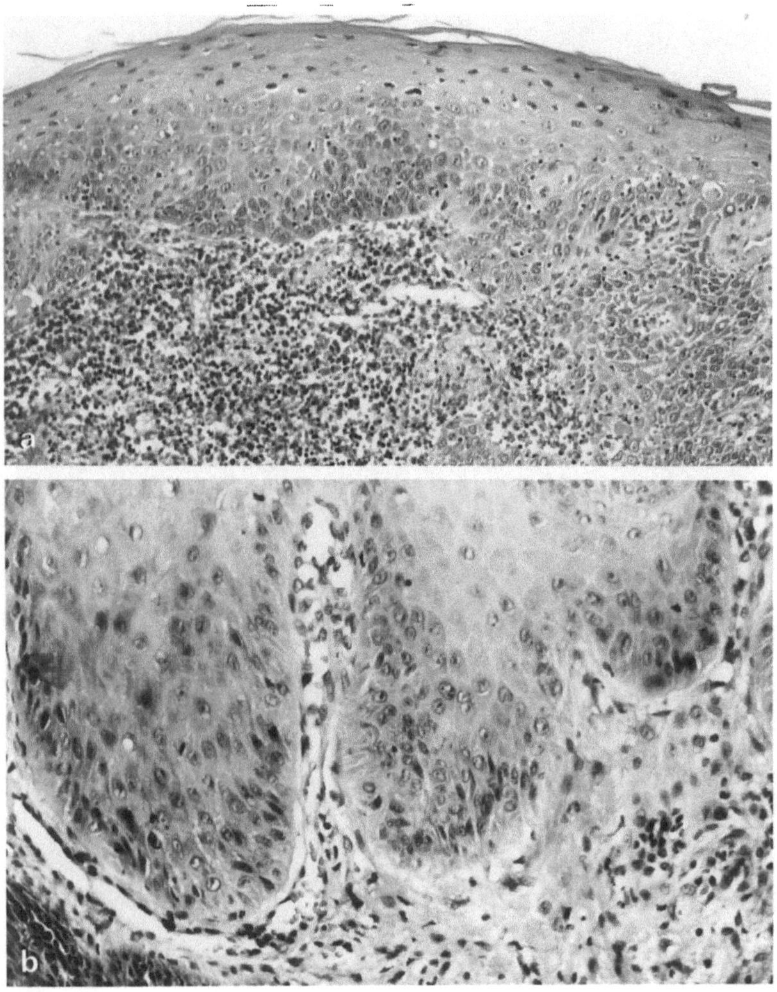

Fig. 4.9 a, b. Epithelial hyperplasia with moderate dysplasia: 76 year old man, glottis. **a** Slightly thickened squamous epithelium with hyperparakeratosis. The stratification of the lower portion of the epithelium is not clearly recognizable, the nuclei show pleomorphism. At the **left**, a single dyskeratosis. Marked inflammatory infiltration of the subepithelial tissue. HE, ×140. **b** The basal cell layer is not clearly delineated and there is variation of size and shapes of nuclei. HE, ×220

Table 4.2. Criteria for a classification of degree of dysplasia and of carcinoma in situ

Degree	Characteristics
Mild	Basal cell hyperplasia Disturbance of basal cell polarity
Moderate	Basal cell hyperplasia Loss of basal cell polarity Moderate cellular pleomorphism Slight increase in mitotic figures Scattered dyskeratoses
Severe	Basal cell hyperplasia and droplet-shaped rete pegs Loss of basal cell polarity Reduction of cellular cohesion Marked cellular pleomorphism Increase of mitotic figures also in suprabasal position Numerous dyskeratoses Disturbance of epithelial stratification
Carcinoma in situ	Characteristics of severe dysplasia enhanced Loss of epithelial stratification No invasive growth

→ dyskeratosis → impairment of epithelial stratification → invasion - is probable.

The same sequence can also be shown in experimental models of carcinogenesis (Grundmann 1973, Burkhardt 1980) where initially basal cell hyperplasia, i.e. thickening of the proliferative zone, and subsequently nuclear and cellular atypia and finally invasion are observed. Giarelli et al. (1977) also see hyperplasia of basal cells or undifferentiated precursor cells at the onset of carcinogenesis, and later epithelial metaplasia, acanthosis and hyperkeratosis which become associated with dysplasia of varying degrees of severity; transformation into carcinoma in situ, microinvasive carcinoma and finally established carcinoma can ensue. The fact that dysplasia occurs on average at an earlier age than carcinoma could similarly reflect the development of carcinoma from dysplasia. Similar sequences have been supposed by other authors (Trentini et al. 1973, Friedmann 1976, Henry

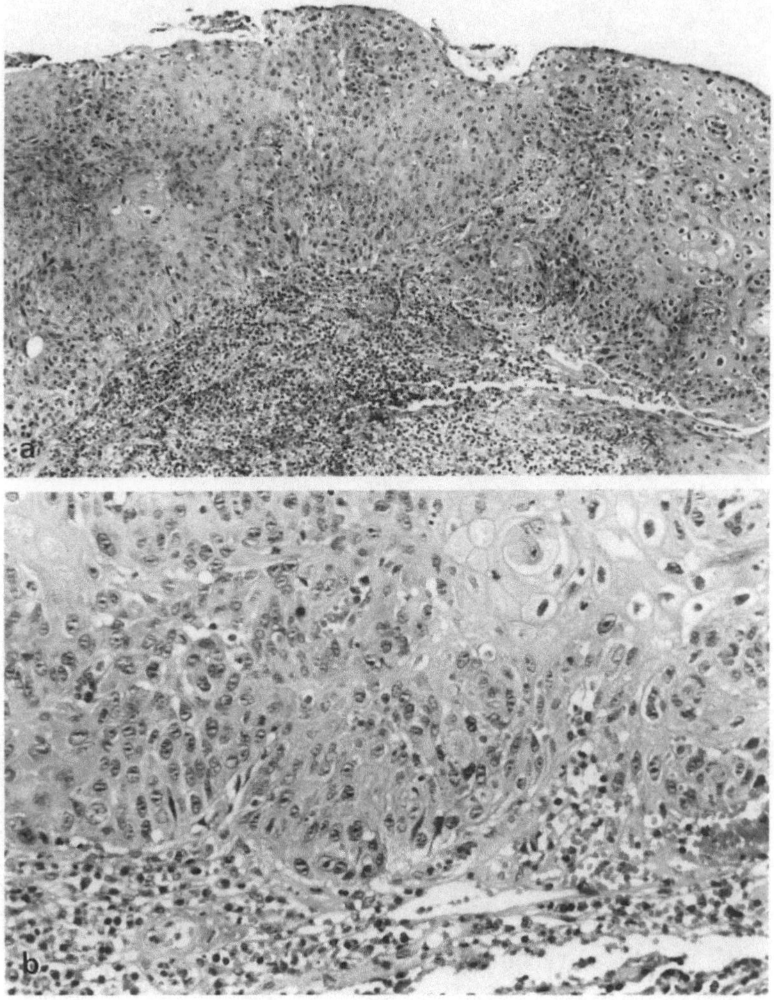

Fig. 4.10 a, b. Epithelial hyperplasia with severe dysplasia: 54-year-old man, supraglottis. **a** Thickened epithelium with marked disruption of stratification, although some maturation to the top is still present. Marked inflammatory infiltration. HE, ×90. **b** A basal cell layer is not recognizable, but the basal membrane is intact. Nuclear pleomorphism and dyskeratosis with formation of a small "keratinous pearl". HE, ×220

1974), although they stress that direct cancerization of normal epithelium is also possible, as is carcinoma development from all stages of dysplasia. The stage of carcinoma in situ may be omitted. Other authors emphasize that epithelial dysplasia does not necessarily undergo malignant transformation (KLEINSASSER 1963b+c, 1983, KAMBIC 1978, FERLITO et al. 1981a).

More recent studies have substantiated the importance of grading of dysplasia in laryngeal lesions.

Using a grading system similar to the one proposed here, CRISSMAN (1979) found mild dysplasia in 55%, moderate dysplasia in 28% and severe dysplasia in 16% of 92 cases. In a 5-year follow-up period three patients (3,3%) - all from the severe dysplasia group - developed carcinoma. LANIADO et al. (1981) found a distribution of 48% mild, 37% moderate and 14% severe dysplasia in 66 patients with leukoplakia of the larynx.

The most impressive data as regards the importance of grading of dysplasia were presented by HELLQUIST et al. (1982). Among 161 patients, 61% presented with mild dysplasia, 15% with moderate dysplasia and 24% with severe dysplasia or carcinoma in situ. Two patients in the group with mild dysplasia (2%), three with moderate dysplasia (12.5%) and nine with severe dysplasia or carcinoma in situ (23%) developed carcinomas in an observation period of up to 13 years.

4.7 Carcinoma In Situ, Microinvasive Carcinoma

Carcinoma in situ is defined as a lesion in which the criteria of dysplasia mentioned above are maximally pronounced in combination with consider-

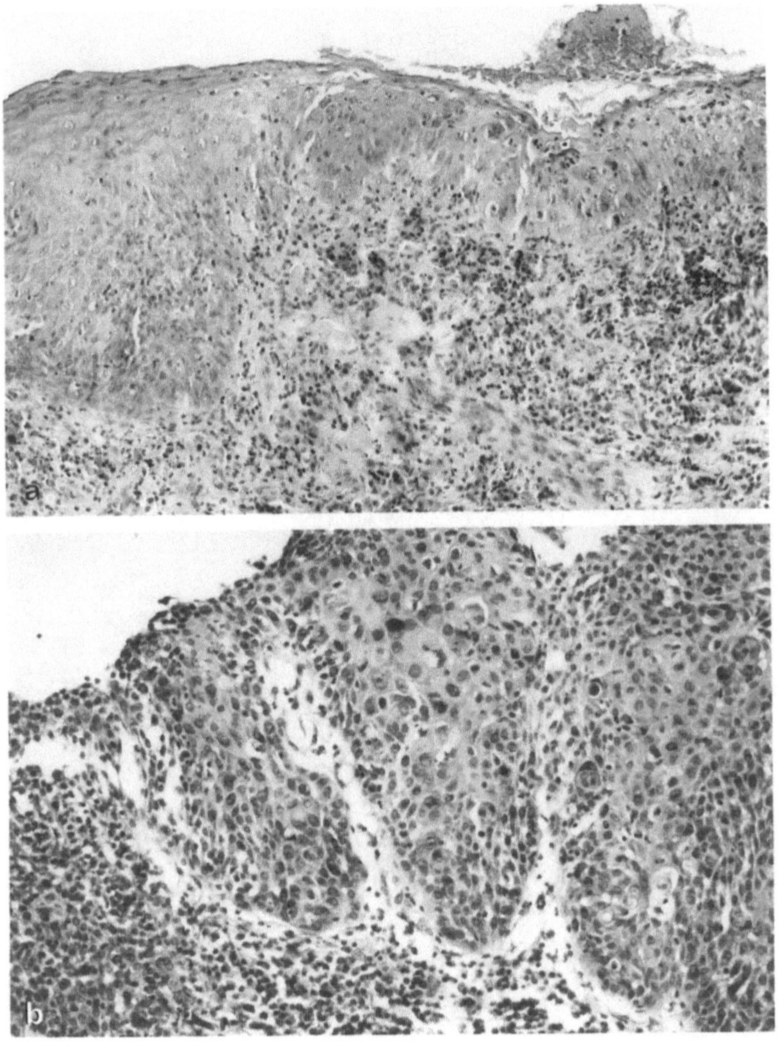

Fig. 4.11 a, b. Carcinoma in situ. 69-year-old man, glottis. **a** At the **left**, hyperplastic epithelium with hyperkeratosis is present. In the **centre**, there is epithelial atrophy with loss of stratification and severe dysplasia. Dense inflammatory infiltration, no invasive growth. HE, ×140. **b** Atrophic epithelium without recognizable stratification or maturation and extreme variation of nuclear size and shape. At the **left**, ulceration has ensued but there is no invasive growth. HE, ×220

able disturbance or complete loss of epithelial stratification, but without invasive growth (Fig. 4.11, 4.12; BRODERS 1932, ALTMANN et al. 1952, STOUT 1953, FISHER and MILLER 1958, KLEINSASSER 1963, KRAMER 1973, FECHNER 1974, ACKERMANN and MCGAVRAN 1978, PESCH and STEINER 1979, BURKHARDT 1980, BURKHARDT and MAERKER 1981, HELLQUIST et al. 1982, GOODMAN 1984). Correspondingly, FRIEDMANN (1976) and FISHER (1976) characterize carcinoma in situ as a lesion in which the entire squamous epithelium has been replaced by cells of the carcinoma type. Mitotic figures can be found in the upper epithelial layers and, by definition, maturation of the epithelium, i.e. lamellar keratosis, should not be detectable (KLEINSASSER and HECK 1959, HYAMS 1976, MCNELIS 1974, KAMBIC 1977). A slight flattening of the upper cell layers (Fig. 4.12), however, does not exclude the diagnosis of carcinoma in situ (FISHER 1974, MICHAELS 1984).

Various authors (FISHER and MILLER 1958, SEIFERTH and GLANZ 1971, FERLITO et al. 1981, KLEINSASSER 1983) make a distinction between an immature, anaplastic, basocellular type (Fig. 4.12), an intermediate type and a mature type (prickle cell type) of carcinoma in situ.

Lesions corresponding to a carcinoma in situ were earlier termed Bowen's disease (KLEINSASSER 1963b, c, GRUNDMANN 1973).

The criterion most often used to exclude invasive growth is an intact basal membrane. The practical value of light-microscopic assessment of the basal membrane is debatable, however, and this method cannot be regarded as absolutely reliable (KLEINSASSER 1959, GRUNDMANN 1973, MCNELIS 1974, KAMBIC 1977, PESCH and STEINER 1979). PESCH and STEINER (1979) report that in 10% of their cases with severe epithelial dysplasia and carcinoma in situ, stromal invasion could not be discounted with

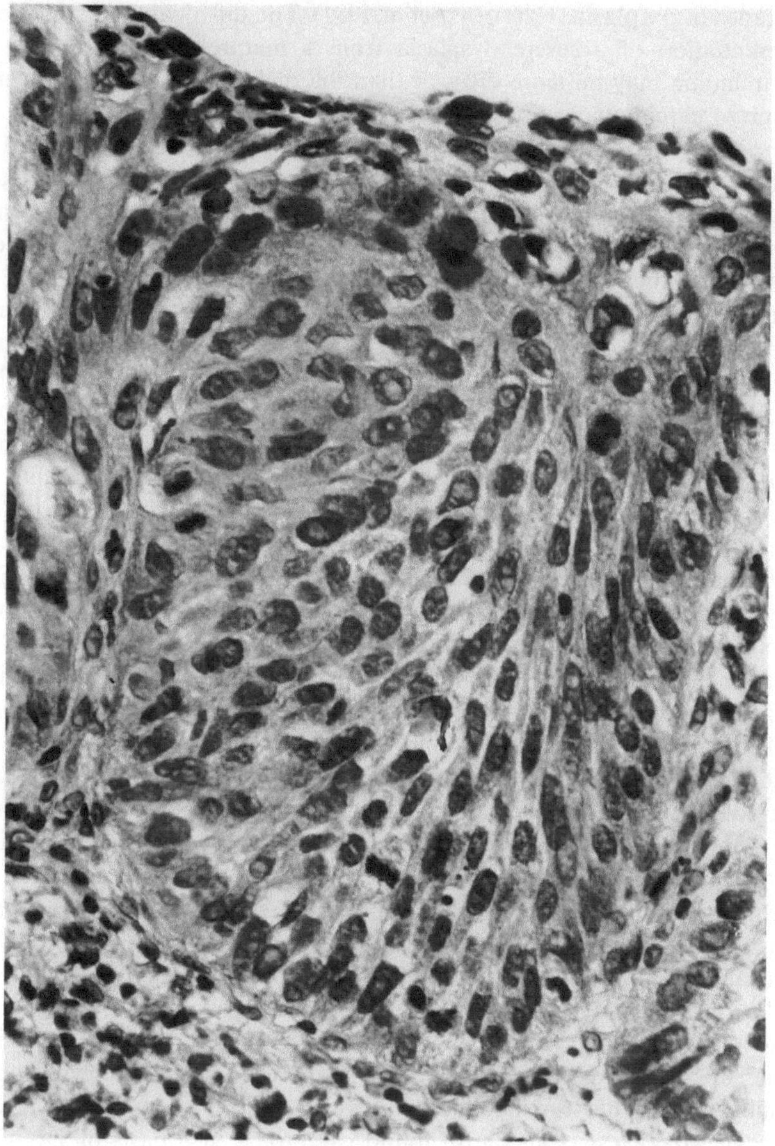

Fig. 4.12. Carcinoma in situ. 56-year-old man, supraglottis. High magnification shows that the entire thickness of the epithelium is replaced by a population of small to medium-sized cells with hyperchromatic nuclei; numerous mitotic figures. At the **top**, slight flattening of the cells as the only sign of maturation. HE, ×350

certainty. Furthermore, spread along the ducts of the mucous gland into depth is possible (STOUT 1953, KLEINSASSER 1983, MICHAELS 1984) and should not be confused with invasion.

Clinically, carcinoma in situ is variable in appearance. It can present as leukoplakia or as erythroplakia (FISHER and MILLER 1958). In addition, finely granular papillomatous and verrucous mucosal changes, erosions and a friable mucosa can be observed (KLEINSASSER and HECK 1959, SEIFERTH and GLANZ 1971, MILLER 1976). Carcinoma in situ is most often seen on the vocal cords, but this is probably due to early symptoms and resultant early diagnosis. In other locations it may progress to invasive cancer without symptoms.

Some authors classify carcinoma in situ as a precancerous lesion which is at least potentially reversible, whereas others regard it as the earliest stage of true carcinoma (ALTMANN et al. 1952, SEIFERTH and GLANZ 1971, FRIEDMANN 1976, BOSSART 1977).

The diagnosis of carcinoma in situ can only be made histologically (GABRIEL and JONES 1976). "Carcinoma in situ" is a term which has come to be accepted worldwide and whose histological definition or recognition is relatively simple (MILLER 1976). Contrary to the assumption made by GABRIEL and JONES (1976), there is broad agreement amongst different pathologists with regard to the definition and diagnosis of carcinoma in situ, and it is more easily defined than are the individual grades of dysplasia (HELLQUIST et al. 1981). The differentiation of a severe dysplasia from a mature carcinoma may be more difficult than the recognition of carcinoma in situ (FRIEDMANN 1976). Today the advantage of the term "carcinoma in situ" is still that "out of the chaos of genetic and prognostically unclear epithelial changes ... a histologically readily definable picture has been separated of which it is known that it is closely related to the development of an invasive carcinoma" (KLEINSASSER and HECK 1959).

The purely theoretical criticism voiced by RYWLIN (1984) against "carcinoma in situ", namely that by definition a neoplasm in situ cannot be diagnosed since the characteristics of malignant cells, i.e. their capacity to invade and to metastasize, are not recognizable at this point of time, is not convincing in light of the wide acceptance and considerable practical value of the term. In the final analysis, most histopathological diagnoses are interpretations based on experience (and also experiments) inferring possible dynamic processes from a static picture. It is thus, of course, simply a forecast on a statistical basis, just like the determination of grades of dysplasia.

The close relationship between carcinoma in situ and invasive carcinoma is underlined by numerous clinicopathological studies. This applies to sex and age distribution (ALTMANN et al. 1952) as well as to location. PESCH and STEINER (1979) were able to demonstrate, in 83 cases, a distribution which corresponded closely to that of T1/T2 carcinomas (glottis 88% of carcinomata in situ, 78% of carcinomas; subglottis neither carcinomata in situ nor carcinomas). AUERBACH et al. (1970) found carcinoma in situ in the glottic region in 11.8% of 942 autopsies on elderly men who died of various causes and in the vestibular ligament region in 4.8%, but none in the subglottic area.

FISHER and MILLER (1958) observed the development of an invasive carcinoma in 10 of 48 carcinomata in situ. SEIFERTH and GLANZ (1971) report a transformation rate of 64,9% in 34 cases of carcinoma in situ which were treated inadequately or not at all at that time. GRUNDMANN (1973) considers 25% of carcinomata in situ to be "reversible" (in fact this process should probably be termed "rejection") and 25% to be persistent, leaving 50% which he presumes transform to invasive carcinomas.

Further support for a connection between carcinoma in situ and invasive carcinoma is provided by almost daily observations and reports by numerous authors: in the periphery of invasive carcinomas, there are often large areas showing changes corresponding to carcinoma in situ and severe epithelial dysplasia (see Sect. 4.5; ROBBETT et al. 1972, GRUNDMANN 1973, BAUER 1976, FRIEDMANN 1976, GLANZ and KLEINSASSER 1976, MICHAELS 1984). KLEINSASSER and HECK (1959) consider carcinoma in situ to be the "herald and companion of cancer" and thus treat it as a warning signal. For the pathologist, this means that he or she must exercise great caution in using the diagnosis "carcinoma in situ" on small biopsy specimens and should always make it clear to the clinician that the tissue could be from the margin of an invasive carcinoma ("false" carcinoma in situ; MARAN et al. 1984, FERLITO 1976, FERLITO et al. 1981). According to BAUER'S (1976) observation, there is an association between carcinoma in situ and 76% of nonkeratinizing carcinomas, but only 26% of keratinizing carcinomas. This might be an indication that the classical, i.e. immature carcinoma in situ is a forerunner of the poorly differentiated squamous cell carcinoma, whereas severe dysplasia with epithelial maturation represents the forerunner of the differentiated keratinizing squamous cell carcinoma. Many authors consider severe dysplasia to have the same malignant potential as carcinoma in situ (HELLQUIST et al. 1981, GOODMAN 1984, MICHAELS 1984); in some cases severe dysplasia may even have a higher malignant potential (HELLQUIST et al. 1982).

CRISSMAN and FU (1986) point out that the classic carcinoma in situ without epithelial maturation, as known from the uterine cervix, is seldom encountered in laryngeal biopsy specimens. On the basis of DNA histograms of six cases with extensive premalignant changes of the laryngeal mucosa, they stress that keratinization as a common reaction to injury does not militate against the diagnosis of intraepithelial neoplastic transformation, as aneuploid DNA values were also found in these lesions.

4.8 Evaluation of Histological Finding

Even though the histological diagnosis provides relatively "hard" data compared to other biological or clinical examinations, nonetheless it is dangerous to overrate histological findings on small biopsy specimens. Whereas the diagnosis of malignancy can often be made on the smallest piece of tissue, it has to be continually borne in mind with a "negative" finding that the biopsy specimen possibly did not contain the lesion, i.e. that the tissue changes are not necessarily representative of the lesion. The pathologist should always point out this possibility. Special caution is necessary if severe dysplasia or carcinoma in situ is found. For his part, the clinician should not hesitate to perform a further biopsy if there is a discrepancy between the clinical findings or course of disease and the histological assessment.

Just how severe the consequences of such misunderstandings between clinician and pathologist can be is well illustrated by the famous example of the German emperor Frederick III, who died of laryngeal cancer. Although nearly 100 years have elapsed since then, the case still has relevance. As is well known, operative treatment of the cancer was postponed by the laryngologist MOREL MACKENZIE because RUDOLF VIRCHOW was unable to find malignant neoplastic tissue in any of three pieces of tissue removed at three different times. His diagnoses read: pachydermia-irritative process. He stressed nonetheless on each occasion that only a superficial piece of tissue could be evaluated. The diagnosis of malignancy was finally made on a slough which had been coughed out. It is undisputed by historians today that a diagnosis made in time could have changed the course of history (for detailed description of the course of the illness, see LINK and PASCHER 1969, MICHAELS 1984).

4.9 Therapy of Dysplasia and Carcinoma In Situ of the Larynx

The principles of treatment of dysplasia and carcinoma in situ of the laryngeal mucosa are elimination of all possible exogenous irritations (exclusion of well-known risk factors, in particular tobacco abuse and alcohol, as well as avoidance of voice stress) and further, if possible, radical surgical removal of the affected mucosal area by excision or mucosal "stripping" (HELLQUIST et al. 1981, 1982, FERLITO et al. 1981, GILLIS et al. 1983, MARAN et al. 1984). Only in exceptional cases should radiation be considered, for example, in multifocal, expansive and recurrent lesions in patients medically unfit or above 60 years of age (MCNELIS 1974). There are a number of reasons to restrict the use of radiation in lesion, that have not yet progressed to invasion. The most important are the difficulty of detecting recurrence or frank malignant transformation in an irradiated larynx and the possible enhancement of malignant transformation (see Sect. 7.3).

Owing to the possibility of synchronous or metachronic multitopical development of cancer, careful life-long follow-up is necessary for patients with severe dysplasia, carcinoma in situ and for those successfully treated for carcinoma.

5 Squamous Cell Carcinomas

Most malignant neoplasms of the larynx and the adjacent regions (hypopharynx and oropharynx with lingual epiglottic surface, valleculae, lower part of the retrolingual region) are squamous cell carcinomas (Table 5.1). In a survey of 1207 patients with malignant tumours of the larynx treated in the Frankfurt University Ear, Nose and Throat Clinic between 1962 and 1986, there were 998 squamous cell carcinomas; including the variants of the squamous cell carcinoma, i.e. the so-called carcinosarcoma, spindle cell carcinoma and verrucous carcinoma, results a good 97%, whereas all other types of malignant neoplasm were seen very rarely.

Age and sex distribution are discussed in Sect. 4.1. The majority (66.3%) of all laryngeal carcinomas observed by us were found in the glottic region; less often affected was the supraglottic region, with 32.9%. This is in agreement with most reports, which state that about 60% of laryngeal carcinomas are found in the vocal cord region and 35%-45% in the supraglottic region (McComb 1967, Martensson et al. 1967, Lott et al. 1972, Schwab and zum Winkel 1975, Bohndorf and Höcker 1976). Pietrantoni et al. (1961) and Taskinen (1969) report a higher proportion of malignant laryngeal tumours originating in the supraglottis. In contrast, Glanz (1984) found only 23.8% supraglottic carcinomas from a total of 189 laryngeal carcinomas. The subglottic region plays a subordinate role as the primary site of carcinomas. The higher figures given for this region in some statistics are most readily explained by the fact that glottic carcinomas with preferred subglottic spread are not uncommonly classified as subglottic. As a rule, however, the proportion of subglottic carcinomas lies below 5% (McComb et al. 1967, Schwab und zum Winkel 1975, Bohndorf and Höcker 1976).

Among the larynx-proximate carcinomas, where squamous cell carcinomas similarly predominate, the piriform sinus is most commonly affected; reports vary between 50% and 85%. The remaining carcinomas are distributed equally between the region of the postcricoid and the posterior hypopharyngeal wall (McComb et al. 1967, Taskinen 1969, Joergensen and Sell 1971, Bryce 1972). According to Bryce (1972), from every 100 new cases of carcinomas of the laryngeal area, 30 are hypopharyngeal. In the period from 1966 to 1982, 64 (69.5%) of the 92 hypopharyngeal carcinomas treated in the Frankfurt University ENT Clinic originated from the piriform sinus, 12 were located predominantly on the posterior wall and six in the postcricoid area. The remaining 10 hypopharyngeal could not be assigned unequivocally to any one site.

In this chapter, the spreading tendencies, the TNM classification and the grading of malignancy of laryngeal and neighbouring carcinomas will be

Table 5.1. Classification and frequency of primary malignancies of the larynx and hypopharynx studied by Ferlito (1976) in Padua and diagnosed in the ENT Department of Frankfurt University (1986)

	Padua 1966–1976 n = 1919	Frankfurt 1962–1986 n = 1220
Carcinoma in situ	54	38
Squamous cell carcinoma	1605	988
Verrucous and papillary carcinoma	71	115
Spindle cell carcinoma	12	8
Lymphoepithelial carcinoma	1	2
Undifferentiated carcinoma	139	33
Oat cell carcinoma	1	0
Carcinoid	1	0
Adenocarcinoma	7	8
Giant cell carcinoma	1	0
Adenosquamous carcinoma	8	0
Mucoepidermoid carcinoma	10	1
Adenoid cystic carcinoma	1	2
Acinous cell carcinoma	1	0
Fibrosarcoma	1	1
Malignant fibrous histiocytoma	1	0
Chondrosarcoma	0	3
Rhabdomyosarcoma	0	2
Haemangiosarcoma	0	1
Malignant lymphoma	5	3
Hodgkin's disease	0	1
Kaposi's sarcoma	0	1

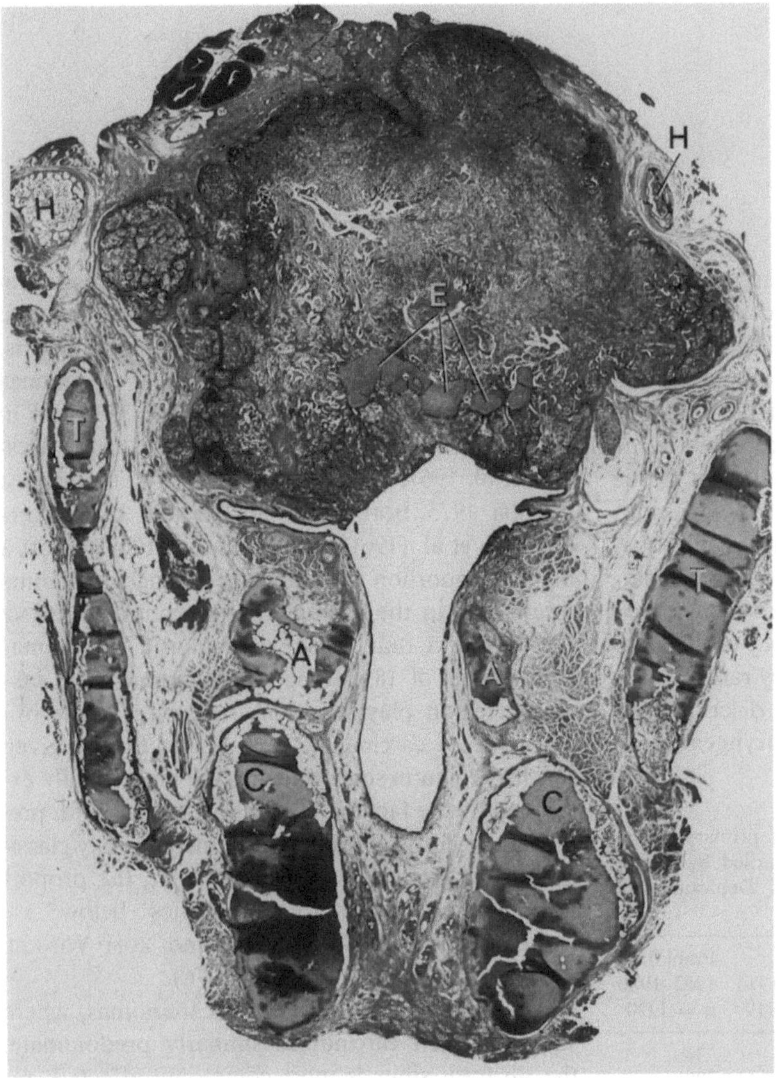

Fig. 5.1. Bulky supraglottic tumour, pushing type: 52-year-old man. The tumour remains within the laryngeal boundaries. Membranes are not infiltrated. *T*, thyroid cartilage; *C*, cricoid cartilage; *E*, epiglottic cartilage; *H*, hyoid bone; *A*, arytenoid cartilage

described and discussed. In the next chapter, the histological findings on partial resection specimens and on tumours treated by irradiation or with cytotoxins will be presented and their importance for future therapeutic concepts evaluated.

5.1 Origin and Spread of Carcinomas

Most laryngeal squamous cell carcinomas are moderately or well differentiated, corresponding to Broders' grades I and II (McGavran et al. 1961, Meyer-Breiting 1981 a, Olofsson and van Nostrand 1973) or to grade I of the WHO grading of squamous cell carcinomas (Wahi et al 1971). The findings of McGavran et al (1961), Kashima (1976) and Meyer-Breiting (1981 a) show that, regarding the degree of differentiation and certain growth characteristics, the invasive growth of carcinoma depends on the tissue involved. Glands, muscles and loose connective tissue virtually serve as guiding tracks for squamous cell carcinomas, including the "pushing type"; bone, cartilage, membranes and ligaments, as well as vessels and nerves, offer higher resistance to tumour infiltration. Bulgy tumours, as illustrated in Figs. 5.1 and 5.2 may not break through the thyrohyoid membrane or the elastic cone but may infiltrate the thyroid cartilage (Fig. 5.2). Only about one-third of 180 laryngeal carcinomas which required total laryngectomy showed infiltration of membranes, blood vessels and/or peripheral nerves. Hence, the anatomical structure of the larynx (described in Sect. 1.4.2) de-

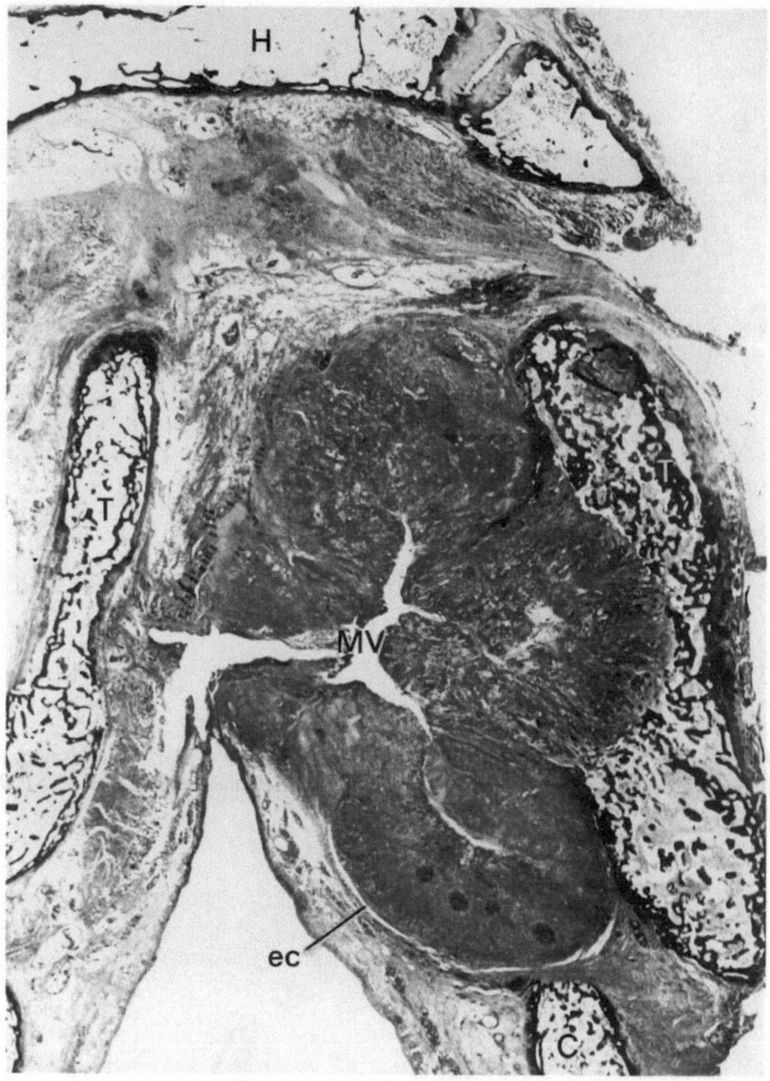

Fig. 5.2. Supraglottic cancer arising from Morgagni's ventricle *(MV)*: 42-year-old man. This type of origin is extremely rare. The carcinoma on the right side was detected 2 years after neck dissection because of cervical lymph node metastases of unknown origin. It completely fills the paraglottic space without penetration of the elastic cone *(ec)*

cisively determines the spread of laryngeal carcinomas depending on the site of origin. The spatial subdivision of the larynx is based on the laryngeal framework, the quadrangular membrane an the elastic cone (Figs. 1.6, 5.3, 5.4). Tumours infiltrate the space of origin in the early stages, and then, sooner or later, depending on the resistance offered, penetrate the bordering membranes or skeletal parts and invade the neighbouring spaces (Meyer-Breiting 1981 a, Lam et al 1983). Here they can expand freely until they impinge once more on boundaries which, for a shorter or longer time, impede their further expansion. A tumour does not necessarily spread faster, however, in a neighbouring space infiltrated at an early stage than in one infiltrated later. Unfavourable nutritional conditions and impermeable separation from other spaces by fibrous tissue, cartilage or bone may delay tumour growth in the space reached earlier, while in a more distant space the tumour may find more favourable conditions and thus spread rapidly. A carcinoma, for example, after finding a complicated path via the paraglottic space caudally through the lateral thyroarytenoid muscle into the preepiglottic space, can expand in the loose connective tissue these more rapidly than it was able to do in the paraglottic space. Different growth ratios can also result from changes in the tumour itself, i. e. formation of cell lines with increased proliferation and anaplastic growth.

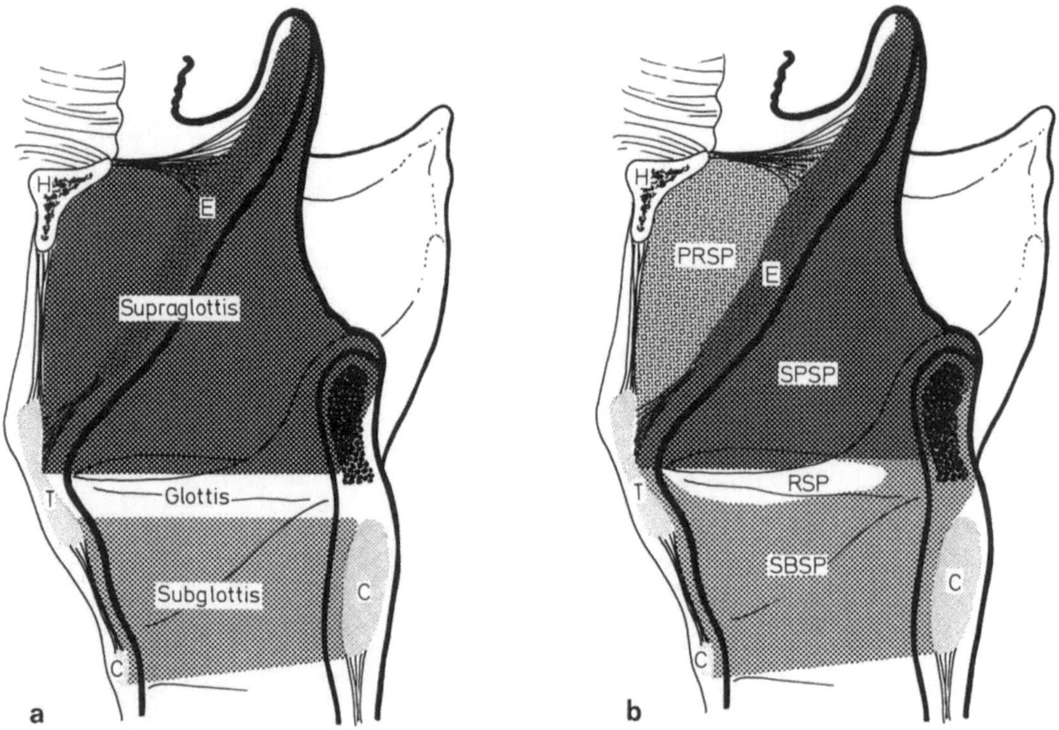

Fig. 5.3a, b. Regional (**a**) and spatial (**b**) subdivision of the larynx: midsagittal sections. *T*, thyroid cartilage; *C*, cricoid cartilage; *E*, Epiglottic cartilage; *H*, hyoid bone; *PRSP*, preepiglottic space; *SPSP*, supraglottic space; *RSP*, Reinke's space; *SBSP*, subglottic space

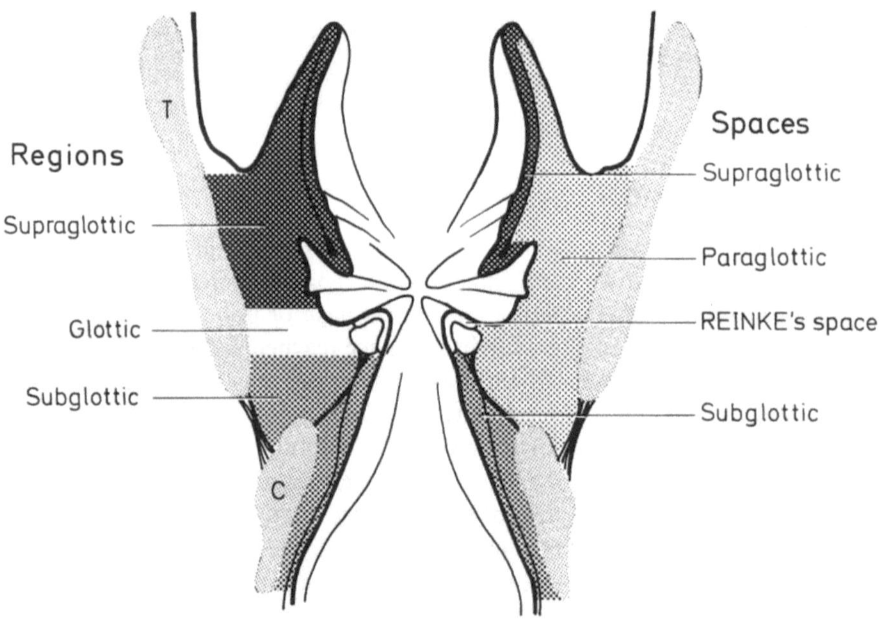

Fig. 5.4. Regional and spatial subdivision of the larynx. Coronal section with frontal mucosal relief. *Left:* subdivision into regions according the ICD-O. *Right:* spatial subdivision based on the anatomy of the laryngeal framework and on the lymphatic drainage system (see Sect. 1.4, Fig. 1.6). *T*, thyroid cartilage; *C*, cricoid cartilage

5.1.1 Supraglottic Carcinomas

As already described, the structure of the supraglottic region is most complicated. HOMMERICH et al (1971) and TUCKER (1974) divided supraglottic tumours according to the site of origin into medial (i.e. ventral) and lateral (i.e. marginal), whereas KLEINSASSER (1967) and HOFFMANN (1968) proposed a division into six areas. MEYER-BREITING and VON ILBERG (1979) compromised and suggested four categories:

1. Ventral carcinoma (epiglottic carcinoma)
2. Lateral carcinoma (vestibular ligament, aryepiglottic fold and Morgagni's ventricle)
3. Ventrolateral carcinoma (so-called "Winkelkarzinom" according to KLEINSASSER (1967)
4. Carcinomas of posterior wall (arytenoid region and interarytenoid space)

This division has been shown to be clinically practicable and has implications for the assessment of the course of the disease, in particular with a view to the tendency to metastasize (MEYER-BREITING and VON ILBERG 1979).

The **ventral carcinomas** of the supraglottic space (Figs. 5.5, 5.7a-d) occur on the laryngeal surface of the epiglottis. From the pars fixa of the epiglottis down to the petiole, these carcinomas can invade the preepiglottic space through the preformed perforations of the epiglottic cartilage without destroying cartilage or bone (Fig. 5.7a). Otherwise they may reach this region either by growing around the lateral edges of the epiglottis or by destruction of the epiglottis (Fig. 5.7b); both routes are diagnostically difficult to assess (OGURA 1955, BOCCA 1968, HOFFMANN 1968, KIRCHNER 1969, OLOFSSON and VAN NOSTRAND 1973, MEYER-BREITING 1981a). The frequency of invasion of the preepiglottic space by ventral carcinomas is more than 80% (KIRCHNER 1969, OLOFSSON and VAN NOSTRAND 1973, WEEDE 1974, KIRCHNER and OWEN 1977, MEYER-BREITING 1981a). The incidence of infiltration of the valleculae and retrolingual region among 20 such carcinomas was reported by WEEDE (1974) to be nine and seven respectively; this appears relatively high, but possibly oropharyngeal carcinomas were included in the series. Since epiglottic carcinomas with infiltration of the valleculae and retrolingual region gain access to the lymph drainage system of this area (retrolingual-lateral oropharynx), this has to be taken into account for therapeutic considerations.

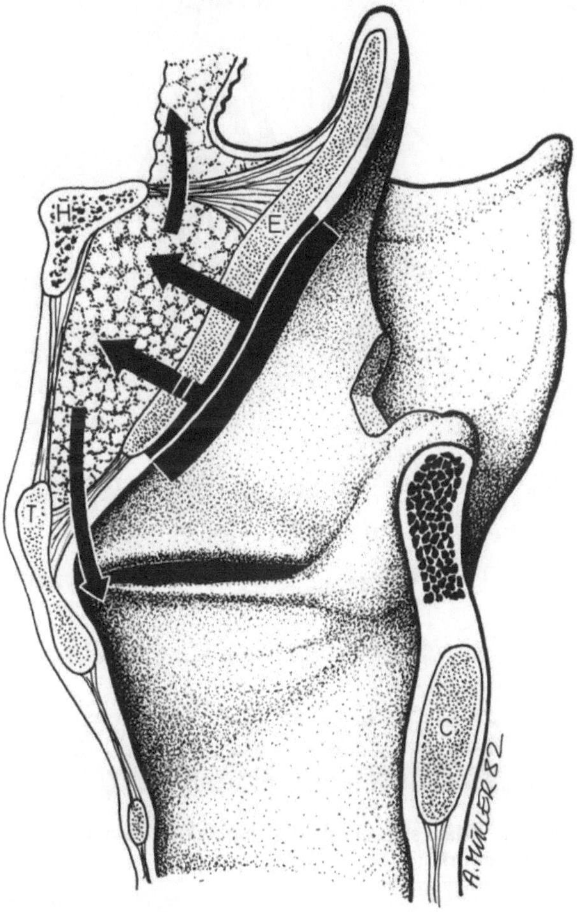

Fig. 5.5. Spread of ventral supraglottic (epiglottic) carcinoma shown by midsagittal section of the larynx. Most supraglottic carcinomas originate in or near the epiglottis, and the majority of them involve the preepiglottic space by penetration of the epiglottic fenestrae or by growing around or destroying the epiglottis. *T*, thyroid cartilage; *C*, cricoid cartilage; *E*, epiglottic cartilage; *H*, hyoid bone

Epiglottic carcinomas reach the glottic region in nearly a quarter of all cases (KIRCHNER 1969, 1977, WEEDE 1974, MEYER-BREITING 1981a). These are predominantly carcinomas originating in the petiole region, whence they tend to descend caudally, as a rule along the mucosal surface via the anterior commissure. This does not exclude the possibility that such tumours may also descend laterally via the paraglottic space into the anterior parts of the glottic-subglottic region. Accounts of the proportion of ventral carcinomas which invade the laryngeal framework have varied between 15% and 50% (MÜLLER 1966, KIRCHNER 1969, 1977, OLOFSSON and VAN NOSTRAND 1973, MEYER-BREITING 1981a). Penetration into the laryngeal framework usually occurs at the transition from the upper edge of the

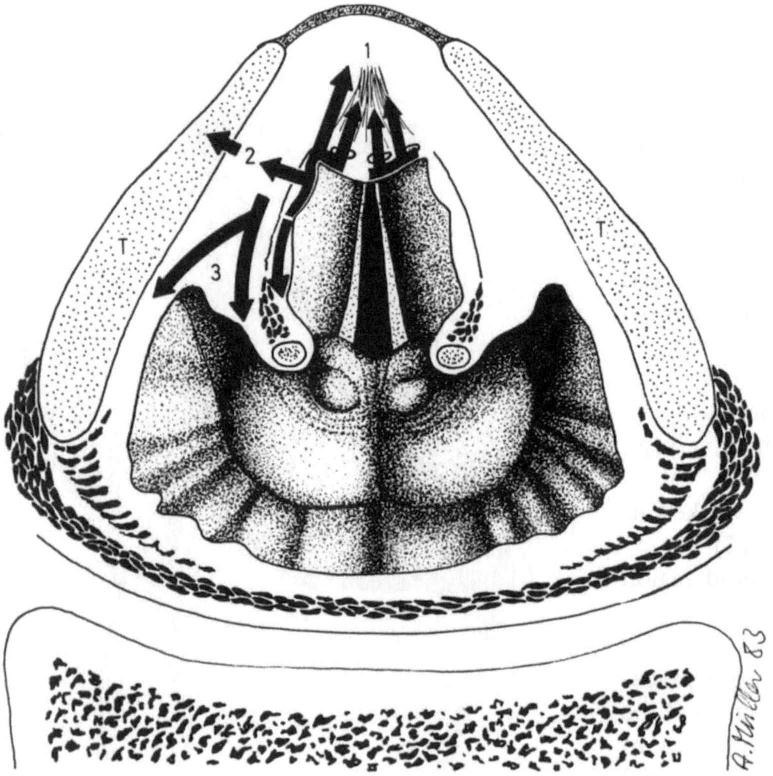

Fig. 5.6. Spread of ventral and ventrolateral supraglottic carcinomas demonstrated by a horizontal section of the larynx showing lower laryngeal and hypopharyngeal relief. Spread ensues preferentially in the preepiglottic *(1)* and paraglottic *(2)* directions. The third route, to the posterior wall of the larynx or to the piriform *(3)*, is seen more often in lateral supraglottic carcinomas

Table 5.2. Main sites of origin of supraglottic squamous cell carcinomas and their tendency to involve or penetrate the laryngeal framework

	Supraglottic sites of origin				
	Ventral n = 10	Ventrolateral n = 23	Lateral n = 23	Dorsal n = 1	Total n = 57
Laryngeal framework					
Hyoid bone	1/1	-	-	-	1/1
Thyrohyoid membrane	-	-	-	-	-
	-	3/3	1/1	-	4/4
Thyroid cartilage					
Upper rim	2/1	-	-	-	2/1
Centre	-	1/0	1/1	-	2/1
Lower rim	1/0	-	1/1	-	2/1
	-	1/1	1/1	-	2/2
Cricothyroid membrane	-	1/1	-	-	1/1
	-	-	-	-	-
Cricoid cartilage					
Ring	-	-	-	-	-
Lamina	-	1/0	-	-	1/0
Total	4/2	7/5	4/4	-	15/11
Involvement	4/10	30%	17%	-	26%
Penetration	2/3	22%	17%	-	19%

The numbers before the slash indicate the frequency of involvement, the numbers after it the frequency of penetration

thyroid cartilage to the thyrohyoid membrane, less commonly at the transition from this membrane to the retrolingual region (Table 5.2) and even more infrequently through the membrane itself.

The **lateral carcinomas of the supraglottic region** (Figs. 5.6, 5.8–5.10) are located predominantly in the area of the quadrangular membrane (Fig. 5.9) and Morgagni's ventricle. As McGavran et al

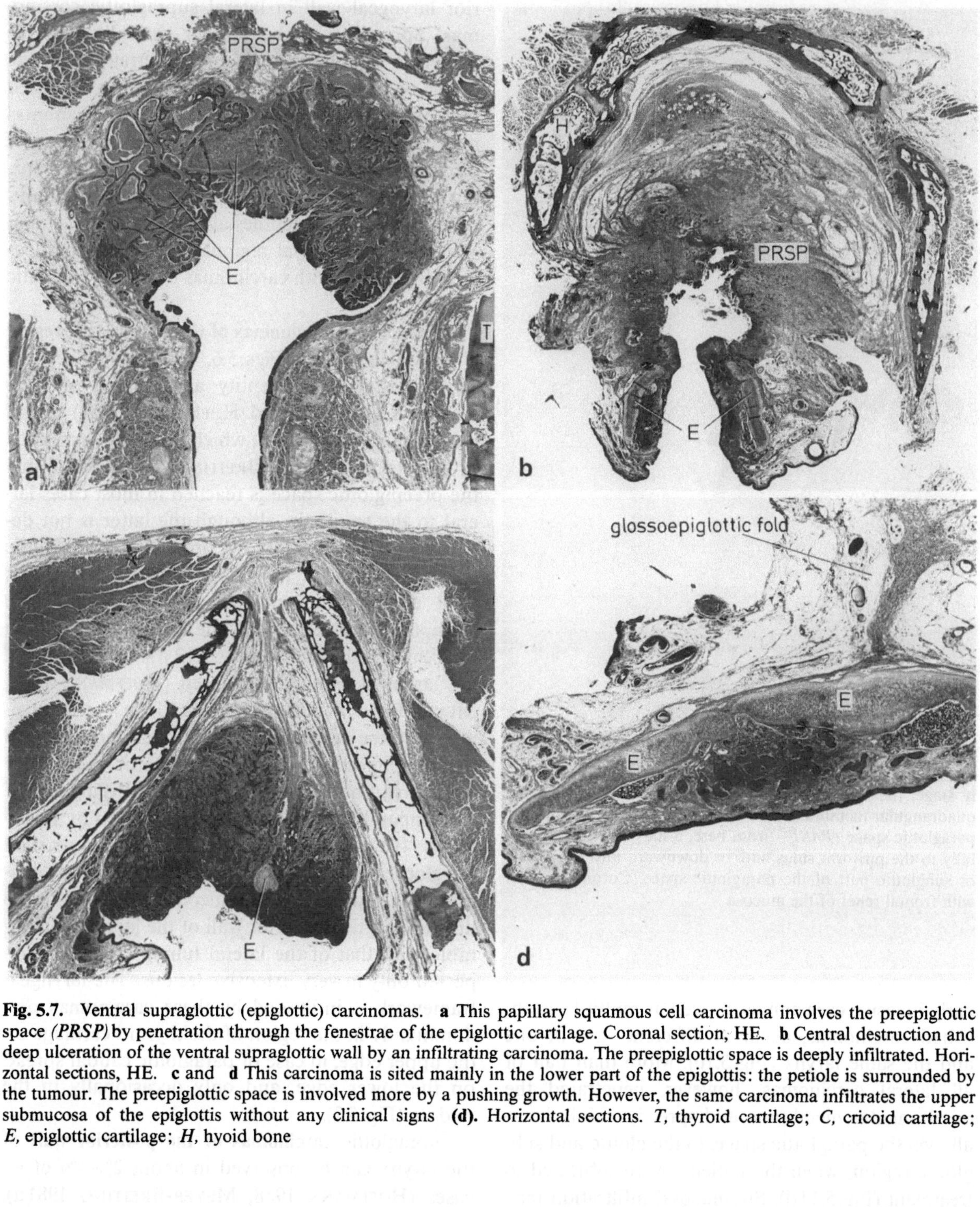

Fig. 5.7. Ventral supraglottic (epiglottic) carcinomas. **a** This papillary squamous cell carcinoma involves the preepiglottic space *(PRSP)* by penetration through the fenestrae of the epiglottic cartilage. Coronal section, HE. **b** Central destruction and deep ulceration of the ventral supraglottic wall by an infiltrating carcinoma. The preepiglottic space is deeply infiltrated. Horizontal sections, HE. **c** and **d** This carcinoma is sited mainly in the lower part of the epiglottis: the petiole is surrounded by the tumour. The preepiglottic space is involved more by a pushing growth. However, the same carcinoma infiltrates the upper submucosa of the epiglottis without any clinical signs **(d).** Horizontal sections. *T,* thyroid cartilage; *C,* cricoid cartilage; *E,* epiglottic cartilage; *H,* hyoid bone

(1961) and KIRCHNER (1969) observed, these carcinomas usually exhibit a persistent superficial growth pattern, which KLEINSASSER (1967) and HOFFMANN (1968) have called "wallpaper-like growth". Such lesions are also characterized by general dysplastic changes of the supraglottic and hypopharyngeal mucosa (see Sect. 4.5). All gradations from dysplasia to early carcinomas are focally distributed throughout this region. The disease proceeds by extension and confluence of these carcinomatous changes (HOFFMANN 1968). This fact explains the observations made by ROSEMANN (1963), HOFFMANN (1968) and MEYER-BREITING (1981 a), that dysplasia, multicentric carcinomata in situ and

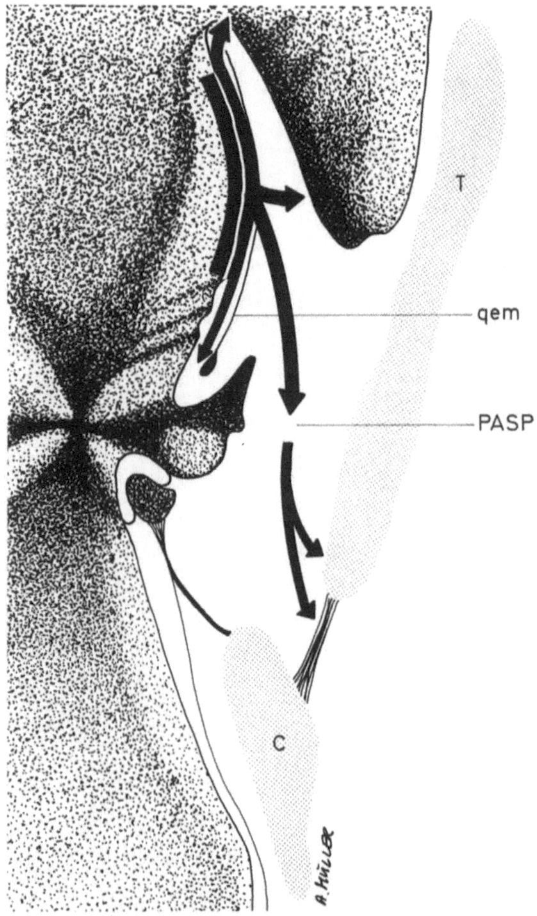

Fig. 5.8. Lateral spread of supraglottic carcinoma. At an early stage, the tumour remains within the boundaries of the quadrangular membrane *(qem)*. It may spread qickly into the paraglottic space *(PASP)*. From here, it may extend horizontally to the piriform sinus and/or downward into the glottic or subglottic part of the paraglottic space. Coronal section with frontal relief of the mucosa

early invasive carcinomas, as well as multiple established carcinomas, occur at different sites in one and the same larynx (Fig. 5.10). More than half of all lateral carcinomas, however, penetrated the quadrangular membrane and spread, mainly laterally via the paraglottic space, to the glottic and subglottic region, when the patients were subjected to treatment (Fig. 5.11 d). Submucosal infiltration may not be present at the initial site of the tumour, but can be demonstrated in the aryepiglottic folds in almost all cases. KIRCHNER (1969) and OLOFSSON and VAN NOSTRAND (1973) point out the frequent involvement of the arytenoid cartilage and the posterior laryngeal wall in lateral supraglottic carcinomas. Spreading of the tumour caudally into the posterior laryngeal wall and infiltration of the upper edge of the cricoid lamina is thus favoured fact. With infiltration into depth, these carcinomas may penetrate into the preepiglottic space just as often as they descend caudally into the neighbouring region. The proximity of the piriform sinuses permits a rapid, sometimes also submucosal, expansion to extralaryngeal regions; this occurs particularly frequently with carcinomas of the aryepiglottic fold.

Ventrolateral carcinomas of the supraglottic region ("Winkelkarzinom", Figs. 5.6, 5.12) have been described as a special entity and treated only by KLEINSASSER (1967) and HOFFMANN (1968) up till now. Their observations, which could be confirmed in our studies (MEYER-BREITING 1981 a) show that the preepiglottic space is reached in most cases lateral to the epiglottis, although the latter is not destroyed for a relatively long time. The preepiglottic space is infiltrated in 70% of Winkel carcinomas (and equally frequently by ventral carcinomas). With the involvement of the valleculae and the pharyngoepiglottic fold (Fig. 5.12 a + b), the limit of the larynx is often transgressed (HOFFMANN 1968, MEYER-BREITING 1981 a). Owing to the special position of these carcinomas at the boundary between the preepiglottic and the paraepiglottic space, they may spread both ventrally and caudally. Fifteen of 43 comparable such carcinomas observed by HOFFMANN (1968) and MEYER-BREITING (1981 a) reached the glottic plane and descended further in the direction of the subglottis. Submucous infiltration in the direction of the posterior wall of the larynx, comparable with that of the lateral tumours, is to be expected only in very extensive lesions. The laryngeal framework is infiltrated by these carcinomas predominantly in the region of the thyroid cartilage on the upper edge, in case of paraglottic caudal spread on the lower edge, and only occasionally in the middle (Fig. 5.2).

Supraglottic **carcinomas of the posterior wall** of the larynx can be observed in about 2%-3% of all cases (HOFFMANN 1968, MEYER-BREITING 1981 a). Similar to the lateral supraglottic carcinomas, they tend to spread subepithelially in a ventral and dorsocaudal direction where they can obtain access to the lower lymph drainage system of the larynx (Fig. 5.11 f).

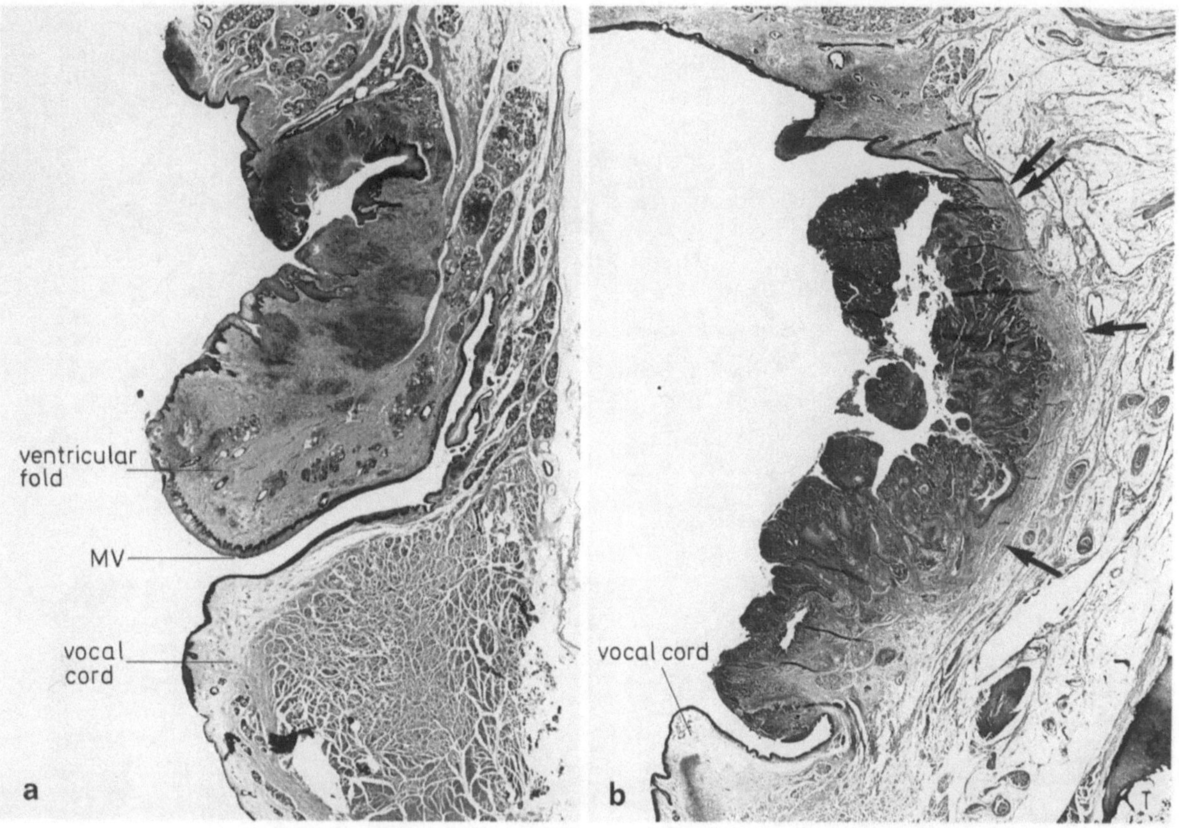

Fig. 5.9 a, b. Early lateral supraglottic carcinomas. **a** Small carcinoma of the ventricular fold (pT_1) resected conservatively: 53-year-old man. The tumour tends to ulceration and infiltration. Coronal section, HE. **b** More superficial spread of a papillary squamous cell carcinoma apparently confined by the quadrangular membrane *(arrows)*

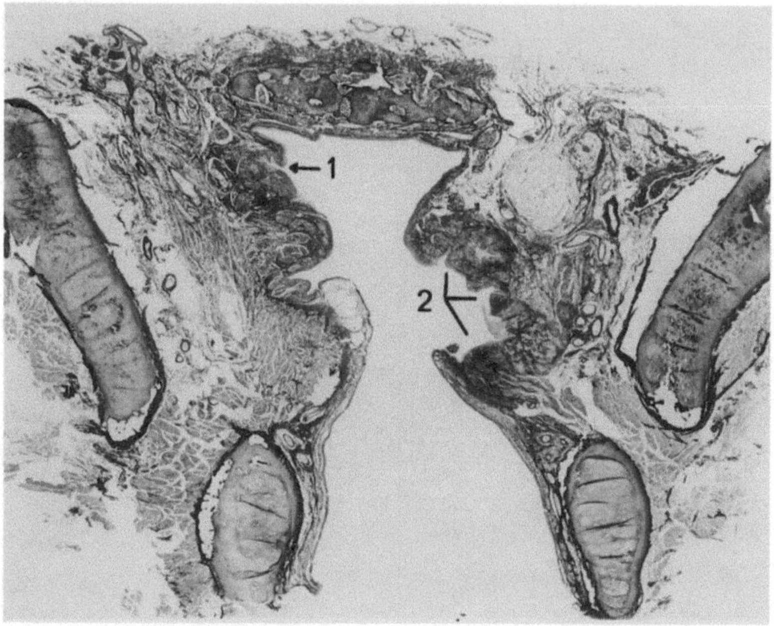

Fig. 5.10. Multiloculated supraglottic carcinomas. Two early isolated carcinomas have originated on different supraglottic sites in this larynx. One is sited on the left lateral wall near the epiglottis *(1)*, the other appears as a transglottic tumour on the right *(2)*. The whole supraglottic mucosa shows squamous epithelial metaplasia with multiple areas of various degrees of dysplasia

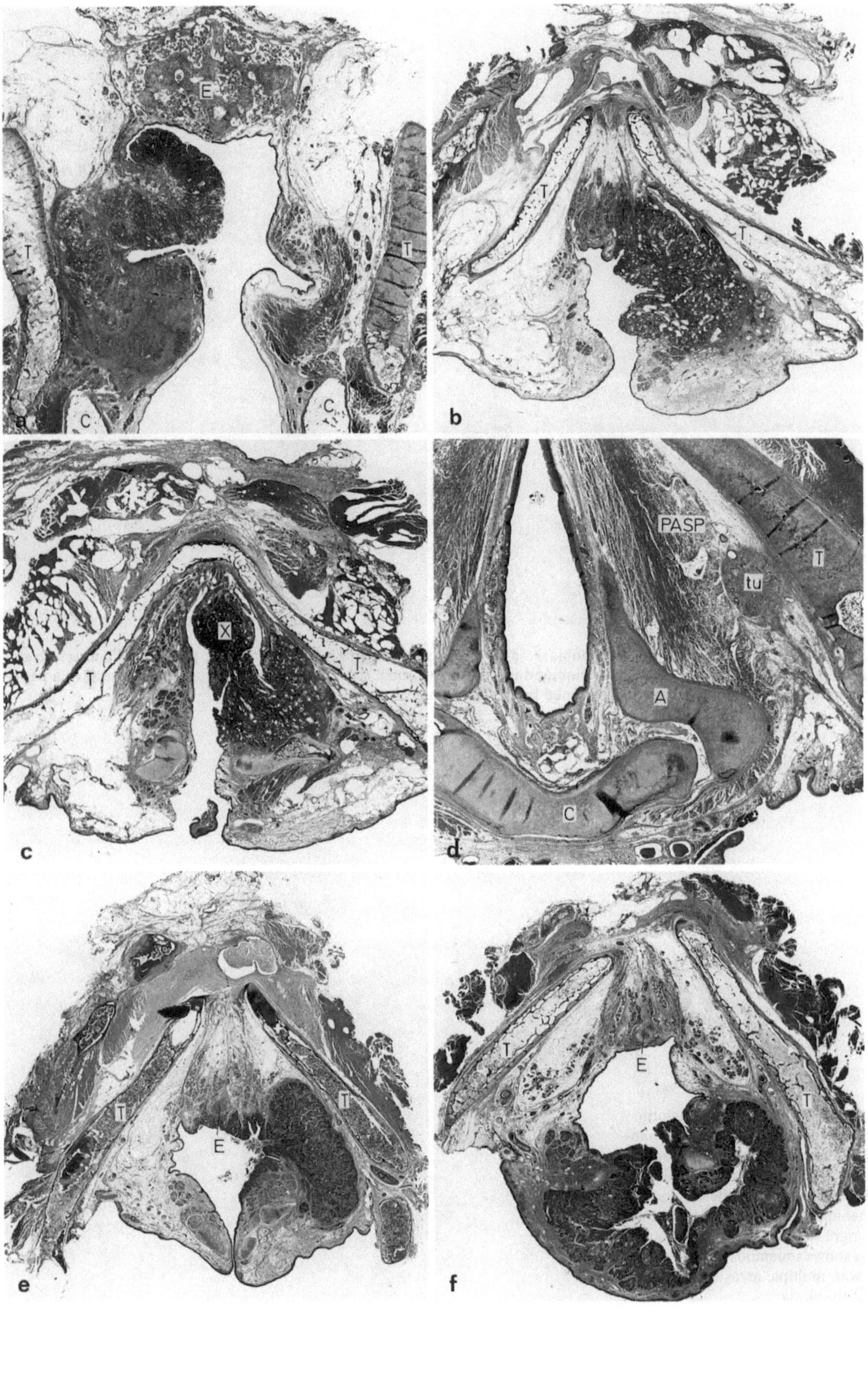
a
E
T
T
C
C
b
T
T
c
X
T
T
d
PASP
tu
T
A
C
e
T
T
E
f
T
E
T

5.1.2 Glottic-Supraglottic Boundary

OGURA (1955, 1958) and BOCCA (1968, 1975), on the basis of embryological considerations, repeatedly postulated a boundary between the supraglottic and the glottic region. Numerous histopathological studies have shown, however, that there is no such barrier (SZLESAK 1966, GÜNNEL and BAERTHOLD 1967, HOFFMANN 1968, HOMMERICH et al 1971, KIRCHNER and SOM 1971, OLOFSSON and VAN NOSTRAND 1973, MEYER-BREITING and von ILBERG 1979, MEYER-BREITING 1981a). Tumours of the supraglottic space of all locations expand via different paths in the caudal direction: lateral and ventrolateral tumours mainly via the paraglottic space and via the posterior wall of the larynx, ventral and ventrolateral carcinomas via the petiole and the anterior commissure. Noteworthy in this connection is the point made by HAST (1974) that even if the supraglottic region arises from different embryological elements than the glottic region, nonetheless one cannot establish exactly where in fact the border between the two regions lies. From this point of view, the horizontal laryngeal partial resection based on embryological considerations appears rather questionable (see Sect. 1.1). From our observations, the descent of supraglottic carcinomas caudally into the glottic and subglottic regions is to be expected in 25%-30% of cases. Also, the argument that the lymph from the paraglottic space drains off in a cranial direction (PRESSMAN et al 1960) does not exclude extension of a supraglottic tumour in a caudal direction. If the special arrangement of the lymph vessels on the posterior wall of the larynx is disregarded, it is hardly conceivable that the slow lymph drainage could offer any real resistance to continual tumour growth. Tumour growth ensues by pushing forward, by expansion and partly by active locomotion of tumour cells and infiltration. A lymph current is therefore forced to come to rest or even to reverse, if, for example, the tumour has reached the lateral wall of the ventricle; such reverse has been shown experimentally by WELSH et al (1961).

5.1.3 Glottic and Subglottic Carcinomas

As already mentioned, most endolaryngeal carcinomas arise in the area of the vocal cords. The extension of these tumours predominantly takes place in two planes namely horizontal and vertical; the former corresponds to the initial spread of glottic carcinomas at an early stage, while the latter prevails during the later course. Nevertheless, unfavourable location can lead to clinical problems even at an early stage. This is the case in carcinomas of the anterior commissure, the vocal cord and the posterior wall in the region of the vocal process of the larynx. This entire area comprises into the glottic region according to the definition of the UICC (1978). Owing to the lack of lymph vessels in the region of the vocal cord, lymphatic spread of carcinomas is possible only in later stages. Also, it is favourable that early signs and symptoms such as hoarseness cause the sufferers to seek medical care much sooner than those affected by lesions of other laryngeal regions. Among 503 patients suffering from glottic carcinomas treated at the Frankfurt University ENT Clinic between 1966 and 1982, 32 had a carcinoma in situ, 247 a T1 and 134 a T2 carcinoma. When such a carcinoma reaches the neighbouring regions, however, the prognosis becomes as poor as that of supraglottic and subglottic carcinomas. In these later stages the tumour, depending on site of origin or extension, may proceed either into only one region or into several neighbouring regions.

In advanced vocal cord carcinomas, the **anterior commissure** is the most frequently affected area (in ca. 70% of cases; OLOFSSON and VAN NOSTRAND 1973, MEYER-BREITING 1981a), of the four problem

Fig. 5.11a-f. Advanced supraglottic cancer of lateral and laterodorsal origin. **a** In the region of its origin, this tumour shows papillary exophytic growth; in the depth, however, it reveals its true character with a surprising paraglottic extension. The paraglottic space, in its subglottic part, is nearly completely infiltrated. Coronal section, HE. **b, c** Horizontal sections of a supraglottic tumour. The tumour has involved a great part of the supraglottic portion of the paraglottic space on the right side. It is infiltrating the ventricular fold **(x)** and growing via the paraglottic space in the caudal direction. **d** Small peripheral infiltration of the lower paraglottic space near the thyroid cartilage on the right side. This tumour originates from the lateral supraglottic part of the paraglottic space. **e** Lateral supraglottic carcinoma tending to grow into the piriform sinus. Horizontal section. **f** Supraglottic carcinomas of the posterior wall are very rare. This example is destroying the interarytenoid muscles and reaching into the hypopharyngeal submucosa. *T*, thyroid cartilage; *C*, cricoid cartilage; *E*, epiglottic cartilage; *PASP*, paraglottic space. Horizontal section, HE

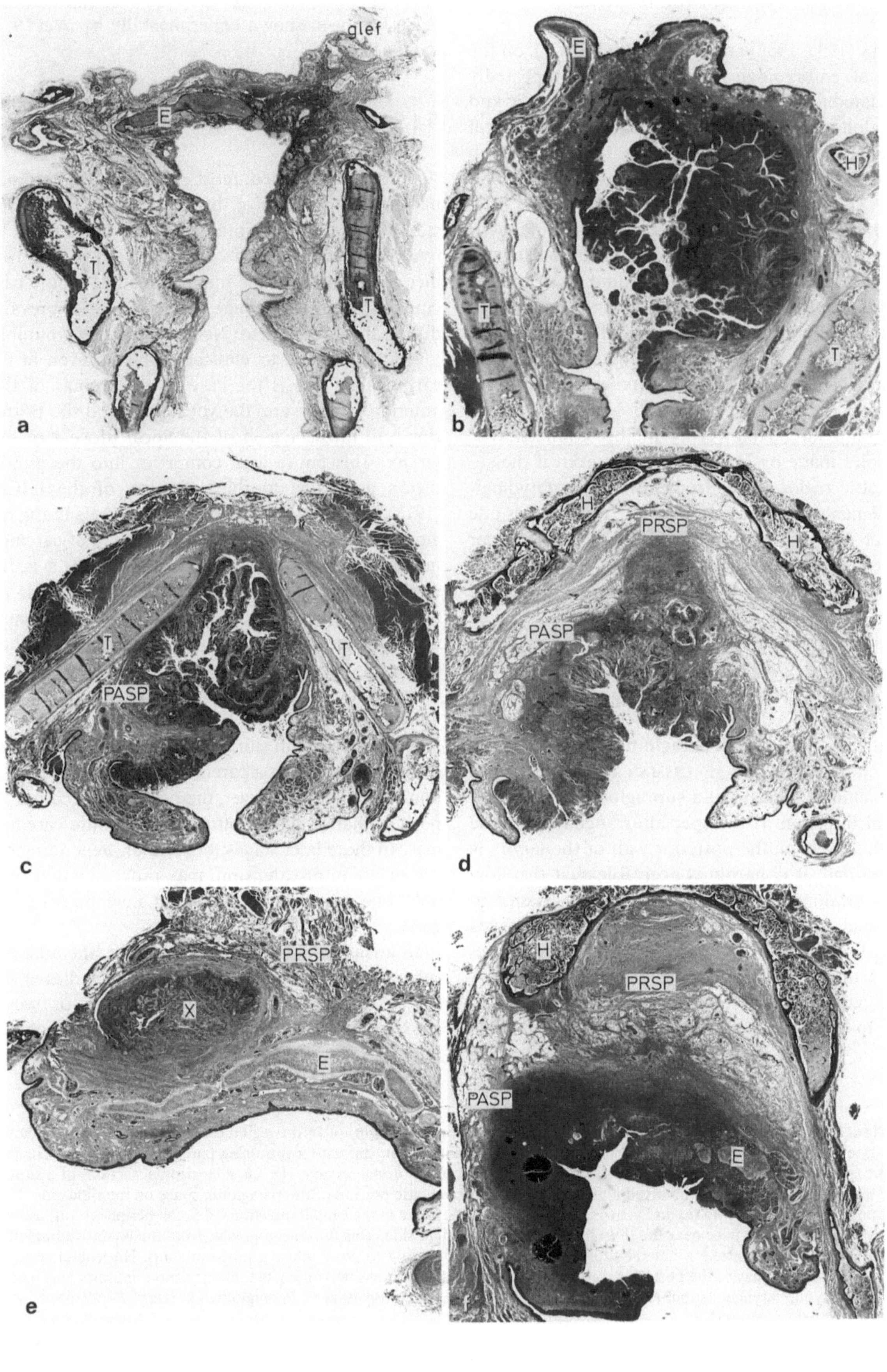
glef
E
T
T
a
E
H
T
T
b
T
T
PASP
c
H
PRSP
H
PASP
d
PRSP
X
E
e
H
PRSP
PASP
E

areas (anterior commissure, posterior wall, ventricle, subglottis). These carcinomas in general adopt a markedly unfavourable course. This is primarily explained by the high penetration rate of such tumours in a prelaryngeal direction (BROYLES 1943, KIRCHNER 1970, OLOFSSON et al 1972, TUCKER 1973, BRIDGER 1974). In our opinion, further dissemination is promoted by a special "distributive" function of the anterior commissure. The particular anatomical structure in this area, i.e. a dense fibrous barrier between the epithelial layer and the thyroid cartilage, hinders tumour invasion into depth (KIRCHNER and FISCHER 1975), as does the radiation of fibres of the so-called "anterior commissure tendon" (so termed by BROYLES 1943) into the thyroid cartilage. As mentioned above, Reinke's space and the vocal ligament narrow in the region of the anterior commissure and end here. Thus the supraglottic and the subglottic space, neither of which possesses a midline separation of its lymphatic system, come as close as 2 mm to one another in this area (Fig. 1.10). This may explain why, just here, the glottic carcinoma can easily gain access to the two neighbouring spaces mentioned and tend to spread multilaterally. As stressed by KIRCHNER and FISCHER (1975) and confirmed by our own investigations (MEYER-BREITING 1981a), invasion and destruction of the thyroid cartilage ensues only after expansion in a subglottic direction. The fact that this happens relatively early, is explained by BRIDGER and NASSAR (1972) in terms of the prevalent tendency of squamous cell carcinoma to infiltrate mucous glands and use them as "guide rails". Mucous glands are found in profusion below and above the anterior commissure, where they branch out below the mucosa, particularly in the subglottic space, which extends to the cricothyroid ligament and the lower third of the thyroid cartilage. The comparison of the glands with guide rails in the spread of squamous cell carcinomas necessitates some considerations. The glands lie, just as in the epiglottic region, in loose fibrous tissue layers which permit the gland to develop here and equally allow the tumour to spread. Such a path is favoured particularly by carcinomas with a more forward-pushing and less infiltrative growth pattern (MEYER-BREITING and SCHNEIDER 1981). Sometimes carcinoma in situ of the surface mucosa can extend far down into the excretory glandular ducts; however, we were not able to observe the development of an invasive carcinoma into depth via the dependent glandular ducts.

Most authors assume that the particularly permeable cricothyroid membrane facilitates penetration in a prelaryngeal direction below the anterior commissure (BROYLES 1943, TUCKER 1971, OLOFSSON and VAN NOSTRAND 1973, TUCKER 1973). Unless squamous cell carcinomas with lymphatic spread are involved, according to our observations the cricothyroid membrane represents, even in the region of the cricothyroid ligament, a solid barrier. Only the preformed openings for the passage of different nerves and vessels through the membrane offer the possibility of penetration. True invasion as a rule takes place at the transition of the lower edge of the thyroid cartilage to the cricothyroid membrane (Table 5.3). In agreement with our observations, OLOFSSON and VAN NOSTRAND (1973) discovered that in most cases penetration through the cricothyroid membrane was associated with a breach at the lower edge of the thyroid cartilage. The locus minoris resistentiae is offered by the ossified lower edge of the thyroid cartilage (Figs. 5.13, 5.14). It is only a short distance from the site of insertion of the cricothyroid ligament to the subglottic mucosal surface. No connective tissue space in which a tumour could expand freely, as in the lateral laryngeal region between the elastic cone and thyroid cartilage, is present. The connective tissue spaces of the subglottic space on the posterior laryngeal wall permit the rapid spread of carcinoma extensions directly onto the thyroid cartilage. The impression that

Fig. 5.12a–f. So-called Winkel carcinoma. Most supraglottic carcinomas originate in the area between the ventricular and the aryepiglottic fold on the one side and the epiglottis on the other side. **a** Here, a small but infiltrating carcinoma spreads into the lateral glossoepiglottic fold *(glef)*. The right margin of the epiglottic cartilage is destroyed. Coronal section. **b** This large Winkel carcinoma is less infiltrative and destructive. Coronal section, **c–e** Horizontal sections of a carcinoma which has its greatest extent in a plane through the thyrohyoid membrane. It originates from the angle between the pars fixa of the epiglottis and the lateral supraglottic wall and infiltrates the preepiglottic and the paraglottic space. Without clinically apparent signs, the tumour extends in the preepiglottic space over the plane of the hyoid bone (x). **f** Winkel carcinoma of the upper supraglottic part of the paraglottic space as seen on horizontal section. The left part of the epiglottic cartilage is destroyed. The tumour reaches both the preepiglottic and the paraglottic space. *T*, thyroid cartilage; *E*, epiglottic cartilage; *H*, hyoid bone; *PASP*, paraglottic space; *PRSP*, preepiglottic space

Table 5.3. Main sites of origin of glottic-subglottic squamous cell carcinomas and their tendency to involve or penetrate the laryngeal framework

	Glottic-subglottic sites of origin				
	Ventral n = 3	Ventrolateral n = 26	Lateral n = 29	Dorsal n = 4	Total n = 62
Laryngeal framework					
Thyrohyoid membrane	–	–	–	–	–
	–	–	2/0	–	2/0
Thyroid cartilage					
Upper rim	–	–	–	–	–
Centre	–	–	–	–	–
Lower rim	2/1	5/3	4/3	–	11/7
	–	6/6	5/5	–	11/11
Cricothyroid membrane	–	1/1	2/2	–	3/3
	–	–	–	–	–
Cricoid cartilage					
Ring	–	1/0	–	2/0	3/0
Lamina	–	1/1	3/3	2/2	6/6
Total	2/1	14/11	16/13	4/2	36/27
Involvement	2/3	54%	55%	4/4	58%
Penetration	1/3	42%	45%	2/4	48%

The numbers before the slash indicate the frequency of involvement, the numbers after it the frequency of penetration

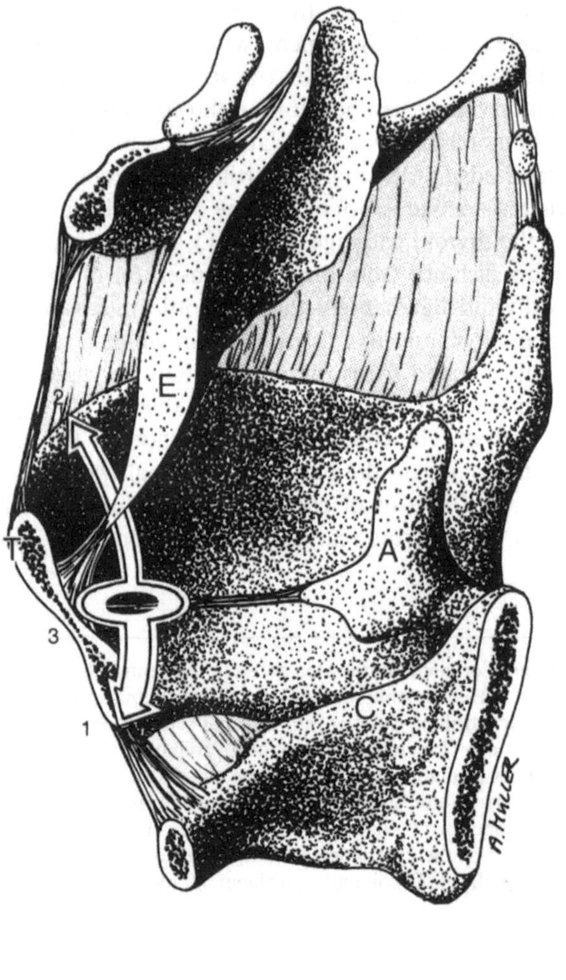

Fig. 5.13. Carcinomas sited near the anterior commissure most frequently spread to the anterior subglottic wall. Hence, the tumour tends to penetrate the lower edge of the thyroid and occasionally the cricothyroid membrane *(1)*. Less frequently, it moves into the supraglottic direction. Growing around the thyroepiglottic ligament, it involves the preepiglottic space *(2)*. Seldom does a carcinoma break directly from the anterior commissure through the thyroid cartilage *(3)*. *T*, thyroid cartilage; *C*, cricoid cartilage; *E*, epiglottic cartilage.

penetration of the cricothyroid membrane is involved is as a rule gained from this secondary involvement.

For this reason, it is really not the infiltration of the anterior commissure but rather that of the anterior subglottic wall which represents the decisive criterion for the tendency of a subglottic or glottic tumour to penetrate in a prelaryngeal direction. More than half of all advanced glottic carcinomas show a tendency to invade or penetrate the laryngeal framework, mostly without clinical evidence (Table 5.3). Tumours which display a primarily vertical subglottic or paraglottic spread (Fig. 5.17) and extend onto the subglottic anterior wall penetrate this region just as often in a prelaryngeal direction as do carcinomas which originated primarily on the anterior commissure, namely in more than one third of cases (Table 5.4). The lateral processes of tumours with predominantly vertical expansion af-

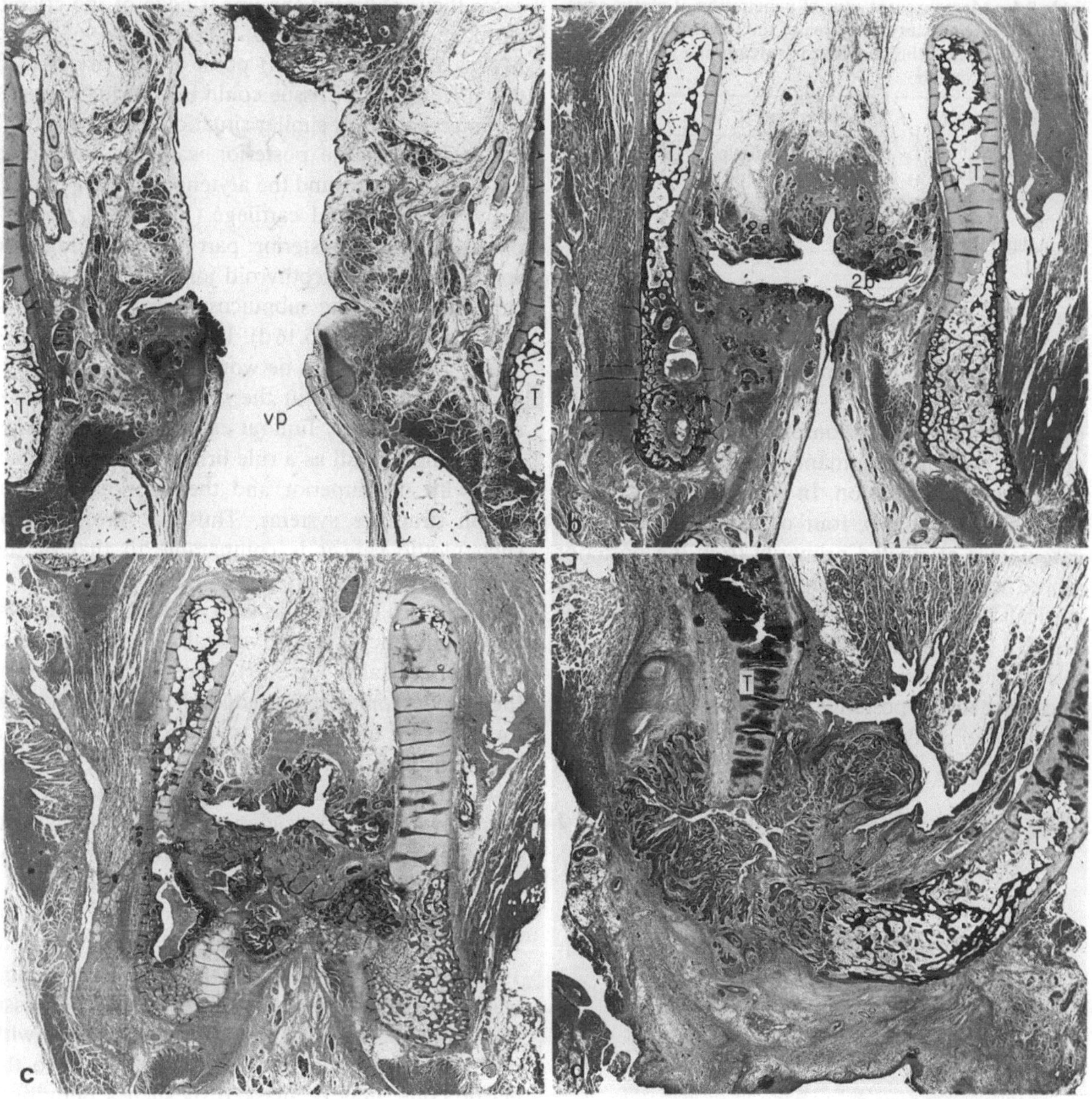

Fig. 5.14a–d. Glottic carcinomas near the anterior commissure. **a–c** Three coronal sections of a larynx with a glottic carcinoma extension from the vocal process **(a)** to the anterior wall **(c)**. Near the anterior commissure **(b)** carcinoma spreads not only in the subglottic direction laterally of the elastic cone *(1)* but also circularly to the supraglottis *(2a)* and to the contralateral parts of the glottic and supraglottic region *(2b)*. Carcinoma involves the lower part of the thyroid cartilage *(arrows)*. **d** Another glottic carcinoma which extends into the subglottic anterior wall, penetrates the lower anterior part of the thyroid cartilage and involves the prelaryngeal structures. *T*, thyroid cartilage; *C*, cricoid cartilage; *PRSP* preepiglottic space

ter infiltration of the paraglottic space preferably grow laterally in a prelaryngeal direction on the lower edge of the thyroid cartilage; but growth in this direction is seen much more often after infiltration of the anterior subglottic wall.

The **posterior wall** of the larynx with the medial surface of the arytenoid cartilage (Fig. 5.15, 5.16), often termed "posterior commissure", is considered a rare primary location of tumours. The region behind Morgagni's ventricle, however, has a tendency to develop dysplasia and subsequent carcinoma (Fig. 5.16a). TUCKER (1963), KIRCHNER (1969), BRIDGER and NASSAR (1972) and OLOFSSON and VAN NOSTRAND (1973) do not describe any carcino-

Table 5.4. Most frequent sites of penetration of glottic squamous cell carcinomas in the area of the lower rim of the thyroid cartilage and the cricothyroid membrane in relation to location and spread

Site of penetration	Type of spread		
	Subglottic anterior	Subglottic lateral	Paraglottic
Frontal	10	4	1
Frontolateral	3	2	2
Lateral	1	-	2

ma with primary origin in the region of the posterior glottic wall. The last-named authors observed only secondary infiltration of this zone in four carcinomas with predominantly vertical supraglottic and subglottic extension. In our study of advanced laryngeal carcinomas, four of 62 subglottic-glottic carcinomas originated primarily from the posterior glottic wall and a further 23 with predominantly vertical expansion had secondarily invaded this area. In 25% of these cases, tumour extensions between and under the interarytenoid musculature had reached the posterior wall of the larynx at the upper edge of the cricoid lamina, and in 22% of

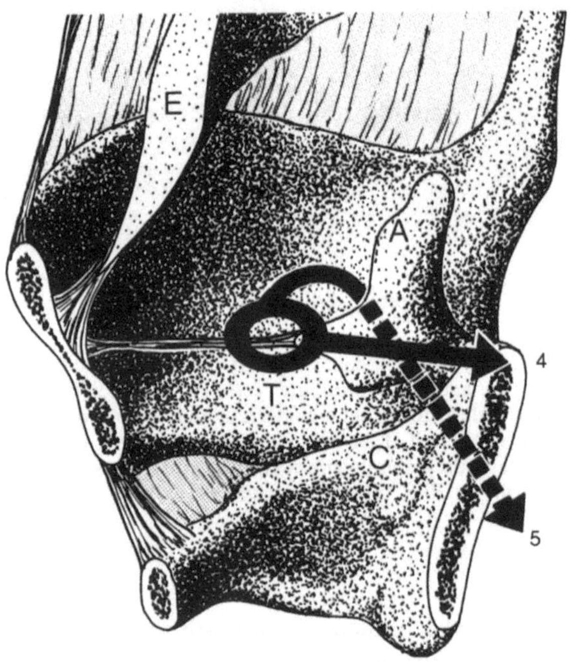

Fig. 5.15. Carcinoma originating in the vocal process area may spread medially into the posterior wall *(4)*, or in the laterodorsal direction, by growing around and/or destroying the arytenoid cartilage *(5)*. *T*, thyroid cartilage; *C*, cricoid cartilage; *E*, epiglottic cartilage; *H*, hyoid bone; *A*, arytenoid cartilage

cases they infiltrated the upper edge of the cricoid cartilage plate (Fig. 5.16). TUCKER (1963) and MEYER-BREITING (1981a) point to the risk that in this region tumour tissue could be left during surgical intervention. A similar situation may arise if, after invasion of the posterior wall, the carcinoma grows laterally around the arytenoid cartilage or destroys the arytenoid cartilage (Fig. 5.16b) and expands into the posterior part of the paraglottic space up to the cricothyroid joint. By this route it can extend into the submucosal parts of the lower piriform sinus (Fig. 5.16d). In contrast to Reinke's space, the lymphatic networks of the supraglottis and subglottis meet in the posterior wall with no anatomical barrier. Tumour extension on the posterior laryngeal wall as a rule brings about a connection with the superior and the inferior laryngeal lymph drainage systems. Thus the prognosis of such glottic cancer is comparable to that of the neighbouring regions.

Vocal cord carcinomas with a lateral location display a tendency towards vertical spread, either cranially or caudally (Fig. 5.17). Depending on whether they grow from the free edge of the vocal cord in the direction of Morgagni's ventricle or rather in a subglottic direction via the lower border of Reinke's space, they extend according to the surface picture, more towards the supraglottis or the subglottis. Lateral expansion along the floor of the ventricle takes place only partly by "transglottic growth" (MCGAVRAN et al 1961, KIRCHNER 1969, MENDONCA and BRYCE 1973, KIRCHNER et al 1974, MITTAL et al 1984) defined as spread on the lateral ventricular wall in a cranial direction (Fig. 5.18a-f). The possibility that such growth can also be associated with infiltration in a subglottic direction, lateral to the elastic cone, may be masked by such a definition. TUCKER (1974) and MEYER-BREITING (1981a) consider it more advisable to speak in these cases of "paraglottic spreading" in order not to implay a particular direction of growth. According to MEYER-BREITING (1981a), a third of all pT3 and pT4 glottic carcinomas (see Sect. 5.3.2) show paraglottic spreading, which in half the cases is associated with caudal infiltration lateral to the elastic cone into the subglottic region. Thus, in half of all cases with the surface picture of transglottic spread, simultaneous infiltration of the tumour in the direction of the lower edge of the thyroid cartilage and the cricothyroid membrane can be expected (Fig. 5.20). From this point of view, the recommendation to term carcinomas which grow laterally

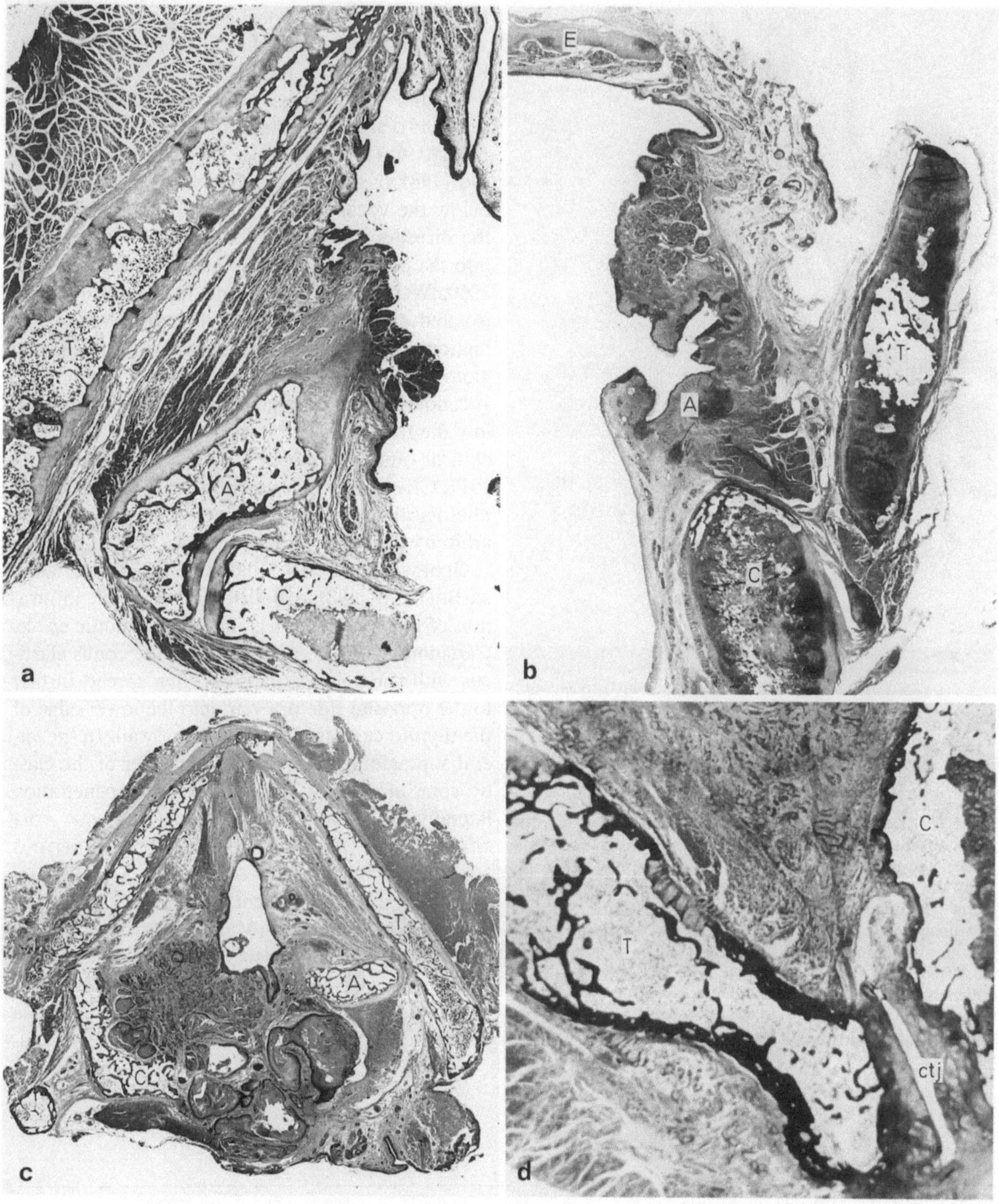

Fig. 5.16a–d. Glottic cancer in the posterior wall. **a** Superficial carcinoma on the vocal process. Horizontal section. HE, × 20. **b** Destruction of the arytenoid cartilage by squamous cell carcinoma. **c** Infiltration of the posterior laryngeal wall with complete destruction of the left arytenoid cartilage and involvement of the cricoid lamina. Tumour reaches the postcricoidal mucosa. **d** Multiple small cell clusters of a moderately differentiated squamous cell carcinoma beneath the cricothyroid joint *(ctj)*. The tumour originates from the glottis and completely infiltrates the paraglottic space in this plane. *T*, thyroid cartilage; *C*, cricoid cartilage; *E*, epiglottic cartilage; *A*, arytenoid cartilage; *MV*, Morgagni's ventricle

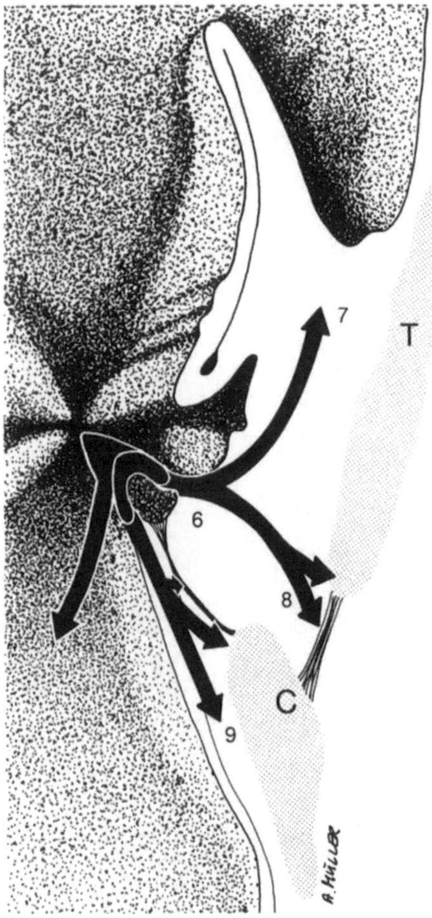

Fig. 5.17. Laterally sited glottic carcinomas spread in two main directions. One route is via the ventricular floor (6). Hence, the tumor may extend to (or, commonly, originate from) the ventricle *(7)*. This type is called "transglottic carcinoma". Its origin should be defined as supraglottic. An undervalued type of spread reaches from the ventricular floor into the lower part of the paraglottic space *(8)*. However, most frequently glottic carcinomas extended in a subglottic direction *(9)*, particularly to the subglottic anterior wall. Frontally sectioned hemilarynx with frontal mucosal relief. *T*, thyroid cartilage; *C*, cricoid cartilage

from the edge of the vocal cord "glottic carcinomas with supraglottic spreading" (Norris et al 1970, Kirchner 1975b) is misleading.

Glottic carcinomas with **subglottic spread** (Fig. 5.19) are, according to Olofsson and van Nostrand (1973), Lund (1974) and Meyer-Breiting (1981a), glottic carcinomas which have spread below the vocal ligament. Here lymph drainage in the direction of the inferior lymphatic vessels and into the paratracheal region begins (Pressman et al 1960, Welsh 1964, Beck and Mann 1980). If an isolated extension into the subglottis leads to formation of a larger tumour mass here than in the glottis, the carcinoma has to be called "subglottic". A caudal boundary of glottic tumours at 15 mm below the free edge of the vocal cord may well be of clinical and prognostic significance (Fleischer 1977, Glanz 1984), but seen in the light of the morphological structure of the larynx, it appears to be arbitrary (see Sect. 1.4.1 and 5.3.2).

Olofsson and van Nostrand (1973) and Meyer-Breiting (1981a) both found frequent infiltration of glottic carcinomas into the subglottic space. Carcinomas which grow medial to the conus elasticus with subglottic expansion often spread further to the opposite side or even onto the lower edge of the thyroid cartilage on the anterior wall. In the lateral supraglottic area, the stable barrier of the elastic cone hinders or retards such early penetration laterally (Tucker 1963, Olofsson and van Nostrand 1973, Fleischer 1977, Meyer-Breiting 1981a). Within the elastic cone, the area immediately below the vocal ligament appears to offer a locus minoris resistentiae (Meyer-Breiting 1981a, Glanz 1984). Metastasis into the paratracheal lymph nodes ensues either via the inferior laryngeal lymphatic vessels or, considerably less often, via a prelaryngeal path.

Fig. 5.18 a–f. Laterally sited glottic carcinomas. **a, b** So-called transglottic carcinomas which cross Morgagni's ventricle. The left tumour shows a pushing growth, whereas the right infiltrates the paraglottic space and its adjacent structures with an irregular tumour-host boundary. In both cases, the ratio of involvement of the glottic and of the supraglottic region leads us to define this type of tumour as supraglottic carcinoma. Coronal sections, HE, × 1.5 **c, d** Glottic carcinoma which originates from the free edge of the vocal cord and the ventricular floor **c.** The tumour infiltrates the lower part of the paraglottic space. Horizontal sections through the ventricular floor and 4 mm below. **e** More advanced glottic carcinoma with the same extension. Note the clear separation of the subglottic and the paraglottic space. Horizontal section 5 mm below the free edge of the right vocal cord. **f** Involvement of the subglottic anterior wall. Carcinoma infiltrates this area without any evident median separation and penetrates the cricothyroid membrane *(ctm)* through a preformed perforation for vessels and nerves *(arrow)*. Horizontal section. HE, ×20 *T*, thyroid cartilage; *C*, cricoid cartilage; *E*, epiglottic cartilage; *A*, arytenoid cartilage; *MV*, Morgagni's ventricle

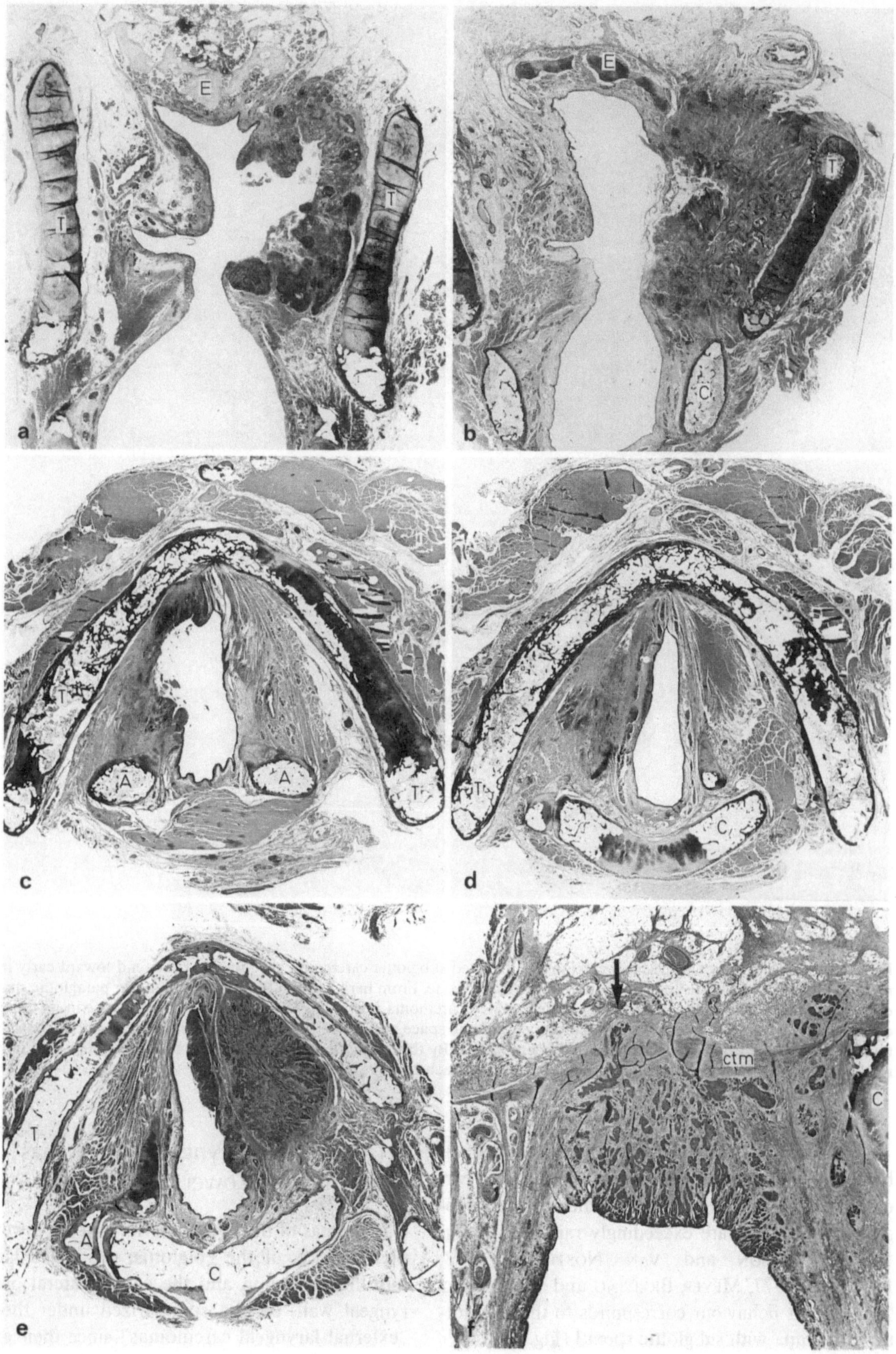
E
T
T
a
E
T
C
b
T
A
A
T
c
T
C
d
T
A
C
e
ctm
C
f

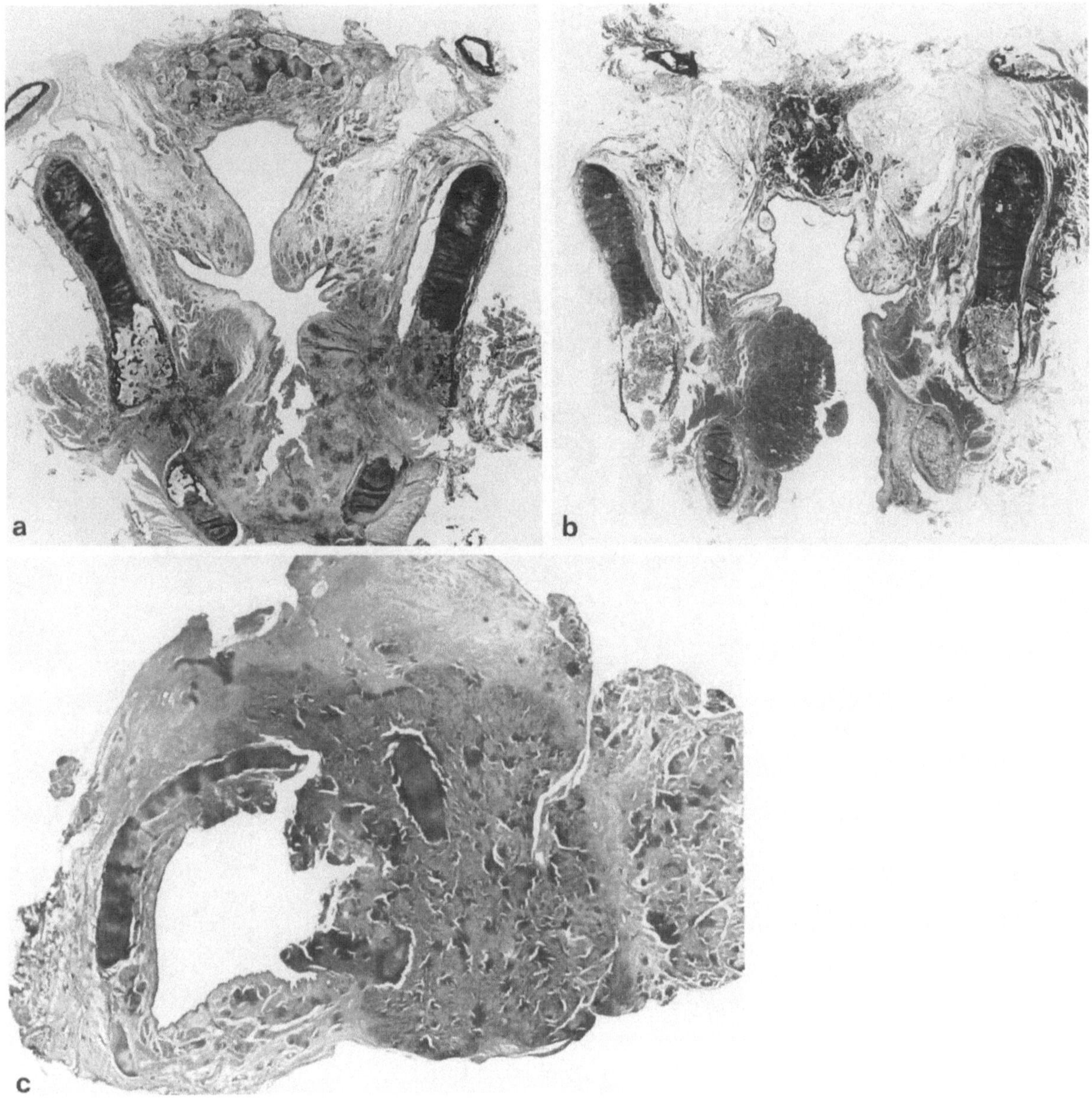

Fig. 5.19a–c. Subglottic and tracheal carcinomas. Isolated subglottic carcinoma are rare. **a** They tend toward early involvement of the cricoid cartilage and penetration of the elastic cone. From here, rapid infiltration of the lower paraglottic space and of the thyroid cartilage follows. **b** Poorly differentiated carcinoma beginning to penetrate the elastic cone in its upper part. **c** Carcinomas of the lower subglottic part of the paraglottic space and of the trachea remain clinically undetectable for a long time. They become evident by dyspnoea and haemoptysis. By this stage, tumour has as a rule broken through and infiltrated the thyroid gland. Horizontal section through the second tracheal ring. HE, ×2

If all laryngeal carcinomas with involvement of both the glottis and subglottis are called glottic carcinoma with subglottic extension, then primary **subglottic carcinomas** are exceedingly rare (KIRCHNER 1969, OLOFSSON and VAN NOSTRAND 1973, FLEISCHER 1977, MEYER-BREITING and VON ILBERG 1979). Their behaviour corresponds to that of glottic carcinoma with subglottic spread (Fig. 5.19).

5.1.4 "External Laryngeal Carcinomas" (Hypopharynx, Lower Oropharynx)

Carcinomas of the hypopharynx and the lower oropharynx, i.e. of the epiglottis, the valleculae, the retrolingual region and the caudal lateral oropharyngeal wall, can be summarized under the term "external laryngeal carcinomas" since their expansion is critically influenced by the morphology of the larynx and its surroundings, and surgery of these carcinomas must take this relationship into consideration. For these reason this group of tumours is included in this treatise.

Squamous cell carcinomas of the valleculae and base of the tongue are easily misinterpretated as supraglottic tumours which have secondarily penetrated the base of the tongue via the preepiglottic space and the valleculae. As a rule such tumours form extensive ulcers at the transition of the base of the tongue to the valleculae. At the base of the tongue invasion of the tumour lateral to the body of the tongue proper, in continuation of the pharyngoepiglottic fold, can reach considerably more deeply than in the tongue musculature itself. Especially with regard to the often conservative method of resection, and owing to the hypoglossal nerves and lingual arteries which course through this section, one must reckon with tumour tissue being left following such surgical resection. Lymphatic metastasis usually takes place via the upper lateral laryngeal wall and the floor of the mouth.

Carcinomas of the piriform sinus predominate among the hypopharyngeal carcinomas (Fig. 5.20) (HARRISON 1972, OLOFSSON and VAN NOSTRAND 1973, KIRCHNER 1975a). True postcricoid carcinomas and carcinomas of the posterior wall of the hypopharynx play, in comparison, only a minor role. Carcinomas of the piriform sinus (Fig. 5.21) have a particularly close relationship to the larynx, evident from the early invasion of endolaryngeal structures. Three major directions of spread seem to be of importance:

1. Penetration medially into the supraglottic lateral and posterior wall
2. Infiltration paraglottically in a ventral direction far into the preepiglottic space (Fig. 5.21b)
3. Submucous growth in a dorsocaudal direction to the cricothyroid joint, the posterior wall of the larynx and from there to the oesophageal inlet (Fig. 5.22a-c).

Penetration of hypopharyngeal carcinomas into the laryngeal framework is more variable than in endolaryngeal carcinomas. Perforations can be observed most frequently at the horns of the thyroid cartilage, less often at the arytenoid cartilages and the cricoid lamina (KIRCHNER 1975a, MEYER-BREITING 1981a). Vocal cord fixation by carcinomas of the piriform sinus is also commonly reported (OGURA

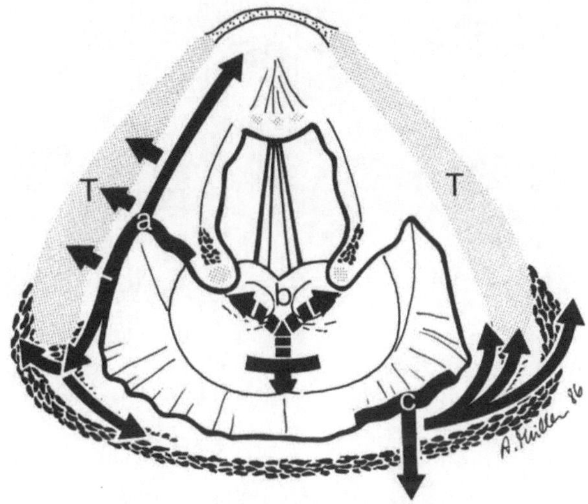

Fig. 5.20. Carcinoma can spread from the piriform sinus *(a)* in three directions: anteriorly, into the paraglottic space; posteriorly, to the posterior edge of the thyroid cartilage and to the posterior hypopharyngeal wall; and distally, to the postcricoid region and the oesophagus. Postcricoid carcinoma *(b)* spreads to both piriform sinuses and distally to the oesophagus. The posterior wall of the larynx is often involved. Carcinomas of the posterior hypopharyngeal wall *(c)* spread to the piriform sinuses, and in a proximal or distal direction. The vertebral column is occasionally involved. Horizontal section with caudal mucosal relief. *T*, thyroid cartilage

1955, OLOFSSON and VAN NOSTRAND 1973, KIRCHNER 1975a). KIRCHNER (1975a) considered the cause of vocal cord fixation to be tumour invasion in the area of the arytenoid cartilage as well as in the cricoarytenoid and interarytenoid musculature. A further cause has been suggested to be infiltration and paresis of the recurrent nerve (OLOFSSON and VAN NOSTRAND 1973, KIRCHNER and OWEN 1977). The thyroid gland can be affected by hypopharyngeal carcinomas, as has often been reported in the literature (OGURA 1955, HARRISON 1972, OLOFSSON and VAN NOSTRAND 1973).

Carcinomas of the postcricoid region gain access relatively quickly to the paraglottic spaces of both sides and expand at the same time caudally in the direction of the oesophageal inlet. Carcinomas of the posterior wall of the hypopharynx tend to spread horizontally to the lateral wall of the piriform sinus, grow round the posterior margin of the thyroid cartilage and penetrate early into the prelaryngeal region. Tumours with a predominantly caudal spread usually grow circularly around the oesophageal inlet. The local and regional extension of carcinomas of the posterior wall of the hypopharynx is highly difficult to assess; these tumours have an exceedingly poor prognosis (MEYER-BREITING

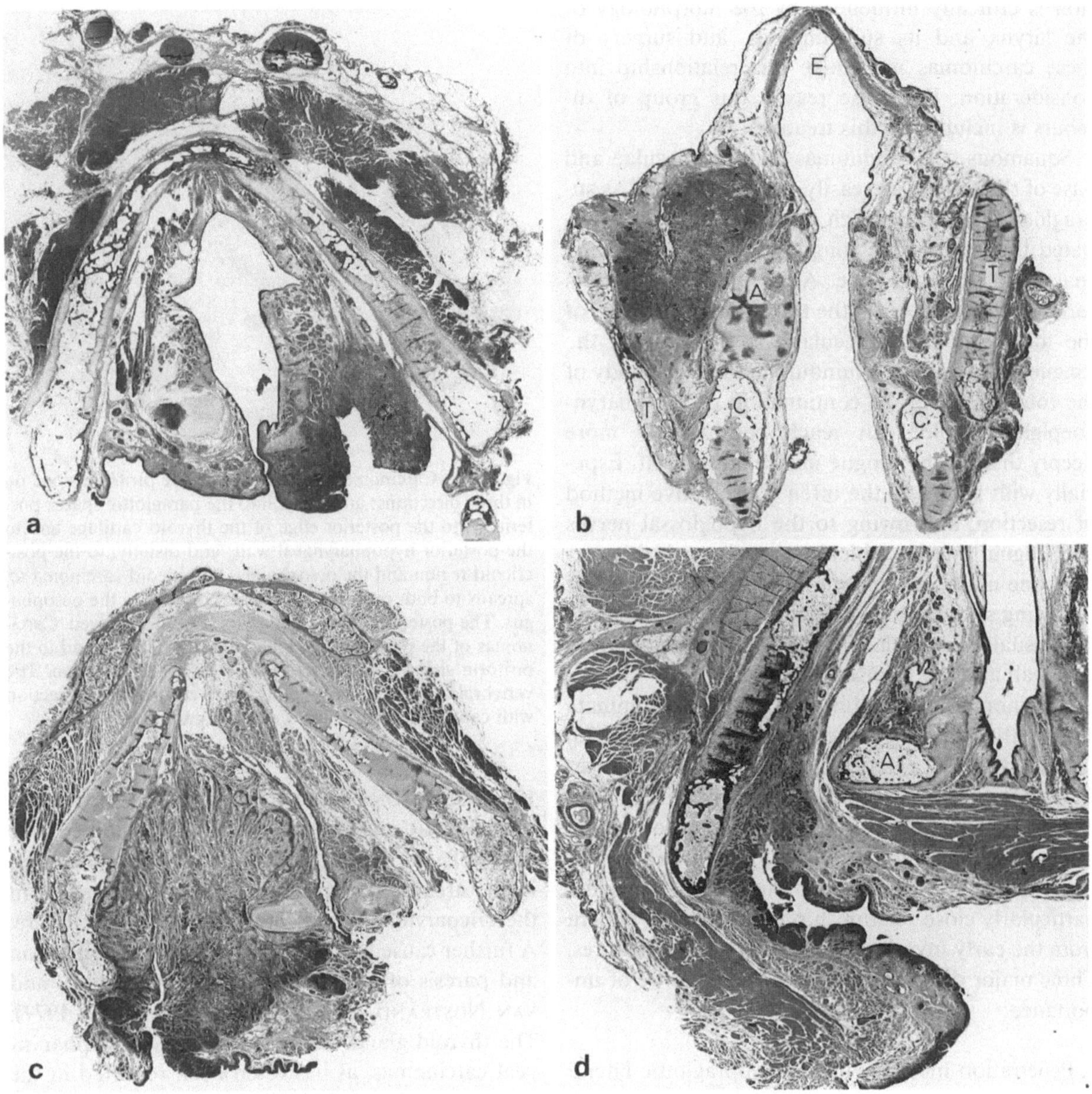

Fig. 5.21 a–d. The piriform sinus is the most frequent location of hypopharyngeal carcinomas. **a** In most cases both parts, lateral and medial, are carcinomatously changed. Horizontal section. HE, ×2. **b** From here, numerous carcinomas infiltrate the paraglottic space and reach just into the preepiglottic space. Coronal section through the vocal processes. HE, ×1.5. **c** Another piriform sinus carcinoma filling the ipsilateral paraglottic space. Endolaryngeal soft tissue is pushed medially. The lumen is nearly obturated. Horizontal section through the thyroid notch and the upper half of the arytenoid cartilages. **d** Some hypopharyngeal carcinomas arise together from the piriform sinus and the posterior pharyngeal wall. This early cancer clearly shows the usual spread of this type: anteriorly and to the posterior edge of the thyroid cartilage

1981 a, Ganzer and Meyer-Breiting 1982). More than 80% of the victims suffer local recurrence, affection of the lymph nodes and/or formation of distant metastasis within 1 year after treatment. Survival of 3 years is extremely rare. Noticeable is the frequency with which second carcinomas are observed in association with squamous cell carcinomas of the hypopharynx. These are found either in the contralateral piriform sinus, in the supraglottic region or in the oesophageal section. Usually they are early invasive carcinomas or carcinomata in situ. In addition, dysplasia of varying grades of severity in all parts of the upper digestive tract is seen in most patients (see Sect. 4.5).

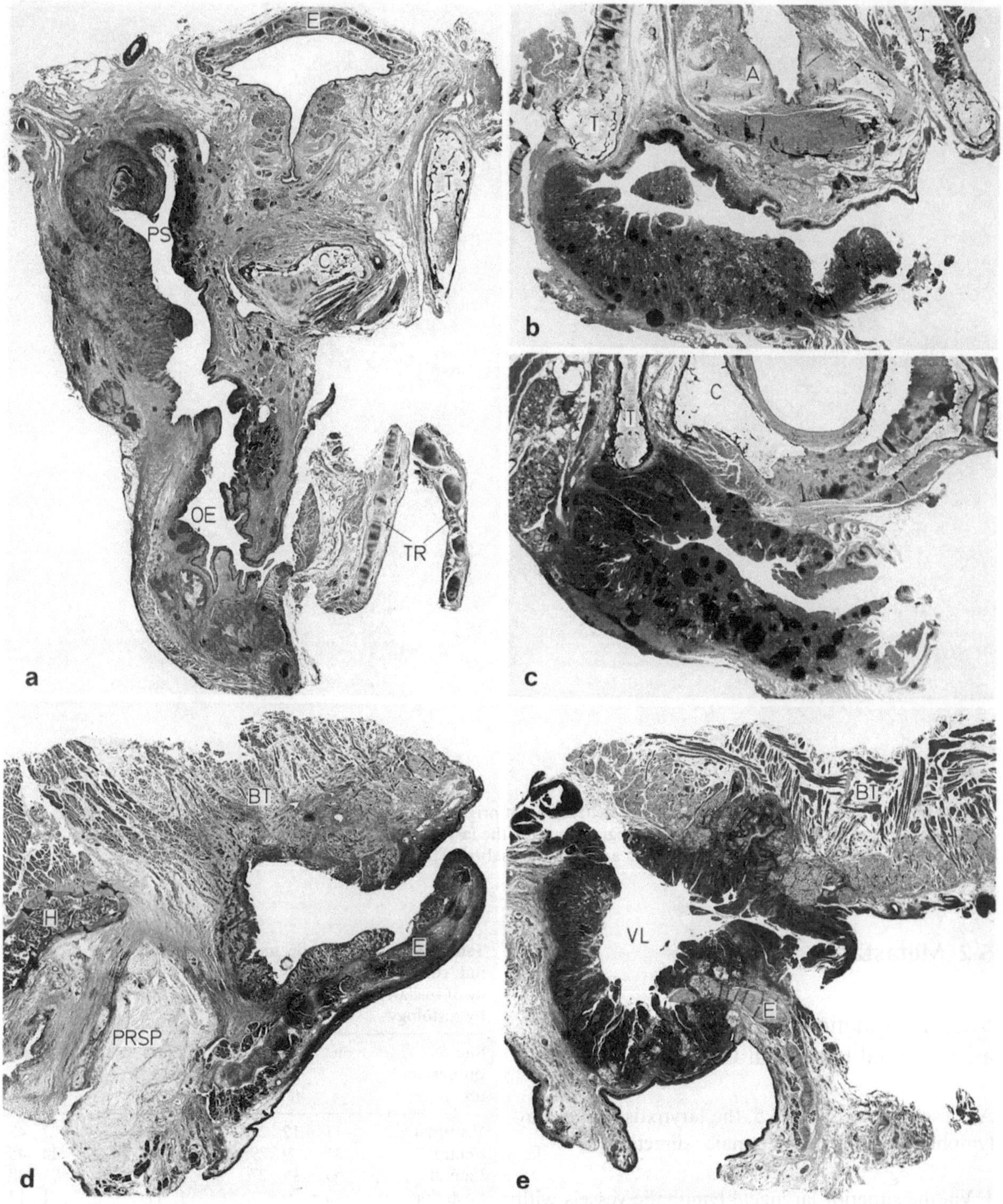

Fig. 5.22 a. Extreme extension of a hypopharyngeal carcinoma which reaches from the left piriform sinus (lateral pharyngo-epiglottic fold) 4–5 cm into the oesophagus. The tumour has involved the thyroid and cricoid cartilages and the thyroid gland (not seen in this section). Coronal section through the posterior laryngeal wall (postcricoidal). *Tr*, trachea. HE, ×1.5. **b, c** Carcinoma of the posterior hypopharyngeal wall. Horizontal sections through the interarytenoid muscles and the centre of the cricoid lamina *(c)*. HE, ×2. **d, e** Larynx-adjacent oropharyngeal carcinomas. Involvement of the base of the tongue *(BT)*, the vallecula and the lingual surface of the epiglottis *(E)*. The tumour has not involved the preepiglottic space *(PRSP)*. **d** Mediosagittal section; **e** horizontal section through the valleculas. HE, ×1.5

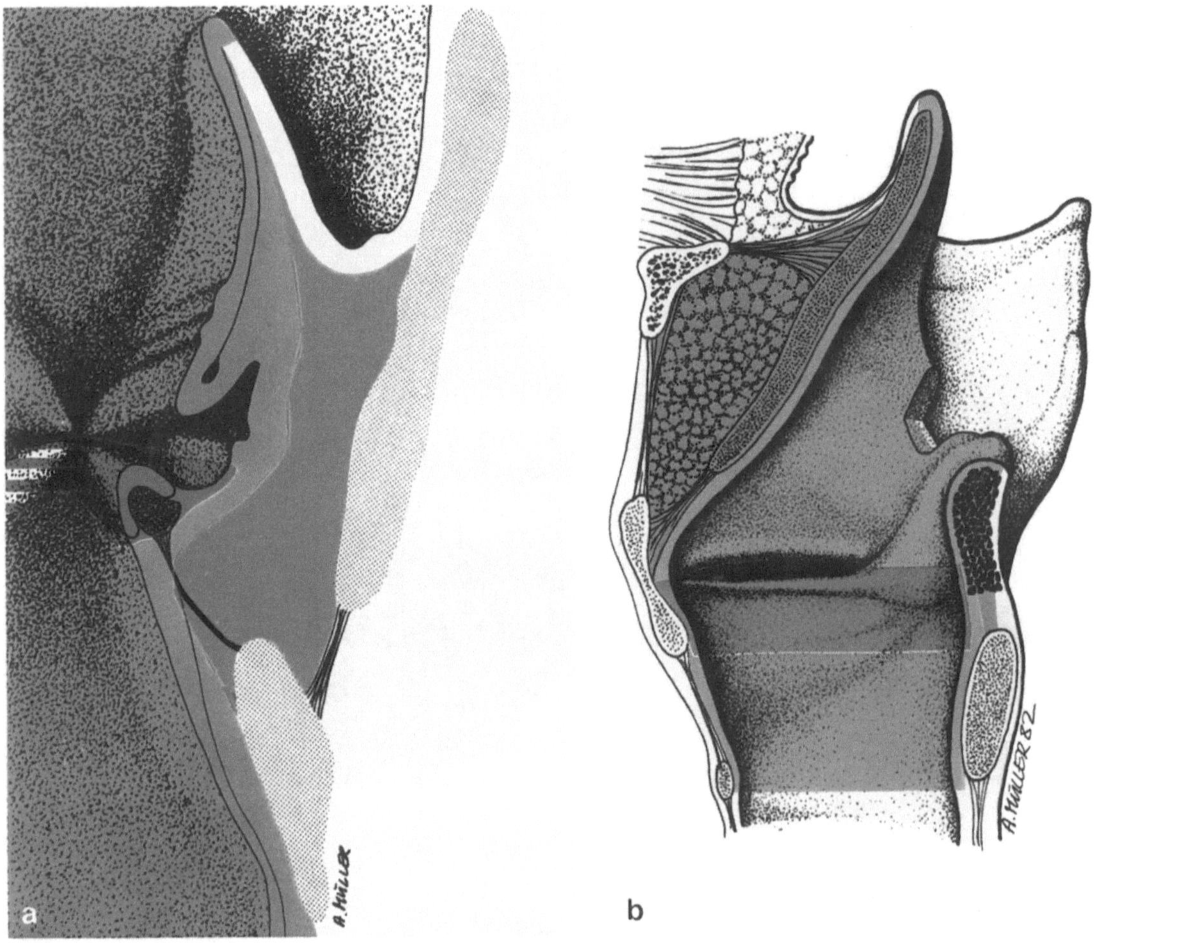

Fig. 5.23 a, b. T classification of glottic cancer. *Red:* region of origin = T_1; *green:* adjacent region = T_2; *blue:* infiltration of the paraglottic or preepiglottic space = T_3; *yellow:* regions outside the larynx = T_4. The *hatched area* displays the extension of a T_{1b} tumour. **a** frontally sectioned hemilarynx with anterior mucosal relief; **b** midsagittal section

5.2 Metastasis

5.2.1 Lymphatic Metastasis of Internal and External Laryngeal Carcinomas

As described in Sect. 1.3.5, the larynx is drained by lymphatic vessels in three major directions:

1. Via the superior laryngeal lymphatic vessels with the drainage areas of the supraglottic, paraglottic and preepiglottic spaces
2. Via the anterior laryngeal lymphatic vessels with the drainage area of the anterior subglottic wall
3. Via the inferior laryngeal lymphatic vessels with the drainage area of the remaining subglottic space and the middle and lower posterior wall of the larynx.

Table 5.5. Lymph node metastasis of supraglottic carcinoma: correlation between site of primary tumour and frequency of ipsilateral, contralateral and bilateral metastasis verified by histology

Site of primary tumor	n	Homolateral n	Homolateral %	Contra- and bilateral n	Contra- and bilateral %	Total n	Total %
Ventrolateral	57	12	21	15	26	27	47
Ventral	31	9	29	5	16	14	45
Lateral	55	15	27	6	11	21	38
Posterior	6	0		1	17	1	17
Total	149	36	24	27	18	63	42

The Reinke's spaces of both vocal cords are only sluggishly drained. A carcinoma generally gains access to the neighbouring lymph drainage systems at later stages by spread into the corresponding

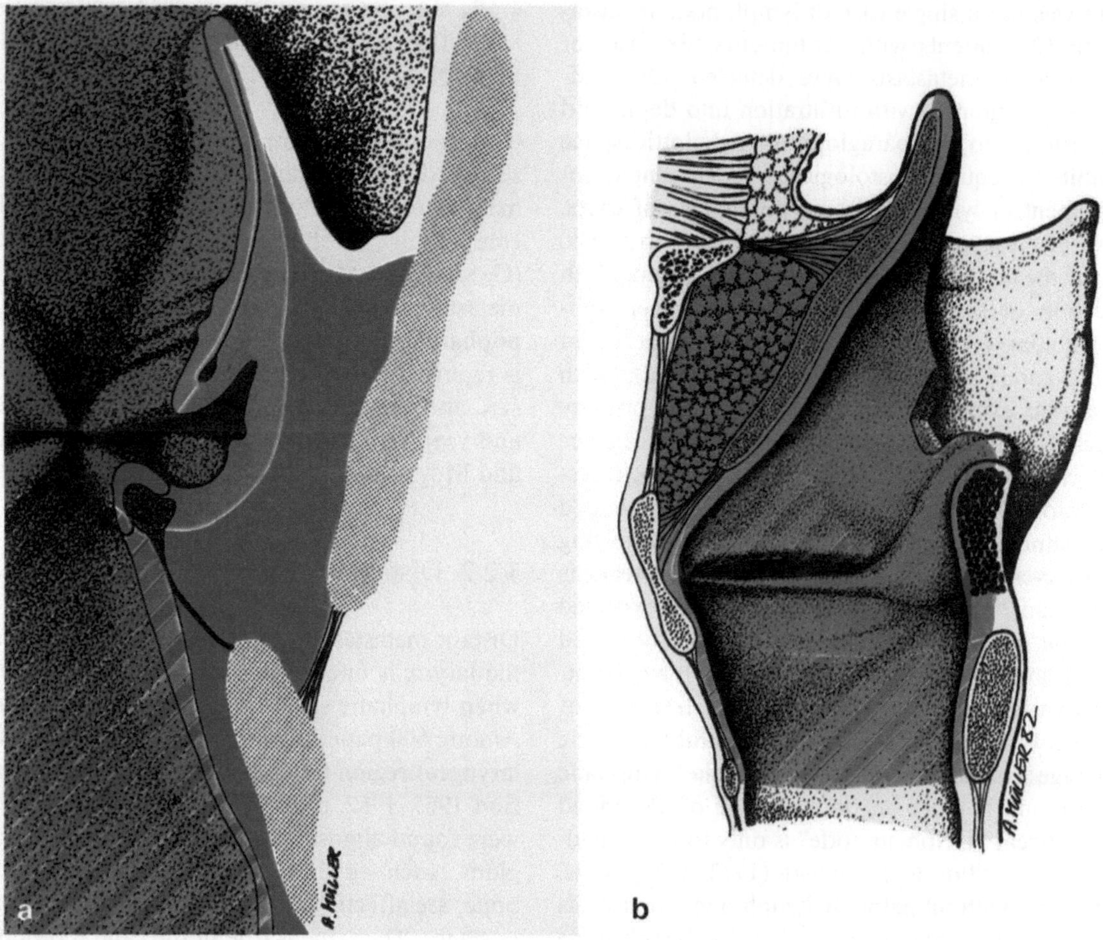

Fig. 5.24a, b. T classification of supraglottic cancer. *Red:* region of origin = T_1; *green:* adjacent region = T_2; *blue:* infiltration of the paraglottic or preepiglottic space = T_3; *yellow:* regions outside the larynx = T_4. The *hatched area* displays the extension of a T_{1b} tumour. **a** Frontally sectioned hemilarynx with anterior mucosal relief representing a ventrally sited (epiglottic) carcinoma. **b** Midsagittal section displaying a laterally sited carcinoma

drainage areas: any of the three drainage systems mentioned can be reached. However, the lymph drainage systems should not be regarded as static and strictly separated. The submucous connective tissue (Fig. 1.6) contains a lymphatic plexus which, to a moderate extent, maintains connections with the neighbouring spaces. Thus a network exists between the subglottic and paraglottic space, especially via the posterior laryngeal wall, and again between the superior laryngeal lymphatic vessels and the submandibular lymphatic system. The "lymph currents" are only weak and can be reversed at any time by local changes (Welsh et al 1961).

In about 30%-40% of cases of **supraglottic carcinoma**, lymph nodes can be palpated before treatment (Meyer-Breiting and von Ilberg 1979, Gudziol and Beleites 1983). Swelling of the lymph nodes is caused by nonspecific lymphadenitis in about 20%-25% of all cases. This is considered a reaction to tumour growth. In a similarly high percentage of cases, however, lymph node metastasis is detected histologically which was not recognized by the clinician (Meyer-Breiting and von Ilberg 1979). In about 18% of all patients with supraglottic carcinomas, particularly in ventral and ventrolateral locations, bilateral metastasis can be reckoned with (Table 5.5). Lymph node metastasis can be expected not only along the major vessels of the neck but also in all three submandibular lymph node groups (Meyer-Breiting and von Ilberg 1979).

Metastasis of **glottic carcinomas** is rarely observed; this is due mainly, however, to the early detection of vocal cord carcinomas. In 247 patients with glottic T1a tumours diagnosed between 1965 and 1982 at the Frankfurt University ENT Clinic, there was not a single case of lymph node metastasis. In 102 patients with T2 tumours, six cases of lymph node metastasis were detected. Only advanced carcinomas with infiltration into depth and expansion into the paraglottic or subglottic space exhibited frequent histologically documented involvement of lymph nodes, in about 25% of cases. Most of these arose on the upper third of the neck, i.e. in the upper jugular lymph node group. With affection of the paraglottic space, however, submandibular lymphatic spread can also occur in glottic carcinoma (MEYER-BREITING 1981a). With subglottic extension of carcinomas or in primary subglottic carcinomas, metastatic spread takes place preferably via the inferior laryngeal lymphatic vessels into the paratracheal lymph nodes, which as a rule cannot be palpated by the clinician. According to FLEISCHER (1977), when subglottic spread is more than 20 mm, such metastasis is to be expected in about 30%-40% of cases, however, we observed paratracheal metastasis also in cases with a subglottic extension less than 10 mm from the free edge of the vocal cord. Metastasis via the ventral lymphatic drainage system into the lower jugular lymphatic node group is more uncommon. The oft-described prelaryngeal "Delphian node" is only formed facultatively according to ROUVIÈRE (1932, 1938); thus, in patients without palpable lymph node metastasis at this site it cannot be concluded that lymph node metastasis via this lymphatic drainage system has not occurred. Incidentally, it is quite possible to misinterpret continuous carcinomatous invasion into the prelaryngeal tissue as metastasis into this lymphatic node. Spreading into the lower jugular lymph node group occurs as a rule via the paratracheal lymph nodes.

Deep **oropharyngeal carcinomas** metastasize mainly along the same lymph drainage systems as the supraglottic carcinomas.

Whereas endolaryngeal carcinomas are generally propagated along only one or two lymphatic paths, **hypopharyngeal carcinomas** can be expected to exhibit multilateral centrifugal lymphatic spreading. They gain access:

1. Via the paraglottic space to the superior laryngeal lymphatic system
2. Via the posterior wall of the larynx, to the inferior laryngeal lymphatics
3. In the lateral pharyngeal wall cranially towards the base of the skull and caudally into the mediastinum
4. Via the pharyngoepiglottic fold to the region of the floor of the mouth and the submandibular lymph nodes

Correspondingly, lymph node metastasis is widely scattered in hypopharyngeal carcinomas. There is a marked tendency to bilateral metastasis, which is comparable to that of supraglottic carcinomas (GANZER and MEYER-BREITING 1982). Lymph node metastasis occurs at an early stage even in small hypopharyngeal tumours. The frequency of metastasis is reported to be between 60% and 70% (JOERGENSEN and SELL 1971, HARRISSON 1972, OLOFSSON and VAN NOSTRAND 1973, KIRCHNER 1975, GANZER and MEYER-BREITING 1982).

5.2.2 Distant Metastasis

Distant metastasis by squamous cell carcinomas of the larynx is uncommon and is usually found only when lymphatic spreading has already taken place. Among 600 patients with carcinomas of the internal laryngeal region treated in Frankfurt during the period 1965–1982, only 13 cases of distant metastasis were found almost exclusively in the lung. Other regions, such as that of the abdominal organs or bone, are affected considerably less often and at later stages. The same is true of the caudal oropharyngeal carcinomas. In hypopharyngeal carcinomas, however, we observed metastasis to bone in the region of the spinal column, the base of the skull and in the endocranium. There is a striking connection between this route of metastasis and the primary location of the tumour on the posterior wall of the hypopharynx.

5.3 TNM Classification of Laryngeal, Hypopharyngeal and Caudal Oropharyngeal Carcinoma

In the 1940s, the French author DENOIX (1944) developed the principles of the TNM system for the staging of malignant tumours. The Subcommittee on the Registration of Cases of Cancer as well as their Statistical Presentation of the WHO proposed for the first time an internationally binding definition of the local extension of malignant tumours for the registration and statistical survey of cancerous lesions. In 1958 the Union Internationale Contre le Cancer (UICC) published the first recommendation for the clinical staging of laryngeal carcinomas (UICC 1958). The classification of laryngeal carcinomas was approved in 1972 and confirmed in 1978, while a new classification for oro- and hypopharyngeal carcinoma was introduced in 1978 (UICC 1978, 1979, 1986). The TNM classification of the American Joint Committee of Cancer deviates slightly in details from that of the UICC (AJCC 1972, 1977, 1983).

5.3.1 Pretherapeutic TNM Classification

The TNM classification for clinical description of the extension of carcinomas is based on the clinical establishment of

T : Extent of primary tumour
N : Involvement of regional lymph nodes
M : Absence or presence of distant metastasis

The addition of numbers to these three symbols describes the degree of tumour spread.

The primary extension is a uniform definition of the pretherapeutic state. The staging is based on clinical, endoscopic and radiological findings in the head and neck region. Experience shows, however, that considerable discrepancies can occur between the pretherapeutic classification and the actual, histologically detectable extent of the tumour spread, depending on the technical facilities available to the clinician and the location of the tumour. Thus for the T4 classification of laryngeal carcinoma, the significant involvement of the laryngeal framework can be established clinically only in a few cases. MEYER-BREITING (1981b) based on multiple serial sectioning of 151 laryngeal carcinomas, found that the pretherapeutic assessment corresponded only in about one-third of all carcinomas to their actual extension. The discrepancy was most impressive in pretherapeutically graded T3 carcinomas: more than half had already affected or broken through the laryngeal framework and thus had to be graded post-therapeutically as T4 tumours.

In order to have more objective data available for appropriate investigations, the so-called pTNM classification was introduced for postoperative classification based on histopathological examination of resection specimens and/or other objective criteria. Its principles had to correspond to the definition of pretherapeutic classification.

Below are set forth the principles of the TNM classification of the tumour locations under discus-

Table 5.6. T-Classification of carcinoma of the larynx

T_X	Minimum requirements to assess the primary tumour cannot be met		
T_0	No evidence of primary tumour		
	Supraglottis	*Glottis*	*Subglottis*
T_{is}	Carcinoma in situ	Carcinoma in situ	Carcinoma in situ
T_1	Tumour confined to the region with normal mobility	Tumour confined to the region with normal mobility	Tumour confined to the region
T_{1a}	Tumour confined to the laryngeal surface of the epiglottis or to an aryepiglottic fold or to a ventricular cavity or to a ventricular band	Tumour confined to one vocal cord	Tumour confined to one side of the region
T_{1b}	Tumour involving the epiglottis and extending to the ventricular bands or cavities	Tumour involving both vocal cords	Tumour with extension to both sides of the region
T_2	Tumour with extension to adjacent sites or to the glottis without fixation	Tumour extending to either the supraglottis or the subglottis with normal or impaired mobility	Tumour confined to the larynx with extension to one or both cords with normal or impaired mobility
T_3	Tumour confined to the larynx with fixation and/or other evidence of deep invasion	Tumour confined to the larynx with fixation of one or both vocal cords	Tumour confined to the larynx with fixation of one or both vocal cords
T_4	Tumour with direct extension beyond the larynx	Tumour with direct extension beyond the larynx	Tumour with destruction of cartilage and/or direct extension beyond the larynx

sion. The deviations of the AJCC system are mentioned. The reader is referred to Sect. 1.4 for regional divisions and definition of boundaries (WHO/ICD-O 1976, 1979).

5.3.1.1 *Larynx*

Table 5.6 shows the currently valid T classification of the larynx. The AJCC (1983) does not recognize the subdivision of the supraglottic T1 into T1a and T1b and thus distinguishes more clearly between T1 and T2 tumours. The T1b tumours of the supraglottis have a special place in the UICC classification (1978, 1979, 1986) owing to its particular location - with the epiglottis, vestibular ligament and ventricle considered as adjacent sites. Both classifications apparently start from the premise that when the subglottic region is affected by a supraglottic tumour and vice versa, there is always infiltration into depth. Otherwise, it cannot be explained why supraglottic and subglottic tumours of stage T2 by definition may involve only the glottis as a neighbouring region. Just how a tumour with pure superficial extension over all three regions of the larynx without fixation of the vocal cords can be classified remains unclear. In any case, classification as T3 group appears to us to overestimate these carcinomas.

5.3.1.2 *Hypopharynx*

The following rules of T classification apply to the hypopharynx:

- TX Minimum requirements to assess primary tumour not met
- T0 No evidence of primary tumour
- Tis Preinvasive carcinoma (carcinoma in situ)
- T1 Tumour confined to one site
- T2 Tumour with extension to adjacent site or region without fixation of hemilarynx
- T3 Tumour with extension to adjacent site or region with fixation of hemilarynx
- T4 Tumour with extension to bone, cartilage or soft tissues

5.3.1.3 *Oropharynx*

Whereas classification of the laryngeal and hypopharyngeal tumours is based on their regional extension, for oropharyngeal tumours (T1-T3) the dimensions discernible on the surface are decisive. The following definitions apply:

- TX The minimum requirements to assess primary tumour not met
- T0 No evidence of primary tumour
- Tis Preinvasive carcinoma (carcinoma in situ)
- T1 Tumour 2 cm or less in greatest dimension
- T2 Tumour more than 2 cm but not more than 4 cm in greatest dimension
- T3 Tumour more than 4 cm in greatest dimension
- T4 Tumour more than 4 cm in greatest dimension with extension to bone, muscle, skin, antrum or neck (or root of tongue)

5.3.1.4 *Regional Lymph Nodes*

Tumours in the entire head and neck region drain into the cervical lymph nodes. Their classification is thus uniform for all areas of origin except for the thyroid gland. In detail (UICC 1986, HERMANEK, SOBIN 1987):

- NX regional lymph nodes cannot be assessed
- NO No regional lymph node metastasis
- N1 Metastasis in a single ipsilateral lymph node 3 cm or less in greatest dimension
- N2a Metastasis in a single ipsilateral lymph node more than 3 cm not more than 6 cm in greatest dimension
- N2b Metastases in multiple ipsilateral lymph nodes, none more than 6 cm in greatest dimension
- N2c Metastases in bilateral or contralateral lymph nodes, none more than 6 cm in greatest dimension
- N3 Metastasis in a lymph node more than 6 cm in greatest dimension

The AJCC (1983) differs markedly from the UICC in the categories N2 and N3. In particular:

- N1 Single, clinically positive homolateral node 3 cm or less in diameter
- N2 Single, clinically positive homolateral node more than 3 cm but not more than 6 cm in diameter, or multiple clinically positive homolateral nodes, none more than 6 cm in diameter
- N2a Single, clinically positive homolateral node more than 3 cm but not more than 6 cm in diameter

N2b Multiple, clinically positive homolateral nodes, none more than 6 cm in diameter
N3 Massive homolateral node(s), bilateral nodes, or contralateral node(s)
N3a Clinically positive homolateral node(s), one more than 6 cm in diameter
N3b Bilateral clinically positive nodes (in this situation , each side of the neck should be staged separately, e.g. N3b: right N2a, left N1)
N3c Contralateral clinically positive node(s) only

5.3.1.5 Distant Metastases

The definitions of the M categories for all head and neck sites are:

Mx Presence of distant metastasis cannot be assessed
MO No distant metastasis
M1 Distant metastasis

The category M1 may be further specified according to the following notation:

Pulmonary	PUL	Bone marrow	MAR
Osseous	OSS	Pleura	PLE
Hepatic	HEP	Skin	SKI
Brain	BRA	Eye	EYE
Lymph nodes	LYM	Other	OTH

5.3.2 pTNM Classification

With their comparative clinical and histopathological studies, Norris et al (1970) influenced the T classification of the larynx decisively. Since 1972, it has been equally accepted by both the AJCC and the UICC. The pTNM classification was designed to permit posttherapeutic control of the pretherapeutically gained TNM classification and a second, more objective, parameter for clinical investigations. This is possible only when the definitions for both classifications, TNM and pTNM, are identical, or at least do not contradict each other. Unfortunately the UICC (1976, 1978, 1979, 1986) demanded for the larynx only that the definitions of the pTNM classification correspond to those of the TNM classification, failing to put forward any more detailed rules.

For T1 and T2 categories there is superficial extension without vocal cord fixation or histologically without discernible infiltration into the depth. In T2, the extent of the surface spreading should be related to all regions of the endolaryngeal mucosa.

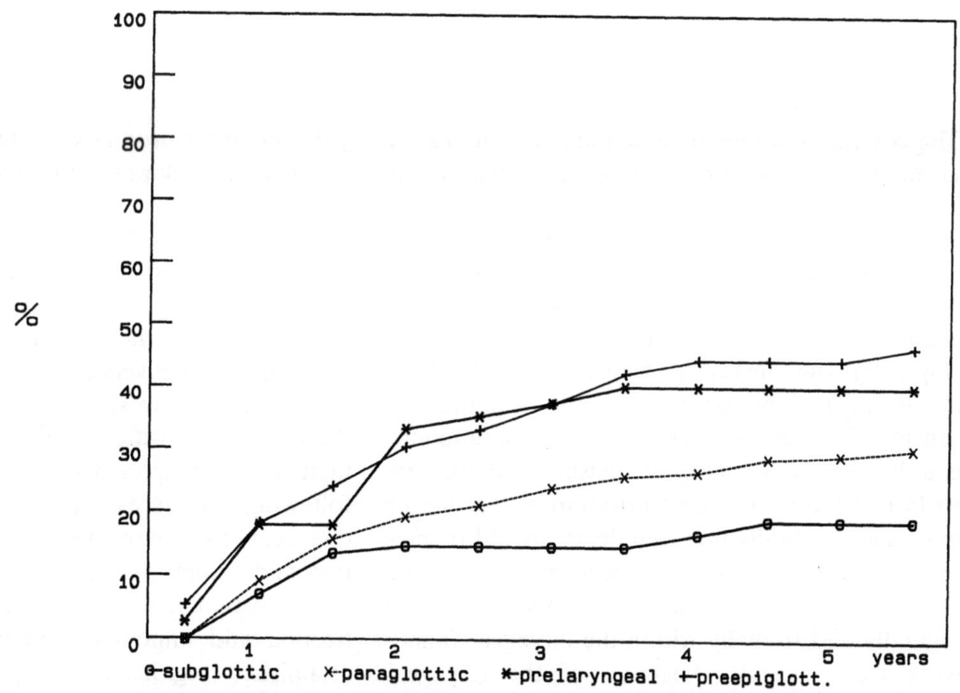

Fig. 5.25. Correlation between on the one hand, involvement of the endolaryngeal spaces and the prelaryngeal extent of carcinoma, and on the other, the 5-year tumour-related death rate

Table 5.7. pT-Classification of carcinoma of the larynx

	Supraglottis	Glottis	Subglottis
pT_X	Minimum requirements to assess the primary tumour cannot be met		
pT_0	No evidence of primary tumour		
	Supraglottis	*Glottis*	*Subglottis*
pT_{is}	Carcinoma in situ	Carcinoma in situ	Carcinoma in situ
pT_1	Tumour confined to the laryngeal surface of one site of the region	Tumour confined to the surface of the region (including 10 mm ventricular and caudal from free edge of vocal cord)	Tumour confined to the surface of the region
pT_{1a}		Tumour confined to one vocal cord	Tumour confined to one side of the region
pT_{1b}	Tumour involving the epiglottis and extending to the ventricular bands or cavities	Tumour involving both vocal cords or crossing anterior commissure and/or posterior wall of region	Tumour with extension to both sides of the region
pT_2	Tumour with extension to adjacent sites or to the glottis involving the epiglottic windows and/or the quadrangular membrane; invasion of paraglottic space less than one-third in depth	Tumour extending to either the supraglottis or the subglottis with infiltration of paraglottic space less than one-third in depth	Tumour confined to the larynx with extension to one or both cords and infiltration of paraglottic space less than one-third in depth
pT_3	Tumour confined to the larynx with involvement of preepiglottic space or extension to involve postcricoid area, medial wall of piriform sinus or deep invasion of paraglottic more than one-third in depth; no infiltration of laryngeal framework	Tumour confined to the larynx with invasion of paraglottic space more than one-third in depth with extension to involve postcricoid area; no infiltration of laryngeal framework	Tumour confined to the larynx with invasion of paraglottic space more than one-third in depth with extension to involve postcricoid area; no infiltration of laryngeal framework
pT_4	Tumour infiltrates or penetrates laryngeal framework and/or involves oropharynx, hypopharynx or trachea	Tumour infiltrates or penetrates laryngeal framework and/or involves oropharynx, hypopharynx or trachea	Tumour infiltrates or penetrates laryngeal framework and/or involves oropharynx, hypopharynx or trachea

The criteria to differentiate between T1 and T2 are given less by the infiltration into depth than by the surface extension. This is particularly important for the supraglottic and subglottic regions. The penetration of the elastic cone and the subsequent involvement of the paraglottic space radically changes the prognosis of the tumour disease (Fig. 5.25). The same is true for cases with any other involvement of the paraglottic spaces. For this reason the T1b classification of supraglottic tumours, is to be viewed as inadequate inasmuch as the ventricle is affected. For categorization as T3 one or more signs of infiltration into depth should be present, but the tumour should not have exceeded the boundaries of the larynx. These boundaries are sagittally and frontally within the laryngeal framework (see Sect. 1.4). Affection of the laryngeal framework or its inner perichondria, or crossing over the boundaries to the trachea, the hypopharynx and/or the oropharynx, characterizes the T4 tumour. In accordance with NORRIS et al (1970) and in general conformity with the AJCC (1972, 1977, 1983) and the UICC (1972, 1978, 1979, 1986), we carried out the pT classification as shown in Table 5.7 and Figs. 5.23–5.24. The larynx specimens from 245 patients with glottic cancer treated surgically at the Frankfurt University ENT Clinic between 1969 and 1980, were investigated by serial sectioning and the tumours classified as described above. All patients had a complete follow-up, and 40 died in the following 5 years as a direct result of the tumour disease. Only few of these had a low pT classification and a high percentage of those with pT4 tumours. A remarkable correlation between pT classification and tumour-related death rate could be established (Fig. 5.26).

GLANZ (1984) undertook a similar investigation for glottic carcinomas; her criteria for these tumours, however, did not correlate with the boundaries of the ICD-O. Thus in GLANZ' study T1 and T2 tumours may have the same superficial extension from the free edge of the vocal cord of 15 mm cranially and 15 mm caudally. In addition it appears to us that including carcinomas with a caudal extension of more than 10 mm in the pT1 category for anatomical reasons is going to far to have any relevance for certain forms of conservative surgery. However, the T1 tumour should not exceed the transition from the ventricular floor to the lateral ventricular wall; because of the above-mentioned prognostically relevant anatomical conditions, it should be confined to the vocal ligaments, Reinke's space and the medial surface of the arytenoid cartilage. According to GLANZ (1984), the glottic pT2 tumour should also be restricted to 15 mm in a craniocaudal direction from the free edge of the vocal cord, but with respect to a deeper infiltration. The T3 tumour of GLANZ' definition may could infiltrate the laryngeal framework. All these points contradict the basic principles set up by the UICC and AJCC and the data cannot be used for comparative studies, although there is a correlation between pT classification according to this definition and the prognosis of the individual patient, as shown in the statistics of the Marburg University ENT Clinic. The publications of NORRIS et al (1970), SMITH et al (1973) and our own results were based on the principles of TNM classification of the UICC and AJCC and showed similarly good correlation (Fig. 5.26).

One of the two real problems in the TNM classification for laryngeal carcinomas as it stands at present is the lack of definition of a clear glottic-subglottic boundary. In our opinion, the extension of Reinke's space, the vocal ligament and the vocal processes of the arytenoid cartilage should define the glottic region. Carcinomas extending beyond this space have a different lymph drainage and a poorer prognosis. Reinke's space, however, in its largest craniocaudal extension, only rarely exceeds a limit of 5-6 mm caudally from the free edge of the vocal cord. This is nearly the same as the extension of Reinke's space in the ventricular floor, i.e as a rule it stops 1 mm before the transition to the lateral wall (MEYER-BREITING and POPESCU 1986). For this reason we consider the appropiate lower boundary for the glottic region to be a plane the same distance below the free edge of the vocal cord as the plane through the ventricular floor is above this edge.

5.4 Histology of Squamous Cell Carcinoma

Squamous cell carcinomas of the larynx do not differ from those of other organ regions as regards their histological and cytological structure. It is well known, however, that particularly in squamous cell carcinomas it is less the tumour type as such that influences the course of the disease but rather the local environment, tumour differentiation and immune responses of the host (manifested as the so-called stromal reaction) (HARRISON 1979). Thus squamous cell carcinomas of the skin in general behave much more favourably than those of mucous surfaces, such as the cervix, the oral cavity and the larynx.

The clinician can only estimate the degree of malignancy, and thus the prognosis, of a malignant tumour from his clinical findings and the course of the disease. Criteria such as demarcation of the tumour, rate of growth, tendency to affect or destroy neighbouring structures, and finally indications of lymphatic blood-borne dissemination are only vague parameters used to assess the progression and prognosis of such a disease - and can only be assessed at all in advanced stages with diminished prospects of cure. When, for example, lymph node metastasis is probable and an aggressive growth is assumed clinically, then, from our experience and that of others authors (COATES et al 1976, MEYER-BREITING and VON ILBERG 1979, GANZER et al 1981), cure can be expected in only 50% of the paients. The prognosis of laryngeal carcinomas accordingly depends critically on the tendency towards lymphatic metastasis, which is by no means dependent only on tumour location, size or local extent. Most publications dealing with the results of treatment of laryngeal carcinomas take only these criteria into consideration. Seldom has it been attempted to establish a relationship between the endogenous determinants of a tumour and its clinical course, but it is a widely acknowledged fact that small tumours are able, under certain circumstances, to metastasize at an early stage, whereas other, exceedingly large tumours grow without any metastasis whatsoever. Naturally the pathologist is challenged by the question of whether it is possible to determine a degree of malignancy and thus give an indication of the prognosis of the tumour disease based on the histological picture. The histological criteria of malignancy, such as cellular and nuclear atypia, increased and abnormal mitotic figures

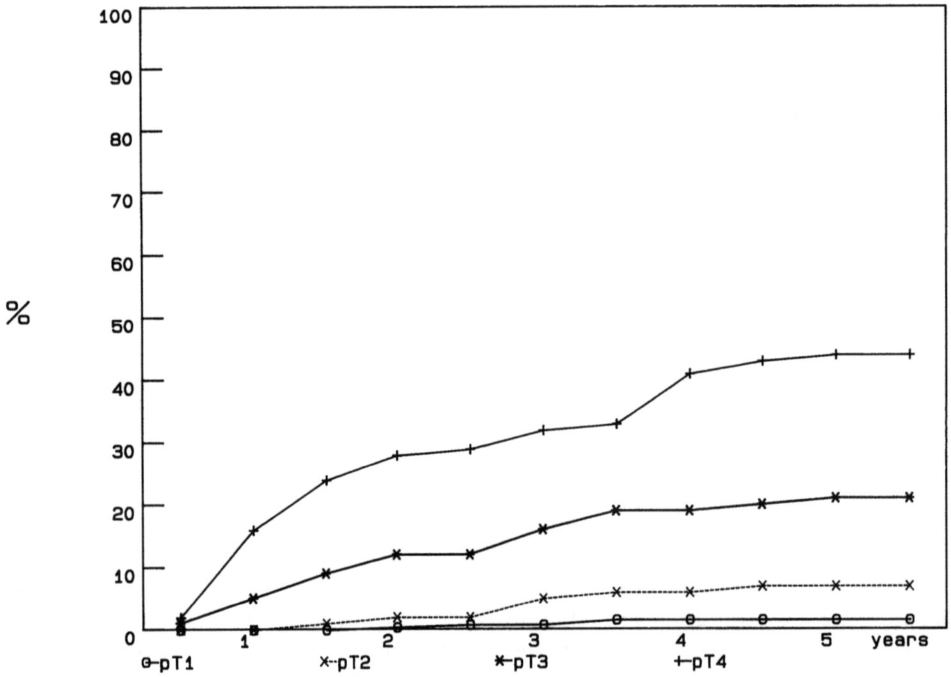

Fig. 5.26. Correlation between pT classification of 245 glottic carcinomas and the tumour-related death rate in a 5-year follow-up. pT_1, 96 cases; pT_2, 52 cases; pT_3 38 cases; pT_4, 59 cases (MEYER-BREITING and SCHORM-EWERS 1987)

and the infiltration of neighbouring tissues (VON ALBERTINI 1974, PARK 1980) also lend themselves to the grading of tumour malignancy.

5.4.1 Degree of Differentiation

HANSEMANN (1890) established the now widely used method of subdividing squamous cell carcinomas according to their degree of differentiation as an indication of the degree of malignancy. He pointed out that malignant transformation is accompanied by different degrees of anaplasia of these cells. BRODERS, based on these considerations, instituted a classification of squamous cell carcinomas (Fig. 2.6) of the lip and skin (1920, 1921) into four grades which he subsequently also applied to other malignant epithelial tumours (1922, 1925, 1932a) (see Sect. 2.2.2). The difficulties involved in this grading start with the fact that numerical counting of differentiated and undifferentiated cells in a routine examination is simply not practicable. Consequently the pathologist more or less has to estimate which grade of differentiation should be assigned to any particular carcinoma. This is a particularly weak point of this system; and the problem is necessarily more marked in a grading into only three groups such as that put forward by the WHO (Sect. 2.2.2).

The histological assessment of the malignancy of a tumour can as a rule be based only on samples taken from the neoplasm. In advanced tumours though, the morphological picture may vary considerably in different regions of the lesion (Table 5.8). For this reason biopsy specimens, especially from the surface, are not necessarily representative for the entire tumour. Table 5.9 shows the correlation between the grade of differentiation determined in 106 biopsy specimens and that found to be pre-

Table 5.8. Grading according to Broders in 142 resected advanced laryngeal carcinomas

Main grading		Additional grading			
Grade	n	I	II	III	IV
I	15	3	9	2	1
II	87	15	43	35	2
III	31	-	20	5	11
IV	9	-	1	7	2

Microscopically, most carcinomas vary in differentiation from one field of view to another. The table shows the quantitively predominant grade of differentiation on the left and the frequency of other grades which are additionally registrable in the respective group.

Table 5.9. Grading according to Broders in biopsy specimens of advanced carcinomas and the resected larynges (n = 106)

Biopsy grading		Grading of the whole carcinoma			
Grade	n	I	II	III	IV
I	11	5	5	1	–
II	57	3	48	5	1
III	31	3	8	18	5
IV	6	–	1	2	3

Two-thirds of the biopsy gradings correspond with the quantitively predominant grade of the whole carcinomas, but the remainder deviate either to a higher or to a lower grade of differentiation

dominant in the serially-sectioned tumour after surgical removal. An analogy can be drawn between tumour grading based on the histological picture seen in a biopsy specimen and the description of a room as seen by an observer through a keyhole. BRODERS (1940) proposed that in the case of different degrees of differentiation being established in one and the same lesion, the lowest should be considered relevant for the biological behaviour of the tumour. Correspondingly, EDMUNDSON (1948) suggested multiple sampling of tumours and determination of the degree of differentiation according to BRODERS. Figures 5.27 and 5.28 show the justification of such a procedure. Figure 5.27 displays the post-therapeutic course of 151 patients with advanced laryngeal carcinomas treated by combined radiosurgery in the Frankfurt University ENT Clinic. Between 1969 and 1978, comparing those who were proved to have died from the tumour disease with those whose cause of death was tumour-independent. If we were to grade tumours according to the quantitatively dominating degree of differentiation then tumour-dependent mortality could not be assessed. But if the tumour-dependent mortality curve is plotted in terms of tumour grade determined according to EDMUNDSON (1948) and BRODERS (1940), then a correlation between survival and tumour grade can be established (Fig. 5.28) (MEYER-BREITING 1981b). Unfortunately the evaluation of biopsy specimens cannot be compared with the investigation of complete tumour, as was done in this study. The preoperative biopsy specimens of the cases studied showed conformity with

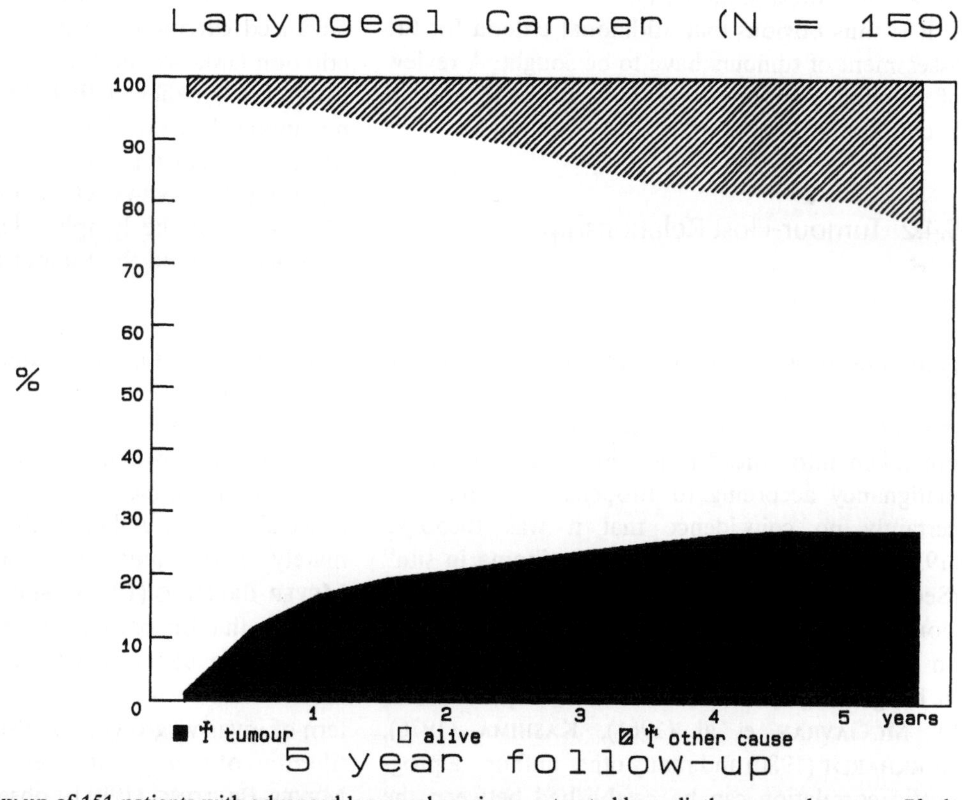

Fig. 5.27. Five-year follow up of 151 patients with advanced laryngeal carcinomas treated by radiotherapy and surgery. *Black area*, death from tumour disease; *lower curve*, tumour-independent death

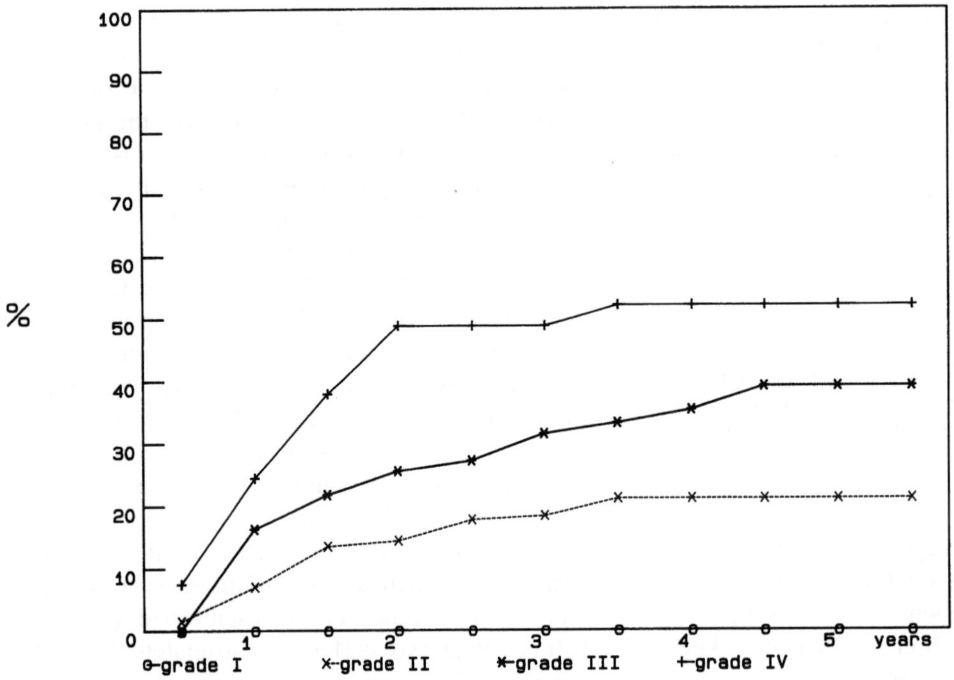

Fig. 5.28. Correlation between the minimal differentiation which can be observed in the carcinoma (Broders grading) and the 5-year tumour-related death rate (same group as in Fig. 5.27)

postoperative histology in 70% of cases if the quantitatively predominant grade was used and only 54% if the lowest grade was taken.

It is thus obvious that additional criteria for the assessment of tumours have to be sought. A review of methods employed so far can be found in Sect. 2.3.

5.4.2 Tumour-Host Relationship

A further important feature of a malignant neoplasm which can be assessed histologically is the pattern of invasive growth and the extent of inflammatory reaction (stromal reaction) of the host. Like the mitotic activity, the tumour-host relationship is not taken into consideration in evaluation of the malignancy according to Broders. It is therefore certainly no coincidence that it was BRODERS (1932b) who defined the term "carcinoma in situ" (Sect. 4.6). This use of the term "carcinoma" in a lesion without invasive growth reflects just as great an underestimation of this criterion as its omission in his grading system. Nonetheless, as pointed out by McGAVRAN et al (1961), KASHIMA (1976), BURKHARDT (1980) and many other authors, a prognostic correlation can be established between the behaviour of tumours at the tumour-host boundary, i.e. the pattern of invasion and the tendency towards lymph node metastasis. The extent of the loss of basal membrane structures in early invasive and advanced carcinomas lends itself as an additional criterion (JAKOBSSON et al 1973). In contrast, HAMPERL (1967) believed that the absence of a basal membrane has no diagnostic or prognostic value. More importance has to be ascribed to the growth pattern (McGAVRAN et al 1961, KASHIMA 1976). The extent of the lympho-plasmo-histiocytic marginal wall around the tumour as a possible expression of host immunological defence can also be drawn upon as a prognostic criterion (review: BURKHARDT 1980, LÖBE and QUADE 1982) (see Sect. 2.3.1.4).

According to GLANZ (1981) and MEYER-BREITING (1981b) the system proposed by JAKOBSSON et al (1973) (see Sect. 2.2.2) is too complicated, especially as a number of the criteria depend ultimately on the same basic features of the tumour. MEYER-BREITING (1981b) and KUS et al (1981) hold the view that the particular behaviour of the tumour towards the connective tissue, possibly related to biochemical factors, determines not only the pattern of invasive growth but also the frequency of infiltration of vascular and neural structures (Fig. 2.7). MEYER-BREITING (1981b) observed that in carcinomas with invasion of vessels, nerves and fibrous

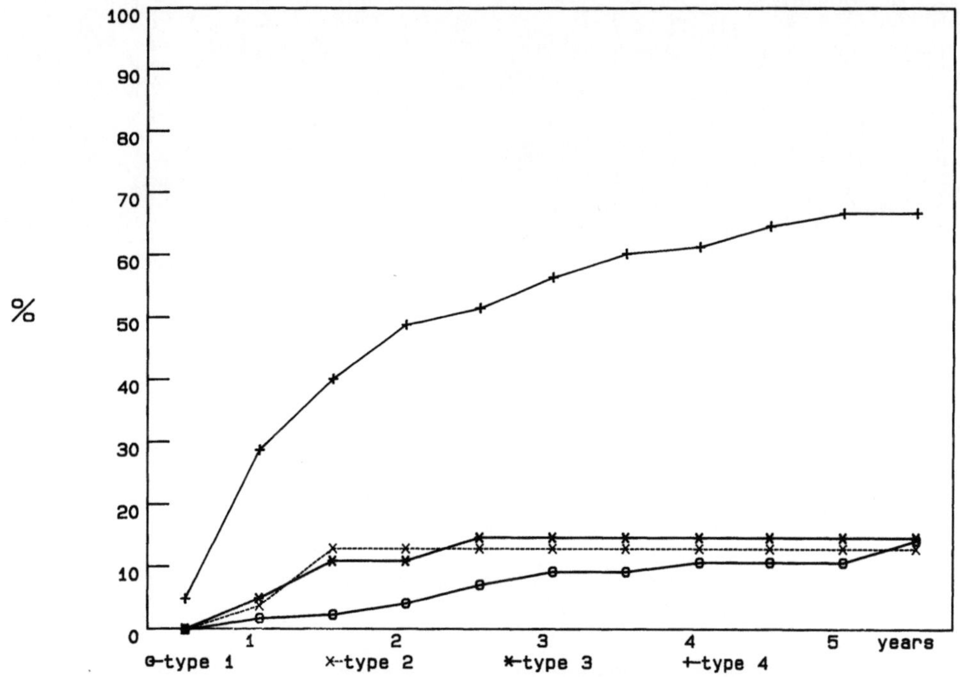

Fig. 5.29. Correlation between different types of infiltration and the 5-year tumour-related death rate (same group as in Figs. 5.27, 5.28). Type 1 infiltrates only soft tissues, i.e. fat, muscles and glands; type 2 also infiltrates cartilage and bone; type 3 can be detected in capillaries; and type 4 infiltrates membranes, larger vessels and nerves, as presented in Fig. 2.7b–c

connective tissue structures such as membranes like the elastic cone, tumour-dependent mortality was more than 5 times as high as in carcinomas not exhibiting these features (Fig. 5.29). As shown in his study, carcinomas of grades II-IV according to BRODERS possess such a destructive potential, whereas he was unable to find this in highly differentiated squamous cell carcinomas (grade I). In the study by MEYER-BREITING (1981) an unfavourable prognosis correlated more with invasion of fibrous connective tissue structures than it had with Broders' grading in the study by McGAVRAN et al (1961). Further subdivision of growth patterns as carried out by KASHIMA (1976), just like the highly detailed method of JAKOBSSON et al (1973), has the disadvantage that subjective variations depending on the observer influence the results more than in the Broders grading. JAKOBSSON et al (1973) found a high degree of coincidence between the degree of malignancy of laryngeal carcinomas determined using their method and the rate of recurrence following radiation therapy; however, their recent attempt to improve the assessment by addition of DNA distribution pattern (HOLM et al 1980) rather suggests that the method has not fulfilled their expectations.

In our view, the grading system proposed by GLANZ (1981, 1984) has eliminated some of the interdependent parameters and the various criteria have been reduced to the essentials. However, on the basis of our own observations we consider that the infiltration of fibrous connective tissue structures merits a higher rating than it has so far been accorded in the GLANZ grading system. Nevertheless we consider this system the most expedient and most suitable standard method yet available for determination of the degree of malignancy of a carcinoma, preferable to the above-mentioned and other proposed methods (HELLWEG-LARSEN et al 1978, GRAEM et al 1980, CHUNG et al 1980).

Although GLANZ and EICHHORN (1985) claim that their malignancy index can discriminate reliably between patients with and without metastasis, independent of site or extension of glottic carcinomas, this statement has to be regarded with scepticism. Time will show whether other investigators can reproduce the same encouraging results.

6 Management of Laryngeal Cancer and Histopathological Inferences

6.1 Diagnosis and Prevention

6.1.1 Diagnostic Procedures, Computerized Tomography

To make a tentative diagnosis, as a rule indirect laryngoscopy using a forehead mirror and a laryngeal mirror in the course of an initial ENT examination suffices. Better diagnostic results can be obtained, however, with a magnifying laryngoscope such as that described by von STUCKRAD and LAKATOS (1975). In all patients with suspected carcinoma of the larynx or lower pharynx, in combination with the appropriate general examination direct laryngoscopy or microlaryngoscopy should be performed in order roughly to determine the tumour spread and to obtain a biopsy specimen (KLEINSASSER 1968). In most cases the TNM classification (Sect. 5.1) and plans for the therapeutic procedure can be made at this point. Concerning the assessment of infiltration into depth, however these methods depend on indirect signs (see definition of T3 in Tables 5.6, 5.7). In our own study, more than a quarter of all laryngeal carcinomas staged as T2 and more than half of all staged as T3 tumours before surgery had to be classified into higher stages after histological examination (MEYER-BREITING 1981).

Recently computerized tomography (CT) has made marked progress in the assessment of advanced laryngeal carcinoma (MANCUSO et al. 1977, MEYER-BREITING et al. 1982, ARCHER et al. 1983). OLOFSSON (1984) achieved a high reliability in detecting penetration of the laryngeal framework. This is of particular importance for the decision between conservative and radical surgery of laryngeal cancer (MEYER-BREITING 1984), as will be demonstrated by several examples. Carcinomatous tissue is generally more hyperdense than all other structures with the exception of the laryngeal framework. Invasion of the preepiglottic space by epiglottic carcinomas can be easily recognized. In Figure 6.1a + b depicts histology and CT of a central plane of a normal supraglottis. In the CT scan shown in Figure 6.1d a hyperdense irregular structure can be seen in front of the epiglottis which has not yet reached the hyoid bone and which corresponds exactly to the carcinomatous spread found in the histological section (Fig. 6.1c).

For the choice of certain techniques of surgery, the preoperative detection of carcinomatous extension into the lower preepiglottic region is of utmost importance. This space can be infiltrated by supraglottic or glottic carcinomas (see Sect. 5.2). In Fig. 6.1f such a distension and displacement of the lower preepiglottic space can be recognized. Owing to the higher density of the ligamentous, membranous and muscular structures, assessment of tumour infiltration is more difficult in their vicinity. Two normally hypodense spaces - a striate area between the thyroid cartilage and the thyroarytenoid musculature and a triangular area in front of the arytenoid cartilage - can provide important information relevant to the question of whether conservative surgery is possible and what technique can be employed. Figure 6.2a shows the CT picture of a carcinoma with extension into the paraglottic space. In spite of vocal cord fixation, this tumour has not affected the hypodense areas mentioned (Fig. 6.2c); conservative surgery is possible. A second case featured impaired mobility of the vocal cord but no fixation: this tumour affected the hypodense field in front of the arytenoid cartilage, as demonstrated by CT and histological section (Fig. 6.2d). Invasion of the laryngeal framework can similarly be depicted by CT (Fig. 6.2e,f), but owing to the variable ossification of the thyroid and cricoid cartilages the risk of misinterpretation is high. Nevertheless, CT is an important aid in clinical diagnosis which helps us to achieve greater accuracy in T classification (Fig. 6.3) and more refined treatment of cancer.

The conclusions from our experience with CT of the larynx can be summarized as follows:

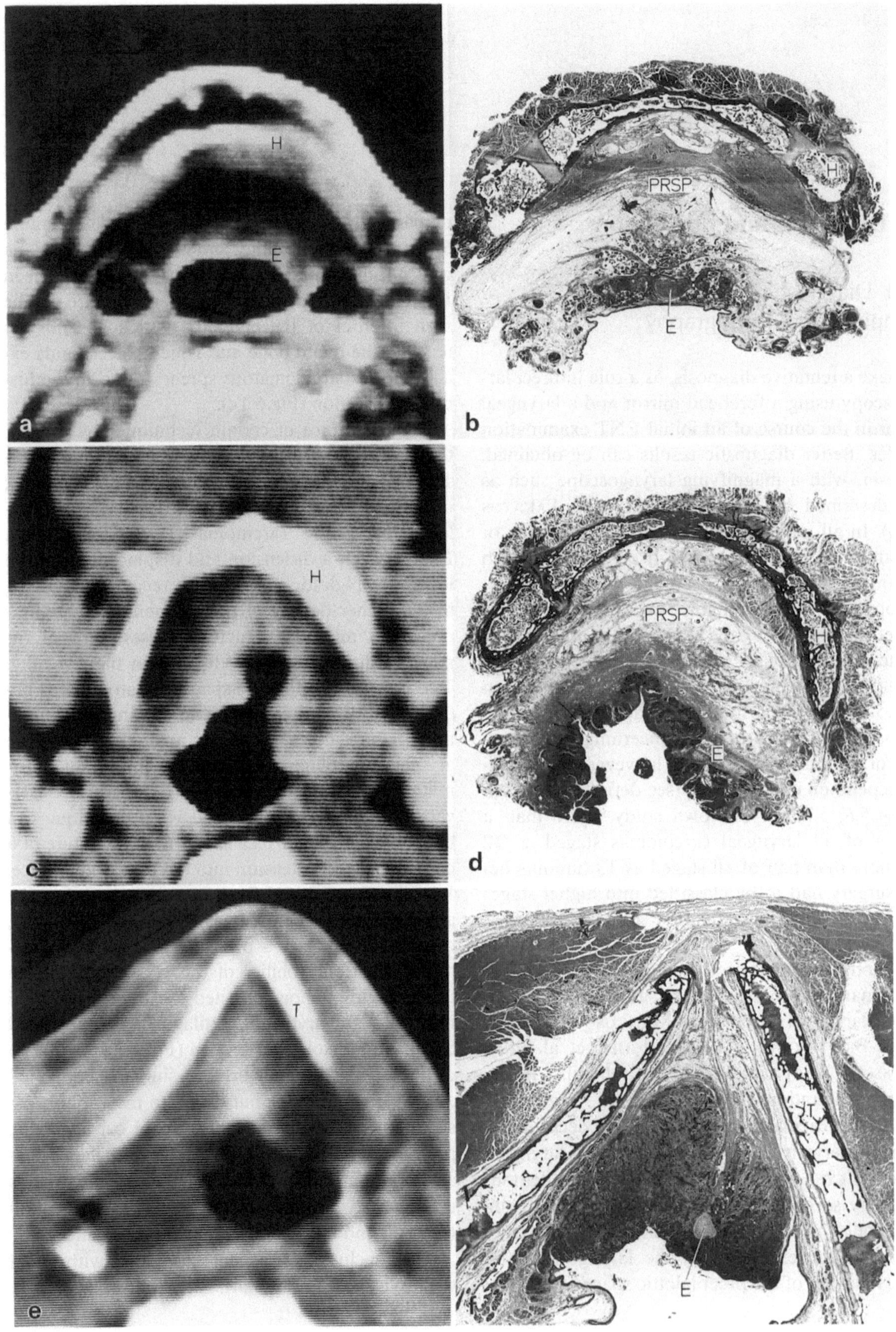
H
E
a
PRSP
H
E
b
H
c
PRSP
H
E
d
T
e
T
E
f

1. CT provides important information regarding the assessment of borderline conditions for conservative surgery.
2. The hypodense areas of the preepiglottic and paraglottic space are critical, revealing early tumour infiltration.
3. To avoid mistakes in CT interpretation particular attention should be paid to the following points:
   a) CT evaluation should not be attempted without exact knowledge of the laryngeal anatomy as well as the behaviour and spread of laryngeal cancers.
   b) CT evaluation should be made only in connection with the laryngoscopic findings.
   c) There should be no evaluation on the basis of one plane of section only.
4. No CT evaluation is possible in cases with preexisting alterations of the larynx.

6.1.2 Prevention

Most laryngeal carcinomas arise in connection with prolonged exposure to inhaled noxaious agents (see Sect. 4.1.4, 4.1.5). The consequences are impairment and loss of voice and eventually death. Prevention must therefore concentrate on three areas:

1. Limitation of exposure to inhaled noxious agents by providing information and protective measures, especially at high-risk work places (Sect. 4.1.4, 4.1.5)
2. Detection of risk groups and their regular monitoring at appropriate intervals (STEINER 1985)
3. Further development of therapeutic measures to retain the voice without increasing the risk of cancer or of death by cancer

6.2 Surgery

The aim of every physician engaged in oncology is to eliminate a life-threatening tumour. Keeping this concept in mind, the surgeon assumes a great responsibility if he decides on conservative surgery in cases of laryngeal carcinoma (TERRAHE 1972). Partial laryngectomy should be performed only after careful consideration whether a more extensive operation or laryngectomy would give the patient a better chance of survival. TERRAHE (1972) pointed out that only the surgeon who determines the extent of resection according to the most stringent standards can protect himself against failure. These standards are provided by our knowledge about the behaviour and spread of carcinomas in different regions of the larynx, based on the observations of LEROUX-ROBERT (1936), ALONSO (1947), OGURA (1955), PRESSMAN et al. (1969), OLOFSSON and VAN NOSTRAND (1973), HOMMERICH et al. (1974), FLEISCHER (1977) and MEYER-BREITING (1981), which are discussed in detail in Chap. 5. These general guidelines find an important supplement in the detailed histological examination of every single resection specimen and active follow-up of each individual patient in order to document success or failure of the therapeutic procedure as completely as possible. After a lapse of more than 10 years, it now seems appropiate to make a critical review of the results obtained with the various techniques.

6.2.1 Conservative Surgery of Glottic Cancer

6.2.1.1 Outline of Techniques

1. Endolaryngeal approach
   a) Microsurgery (LORÉ 1962, KLEINSASSER 1968)
   b) Laser (STRONG 1975, VAUGHAN et al. 1980, STEINER 1982, 1984)
2. Thyrotomy (LORÉ 1962, MONTGOMERY 1973, NAUMANN 1972, DENECKE 1980)
   a) Cordectomy
   b) Extended cordectomy
3. So-called hemilaryngectomy
   a) LEROUX-ROBERT technique (LEROUX-ROBERT 1957, NAUMANN 1972, DENECKE 1980)

Fig. 6.1 a–f. CT and histology of normal supraglottis and supraglottic carcinomas. **a + b** Normal supraglottis. Between the hyperdense structures of the hyoid bone and the epiglottis lies the fat-filled hypodense preepiglottic space *(PRSP)*. In this space infiltrations by carcinoma can be detected very easily by CT. **c + d** Destruction of the central part of the epiglottis and involvement of the preepiglottic space. **e + f** The situation in the lower preepiglottic space is very important in the decision on supraglottic laryngectomy. CT and histology show a carcinoma originating from the pars fixa of the epiglottis. Below, carcinoma has deeply infiltrated the space in front of the petiolus and the thyroepiglottic ligament. Successful eradication of the tumour by conservative surgery seems to be doubtful

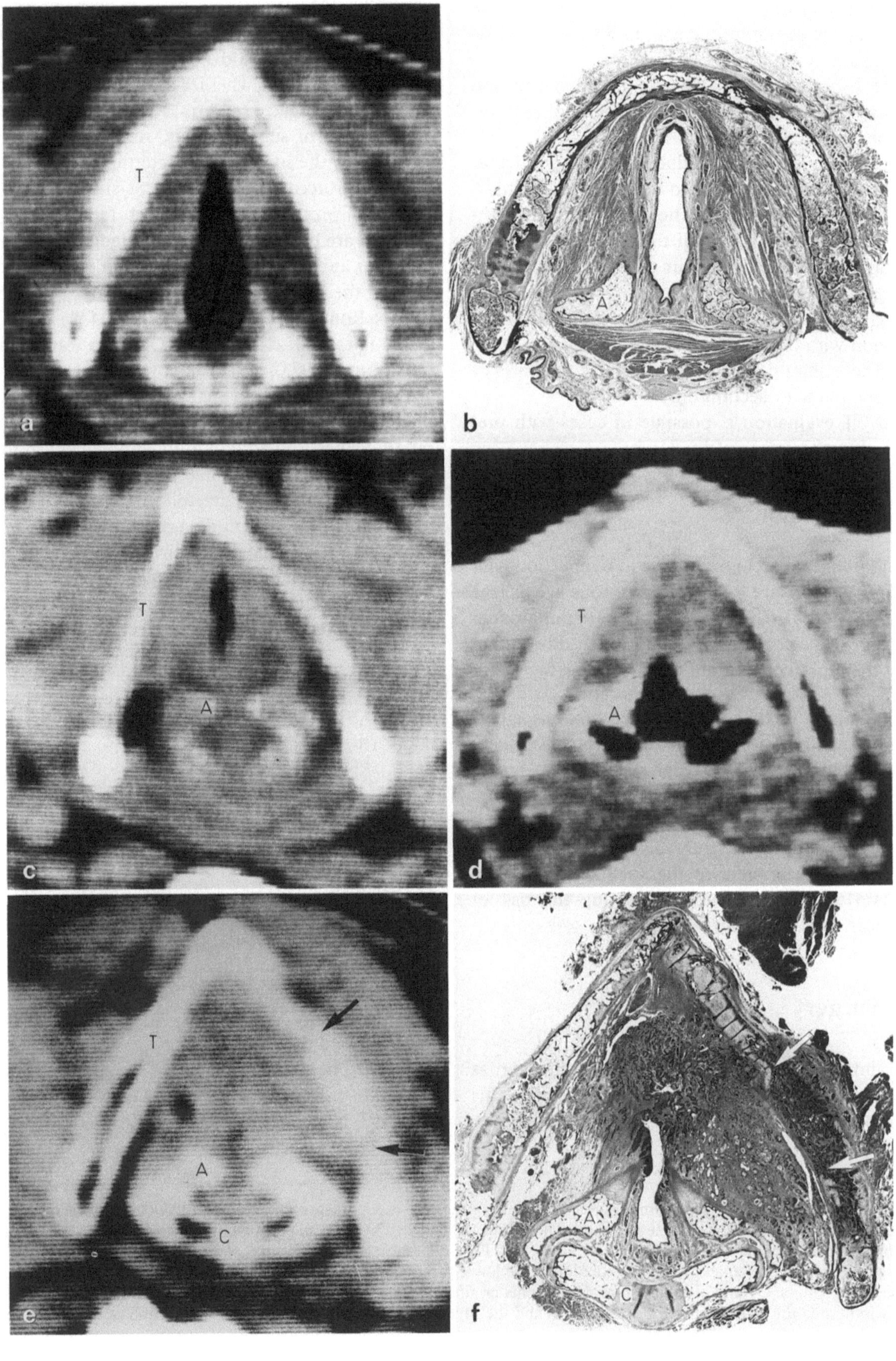
T
a
T
A
b
T
A
c
T
A
d
T
A
C
e
T
A
C
f

b) Hemilaryngectomy [partial lateral laryngectomy (SOM 1975, SILVER 1977, NUSSBAUM et al. 1981)]
c) Anterior hemilaryngectomy (SOM 1951, SOM and SILVER 1968, MONTGOMERY 1973)
4. Extended techniques of hemilaryngectomy
a) Hautant technique (OMBRÉDANNE 1930, NAUMANN 1972, DENECKE 1980)
b) GLUCK-SOERENSEN technique (GLUCK und SOERENSEN 1922, NAUMANN 1972, DENECKE 1980).

For further details, we refer to the literature cited, as well as to **Reports from the Course of Conservation Surgery for Carcinoma of the Larynx** (WIGAND et al. 1984).

Most of the methods listed above are performed in our clinic and the resected specimen are subjected to thorough histological examination. The combination of diagnostic, surgical and histological information and finally the results of follow-up, has made it possible to compile important data regarding the advantages and disadvantages of the different operative techniques.

From January 1966 to June 1982 a total of 390 patients (365 male, 25 female) with glottic carcinomas were treated by conservative surgery at Frankfurt University ENT Clinic. All tumours were classified retrospectively according to the UICC system for malignant tumours (UICC 1978), the principles of which are shown in Table 5.6. In order to record the location and extent of the tumours as accurately as possible and to arrive at a definite indication for the respective partial resection, direct supported laryngoscopy with the aid of different viewing angles was employed in addition to indirect laryngoscopy.

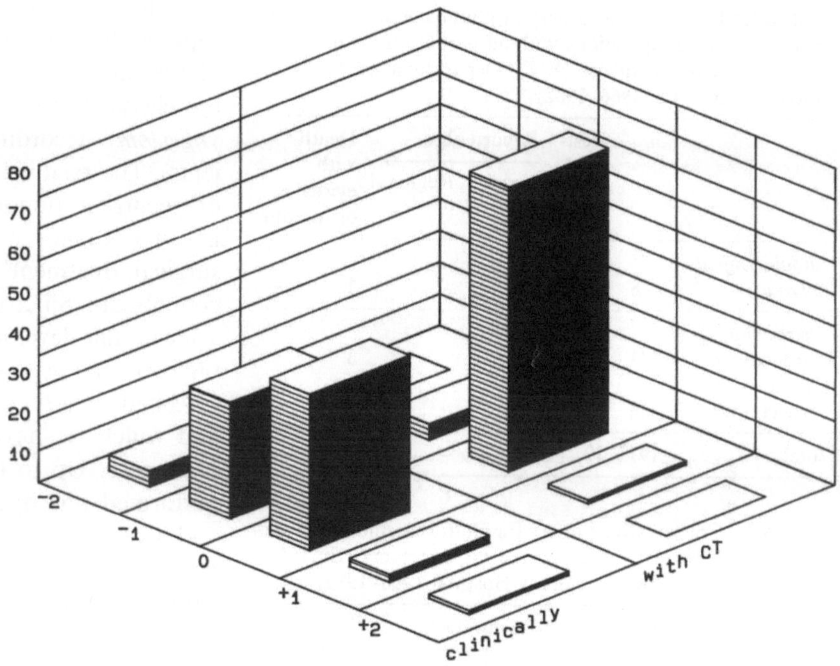

Fig. 6.3. Normal T classification vs CT-supported T classification. The numerals on the *bottom line* represent the degree of deviation of the respective T classification from the pT classification

Fig. 6.2 a–f. CT and histology of normal glottis and glottic carcinomas. **a, b** A section through the vocal cord shows that the neighbouring soft tissue consists of hyperdense structures, e.g. muscles and ligaments. But there are also hypodense areas which can help to discern the extension of early glottic carcinoma: between the thyroarytenoid muscles and the thyroid cartilage, there is a small hypodense stripe which ends 5–10 mm before the anterior commissure, and in front of the arytenoid cartilages the thyroarytenoid muscles part, leaving a hypodense triangular field. **c** CT of an early glottic cancer. Irregularity of the surface of the right glottis and a neighbouring small hyperdense field are shown, representing the carcinoma. The above-mentioned hypodense areas are not involved. **d** Glottic cancer involving the hypodense triangular field in front of the right arytenoid cartilage. **e, f** Advanced glottic cancer filling the paraglottic space and involving the thyroid cartilage

The principle "no partial laryngectomy without previous microlaryngoscopy" should be mandatory. The TNM classification of the 390 glottic carcinomas based on these diagnostic measures is presented in Table 6.1.

Conservative surgery as listed in Tables 6.2 and 6.3 was employed in the patients included in our study. More than 50% of the patients treated are still being seen regularly and cared for in our tumour clinic. We lost track of some of the patients temporarily after the initial treatment, and it was only after extensive inquiries that we were finally able to trace them again and learn about their fates. This time-consuming search is the explanation for the small number of unknown courses of disease in the first 3-5 years (Fig. 6.4).

Table 6.1. TN classification of early glottic cancer treated by conservative surgery in the ENT Department of Frankfurt University Hospital (1966-1982)

	Tis	T1a	T1b	T2	T3	Total
N0	32	147	100	96	9	384
N1	–	–	–	6	–	6
Total	32	147	100	102	9	390
Death due to tumour within 5 years			6	12		18

Table 6.2. Conservative surgery of glottic carcinoma: results of minor surgical operations without partial resection of thyroid and cricoid cartilage (ENT Department of Frankfurt University Hospital 1966-1982)

	n	Residual tumour	Recurrences		Death with evidence of tumour
			Local	Regional	
Endolaryngeal approach	8	2	3	–	1
Thyrotomy:					
Cordectomy	143	11	8	–	3
Extended cordectomy	44	6	8	–	3
Total	197	19	19	–	7

Table 6.3. Conservative surgery for glottic carcinoma: results of various types of vertical partial laryngectomy (ENT Department of Frankfurt University Hospital 1966-1982)

	n	Residual tumour	Recurrences		Death with evidence of tumour
			Local	Regional	
Leroux-Robert	63	5	6	1	5
Hemilaryngectomy Som, Ogura	81	4	0	5	2
Extended hemilaryngectomy Hautant,	44	8	5	1	3
Gluck-Soerensen	20	5	4	0	1
Atypical	3	0	0	0	0
Total	211	22	15	7	11

Vocal cord stripping or superficial resection of vocal cords areas for curative purposes was carried out via the supported laryngoscope in seven patients in early 1966, but was abandoned thereafter. One hundred and forty-three *cordectomies* were done by the known technique for T1a carcinomas of the glottis. Up to the early 1970s, *extended cordectomies* (classic cordectomy and additional resection of endolaryngeal soft parts) were occasionally carried out in patients with carcinomas extending from the vocal cord to the anterior commissure and the lateral wall of the ventricle (44 cases). In Europe, glottic carcinomas with marked involvement of the anterior commissure are today regarded as the classical indication for *frontolateral partial laryngectomy* according to Leroux-Robert (63 patients). The relatively high number of residual and/or recurrent tumours after surgery according to Leroux-Robert motivated us to look for a safer surgical treatment of carcinomas of the anterior commissure. Since the early 1970s we have adopted a technique developed by Ogura which in principle corresponds to the procedure of Som (1951), the so-called *lateral and anterior hemilaryngectomies*, and which we have modified into a more radical procedure. Up to the end of the study period we performed this operation on 81 patients with T1a and T2 tumours. *Vertical partial laryngectomies according to* Hautant were carried out in 44 patients with subglottic involvement. *Hemilaryngectomy according to* Gluck *and* Soerensen was performed in 20 patients with subglottic and/or supraglottic or dorsal extension, including all nine patients with T3 tumours.

6.2.1.2 Results of Different Surgical Procedures

Vocal cord stripping. This operation was performed on seven patients. In two of them it was found that the tumour had not been removed with a margin of normal tissue. Three other patients had local recurrences, and one of these later died as a consequence of the tumour disease.

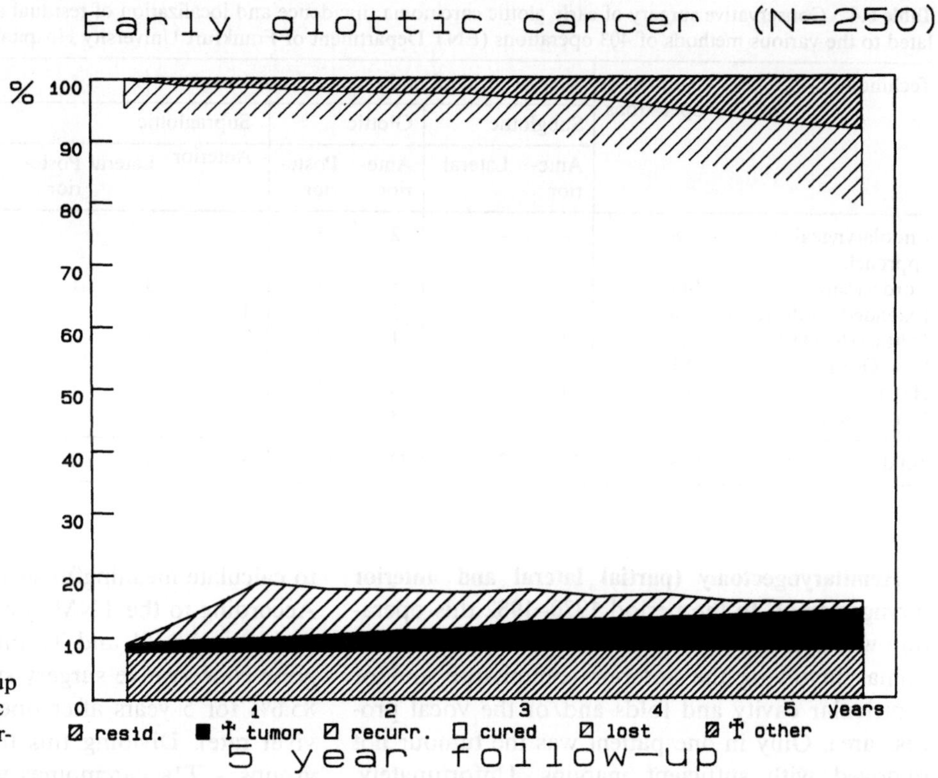

Fig. 6.4. Five-year follow-up of patients with early glottic carcinoma treated by conservation surgery

Classical cordectomy. More than two-thirds of all cases of conservative surgery in the vocal cord area concerned patients with carcinomas classified as T1a tumours, i.e. the carcinoma was strictly limited to the vocal cord itself, did not reach the anterior commissure, and at the most touched the anterior portion of the vocal process area. The distance from the lateral wall of Morgagni's ventricle was at least 2–3 mm. Of the 143 carcinomas in this category, 11 proved to have been resected without sufficient margin of normal tissue. With subsequent more extensive partial resection and laryngectomy the disease could be controlled in all these patients. Among eight patients with late local recurrences, three ultimately died as a consequence of the tumour disease. The cumulative 5-year survival rate for patients treated by cordectomy with the abovementioned indication was 96%.

Extended cordectomy. This was usually performed for tumours which either reached the anterior commissure or apparently had just invaded the subglottic or supraglottic space. Surgery in these 44 patients, consisting of only soft tissue resection via laryngofissure, had a particularly high rate of failure. In five patients the tumour had not been removed with a sufficient margin and there were local recurrences in eight patients (see Table 6.2).

Histology after operations via thyrotomy. The review of the histological specimens showed that after operation via thyrotomy residual tumour tissue was most frequently left in the area of the anterior commissure and its surrounding. In 10 cases the cancer had not been completely removed and residual tumour tissue was detected near the anterior commissure, towards the posterior wall at the vocal process, and contralaterally. In only one case was there failure to correctly assess and remove subglottic extension (Table 6.4).

Frontolateral partial laryngectomy. This operation was performed in 63 patients with tumours of the anterior commissure. In two cases histological examination revealed that the tumour had not been completely removed. Of five local recurrences, four could not be controlled by any treatment. One patient suffered from late lymph node metastasis. The histological examination of the specimens removed after recurrence revealed that a tendency of carcinomas treated by this method to recur in the subglottic area. In two cases there were recurrences in the supraglottic region.

Table 6.4. Conservative surgery of early glottic carcinoma: incidence and localization of residual and recurrent carcinoma related to the various methods of 403 operations (ENT Department of Frankfurt University Hospital 1966–1982)

Technique	Number of operations	Sites of residual and recurrent tumours									
		Subglottic		Glottic		Supraglottic			Contralateral	Multiloculated	
		Anterior	Lateral	Anterior	Posterior	Anterior	Lateral	Posterior		Carcinoma	Precancer
Endolaryngeal approach	8	–	–	2	3	–	–	–	1	1	1
Cordectomy	143	1	–	5	1	–	3	1	3	1	–
Extended cordectomy	44	–	–	5	4	1	–	–	3	2	–
LEROUX-ROBERT	63	4	2	1	2	2	1	–	2	–	–
SOM, OGURA	81	1	–	2	–	–	–	–	2	1	1
HAUTANT	44	4	–	4	1	–	–	1	1	–	–
GLUCK-SOERENSEN	20	2	–	3	–	–	–	–	3	–	–
Total	403	12	2	22	11	3	4	2	15	5	2

Hemilaryngectomy (partial lateral and anterior laryngectomy). In the period 1970–1982 this operation was performed in 81 patients with glottic carcinomas involving the anterior commissure and/or ventricular cavity and folds and/or the vocal process area. Only in one patient was the tumour not removed with sufficient margins. Unfortunately, however, this group included four patients with carcinomas which despite minimal local extension – subglottically less than 10 mm – showed early metastasis in the paratracheal and inferior jugular lymph nodes. In two instances tumour growth could be controlled, but two patients died from the sequelae of metastatic disease (Table 6.3).

Extended Hemilaryngectomies: The HAUTANT and GLUCK-SOERENSEN techniques, in both of which part of the cricoid cartilage is included in the resection, were employed in 44 and 20 patients respectively. In seven cases the tumour was not removed primarily with sufficient margins and local recurrences ensued, in one case associated with lymph node metastasis. Three of the patients operated on according to HAUTANT's method and one of those operated on according to the method of GLUCK and SOERENSEN later died from their tumour disease.

Histological examination revealed that the two surgical techniques failed most frequently in tumours infiltrating the glottic and subglottic anterior wall: in seven cases there was residual tumour tissue in the glottis, in four in the contralateral part of the larynx, and in six at the anterior subglottic wall (Table 6.4).

Except for the group of patients treated by classical cordectomy we considered the groups too small to calculate meaningful **survival rates** (UICC 1976). According to the TNM system (UICC 1976) 90.7% patients with T1 and T2 tumours who had undergone conservative surgery survived for 3 years and 85.6% for 5 years after operation (cumulative survival rate). Dividing this total collective into two groups – T1a carcinomas vs T1b carcinomas and higher categories, we calculated for the first group, treated by vocal cord stripping or classical cordectomy, a 3-year survival rate of 96.5% and a 5-year survival rate of 94.7%, and for the second group, which underwent more extensive surgery (extended cordectomy, vertical partial laryngectomies), a 3-year survival rate of 86% and a 5-year survival rate of 77.9%.

6.2.1.3 Comment and Conclusion

As already mentioned, we abandoned an endolaryngeal approach with excision of early glottic cancer and carcinoma in situ of the vocal cord as a curative procedure near the beginning of the 1966–1982 study period. As recommended by KLEINSASSER (1968), however, this technique is still being used as a diagnostic procedure in cases of irregular changes in the whole vocal cord without definite proof of invasive cancer, in order to detect a carcinoma in situ or early invasive carcinoma within a dysplastic region by means of serial sections. KLEINSASSER (1980) himself has recommended extreme caution in using this technique for curative purposes. If a carcinoma is histologically verified, appropriate, more extensive conservative surgery should be performed. We do not consider laser treatment a procedure which could make endolaryngeal resection more successful.

The curative results obtained with classical cordectomy are evident and do not need additional interpretation. The frontolateral partial laryngectomies according to LEROUX-ROBERT and TAPIA, as well as extended cordectomy, do not seem to be completely adequate in the control of tumour growth at the anterior commissure and the adjoining supraglottic and subglottic spaces as judged from the frequency of recurrences. Considering that LEROUX-ROBERT, in his statistical review (1961) on conservative surgery of laryngeal carcinomas, lists 41 cordectomies as compared to 123 frontolateral partial laryngectomies, it could hardly be assumed that we chose the frontolateral operation for cases which overstressed this method. On the contrary, we feel it more likely that LEROUX-ROBERT used the frontolateral approach in situations where we employed cordectomy. However, the cure rate of 72% achieved by LEROUX-ROBERT with frontolateral partial laryngectomy approximately corresponds to our own results. The technique of vertical partial laryngectomy according to OGURA (1970) and SOM (1951) seems to be more suitable to control squamous cell carcinomas of the anterior laryngeal wall. The above-mentioned case in which the tumour turned out histologically not to be completely resected, there was extensive deep infiltration of the tumour in the area of the lateral thyroarytenoid muscle which was not made apparent by impaired motility of the vocal cord at the preoperative examination. Fifty percent of the cases of histologically proven lymph node metastasis occurred in the group of patients treated by this technique; this must be considered as incidental in a total collective of 390 cases, but gives rise to reflections about the indication for neck dissection in patients with T1b and T2 carcinomas.

Obviously, the extended vertical partial laryngectomies according to HAUTANT and to GLUCK and SOERENSEN cannot completely control multilateral supraglottic and subglottic spread of carcinomas. With only one exception, the residual tumours observed in these cases were located in the anterior laryngeal wall. One of them extended into the supraglottic region. In the remaining 17 cases the tumour extended beyond the resection line into the anterior subglottic wall and the contralateral vocal cord area. The reason may be the paramedian incision which runs close to the midline in both techniques. Our morphological studies (MEYER-BREITING and SCHNEIDER 1981) have shown that carcinomas at the anterior subglottic wall have a much earlier tendency to involve the laryngeal framework at the lower rim of the thyroid cartilage and the adjacent areas of the cricothyroid membrane. Thus the possibility of prelaryngeal penetration must always be taken into consideration when endolaryngeal extension of the tumour necessitates resection of part of the cricoid cartilage. In these cases, in which clinical staging may be problematic, the tumour has reached the T4 category and can be safely controlled only by laryngectomy, an opinion we share with other authors. This holds all the more true since the extended vertical partial laryngectomies completely fail to consider the structure and function of the endolaryngeal lymphatic system. According to MOST (1899), PRESSMAN et al. (1960), WELSH et al. (1961) and BECK and MANN (1980), lymphatic drainage in the subglottic area, especially at the anterior wall, has a more horizontal course without separation at the midline. According to our observation, this favours the multilateral submucosal spread of carcinomas from the anterior commissure and their growth from the free edge of the vocal cord into the subglottic space. HARRISON (1979) has pointed out the risk of underestimating intrinsic factors of laryngeal carcinomas when the TNM system is used exclusively. In 12 of 390 patients we were able to verify lymph node metastasis histologically. In four of these cases metastasis was suspected clinically before surgery, whereas in 8 cases metastasis was discovered postoperatively by histology. Apart from the fact that the tumours were T2 carcinomas with mostly subglottic extension, it seems to be of interest that they either had a low degree of differentiation (BRODERS' grade III) or showed a distinctly more aggressive growth than most of the other squamous cell carcinomas. Grade II carcinomas of this group had a striking tendency towards infiltration of lymphatic clefts and vessels. Our observations are in accordance with the findings of MCGAVRAN (1961) and GLANZ (1981, 1984).

Control of the tumour must be the paramount objective of oncology. Function-preserving aspects must rank second. Accordingly, the results of our conservative surgery of the larynx have to be measured by the yardstick of whether another procedure, in particular total laryngectomy, could have saved the patient's life. Furthermore in each individual patient the decision has to be made which technique of partial laryngectomy is appropriate. From the clinical data and histological examination in our patients we come to the following conclusions:

1. Cordectomy is the classical operations for T1a carcinomas.
2. T1b and early T2 carcinomas of the vocal cord require partial vertical laryngectomy (modification of the method of Som 1951 and Ogura 1970). All tumours that are more extensive should be treated by total laryngectomy.
3. Since the chances of cure are distinctly poorer in patients with residual tumour tissue and/or local recurrences, conservative surgery of the larynx should be performed only if thorough histological examination of the surgical specimens in serial sections is possible.
4. The cytological and histological features of a tumour, i.e. degree of differentiation, aggressiveness and tumour-host relationship, like pattern of invasion, should receive greater attention. If aggressive behaviour must be expected, possibilities for a more radical therapeutic approach, in particular preventive neck dissection, should definitely be considered.

Laser therapy of glottic carcinomas, described more frequently in the past few years (Strong 1975, Vaughan et al. 1980, Steiner 1980, 1984), can at the most be accepted for very small tumours situated on the free edge of the vocal fold (Rudert 1985). This method is technically no better than the commonly used endolaryngeal surgery, simply more spectacular. The view that papillary squamous cell carcinomas present a particular indication for laser surgery owing to their histological characteristics (Grossenbacher 1985) is not justified; this type of carcinoma often shows true aggressive growth in the depth and then does not differ from other squamous cell carcinomas. Under the premise made at the beginning, namely that each death from carcinoma which could have been prevented by the next more extensive surgical procedure is one too many, we reject at present every form of endolaryngeal resection of glottic carcinomas, with the occasional exceptions of very small carcinomas.

6.2.2 Conservative Surgery of Supraglottic Cancer

6.2.2.1 Techniques

From January 1966 to June 1982, 48 patients with supraglottic carcinomas, about a fifth of all patients with tumours in this location, were treated at the Frankfurt University ENT Clinic by conservative surgery of the larynx. This is only a small part of all supraglottic carcinomas treated by us (Table 6.5). The techniques used were:

1. Epiglottectomy
2. Lateral pharyngotomy
3. Subtotal supraglottic horizontal laryngectomy (Alonso 1947, Bocca 1968, 1975, Montgomery 1973, Naumann 1972, Denecke 1980)

6.2.2.2 Surgical Procedures and Results

Epiglottectomy was performed in only four patients, all in the early years of the study, being abandoned in favour of horizontal supraglottic laryngectomy on the basis of the treatment failures (Table 6.6). Very small cancers of the aryepiglottic fold were locally resected via **pharyngotomy** in three patients. One of them died due to tumour recurrence, and one residual tumour verified by histology could be controlled by total laryngectomy and postoperative irradiation. These two techniques are not to be recommended and will not be discussed further. The same applies to endolaryngeal laser therapy of supraglottic carcinomas.

Our indications for **supraglottic horizontal laryngectomy** were, up to 1979, very restrictive; this technique was applied only for purely epiglottic carcinomas (T1 and T3 with invasion of the preepiglottic space). Only in the past few years has our approach changed to include neighbouring areas (Table 6.6).

Table 6.5. TNM classification of 250 patients with supraglottic carcinoma who underwent combined radiosurgical treatment (ENT Department of Frankfurt University Hospital 1966-1982)

	T1	T2	T3	T4	Total
N0	17	33	67	26	143
N1	3	9	26	20	58
N2	1	4	20	14	39
N3	0	0	5	5	10
Total	21	46	108	65	250
N1-3	19%	28%	43%	60%	43%

Table 6.6. Conservative surgery of supraglottic carcinoma: results of treatment by radiosurgical combination therapy in 49 patients (ENT Department of Frankfurt University Hospital 1966–1982)

	Number of operations	Residual tumour	Recurrences		Death with evidence of tumour
			Local	Regional	
Epiglottectomy	4	3	0	0	0
Pharyngotomy	3	1	1	0	1
Supraglottic laryngectomy	37	5	5	1	6
Including base of tongue	3	0	0	0	0
With arytenoid cartilage	1	0	0	0	0
Total	48	9	6	1	7

Four patients died without evidence of tumour and one is lost to follow-up

In five patients, residual tumour tissue was located in front of the arytenoid cartilage and in the oropharyngeal wall (lateral glossoepiglottic fold). Recurrences were primarily in the lateral retrolingual region and the lateral pharyngeal wall. The analysis carried out by SERAFINI (1984) of 16 local recurrences among 180 patients treated by supraglottic horizontal laryngectomy, where the indication in patients with caudal extension was apparently more generous than was the case with our patients, showed that recurrences can be avoided if the extension of the tumour in this area is correctly assessed. The extension of the supraglottic horizontal laryngectomy to include the arytenoid region and the base of the tongue in cases with involvement of these areas had no detrimental aspects. Adding together the cases with residual tumours detected by serial section and the cases with later recurrence, the recurrence rate in our patients is similar to that reported by other authors for this surgical procedure (COATES et al. 1976, VEGA 1984, STEINER 1984). But since in our study only patients with recurrences succumbed to the tumour, not those with secondary surgery for residual tumour tissue, it is clear just how essential a careful and painstaking histological examination of the resected material is. Unfortunately local lymphatic dissemination is not detectable by this means. The location of the recurrences in the lateral pharyngeal wall and the base of the tongue, both rich in lymphatic tissue, leads to the conjecture that lymphatic spread may have been involved.

6.2.3 Radical Surgery of Laryngeal and Laryngopharyngeal Cancer

Advanced carcinomas of the larynx and all hypopharyngeal carcinomas are treated by laryngectomy or laryngopharyngectomy, usually combined with neck dissection and with radiotherapy. Early carcinomas in unfavourable locations, for example supraglottic T2 tumours or glottic T1 tumours with affection of the posterior wall, also require laryngectomy, as a rule, but no neck dissection or radiotherapy is necessary in these cases. For further details of laryngectomy and pharyngolaryngectomy we refer the reader to the appropriate surgical manuals (LORÉ 1962, MONTGOMERY 1973, NAUMANN 1972, DENECKE 1980, STELL 1981, SHAW 1981, WHITTAM and WILKINSON 1981).

From 1966 to 1982, 461 laryngectomies and 11 laryngopharyngectomies were performed at the Frankfurt University ENT Clinic. Of these, 83 were operations following unsuccessful conservative surgery of the larynx and radiotherapy (Table 6.7). Figure 6.5 illustrates the most frequent areas in which recurrences may occur after partial and total laryngectomy.

In patients with **supraglottic carcinomas** complete resection of the tumour was not accomplished in 14 cases. Residual tumour tissue was detected on the lateral portion of the base of the tongue in six and on the lateral oropharyngeal wall in five cases. These were all T4 tumours with extension into the oropharnyx or Winkel carcinomas (see Sect. 5.2.1) which extended cranially via the pharyngoepiglottic fold. In three cases with a more laterodorsal spread, the tumour extensions reached down as far as the cricothyroid joint and there led to local recurrences in the hypopharynx. Recurrences in the oropharynx in cases with tumour-free resection lines were estab-

Table 6.7. Indications for 472 laryngectomies and laryngopharyngectomies performed between 1966 and 1982 (ENT Department of Frankfurt University Hospital)

	Main location of cancer			
	Glottic	Supraglottic	Subglottic	Hypopharynx
Primary therapy	103	202	6	68
Salvage after				
Conservative surgery	51	15		
Radiotherapy	21	6		
Total	175	223	6	68

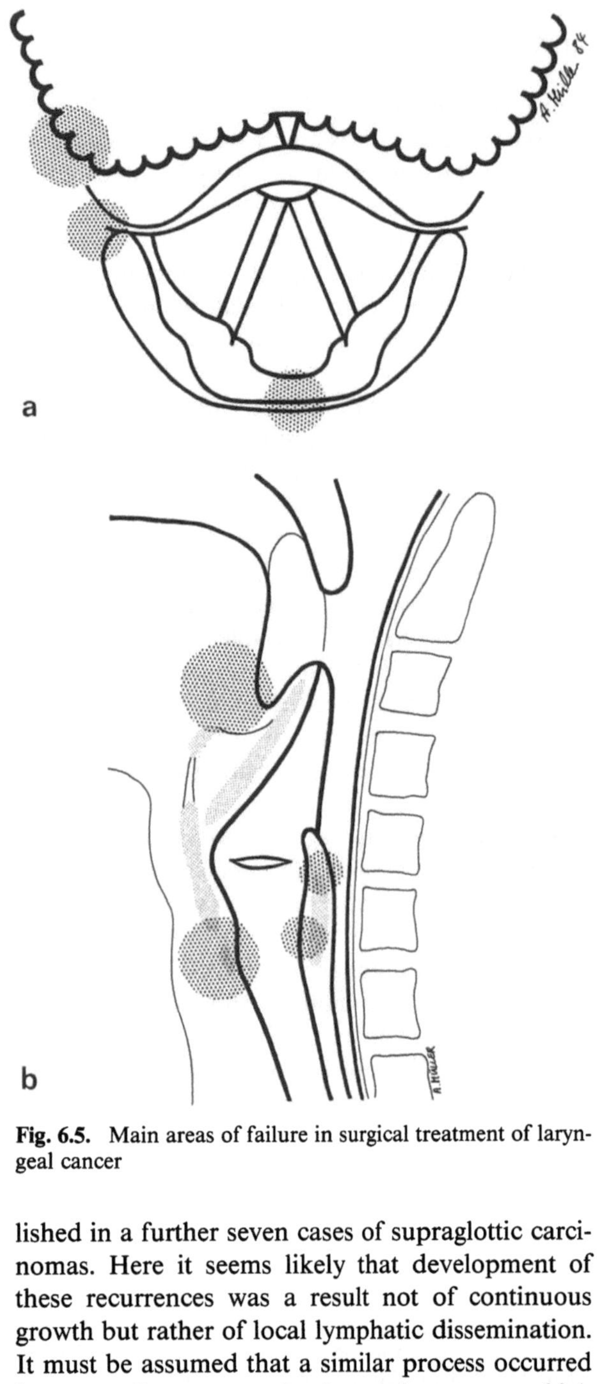

Fig. 6.5. Main areas of failure in surgical treatment of laryngeal cancer

lished in a further seven cases of supraglottic carcinomas. Here it seems likely that development of these recurrences was a result not of continuous growth but rather of local lymphatic dissemination. It must be assumed that a similar process occurred in cases of recurrence in the tracheostoma, which likewise developed without any indication of residual tumour tissue in the surgical specimen.

Glottic carcinomas tend to local recurrence only when there is extensive spreading in a craniocaudal direction or when spreading extends to the posterior laryngeal wall. The preferred location of recurrence was the tracheostoma. Nevertheless, only in two of five cases were we able to demonstrate an incomplete resection of the tumour. In the other three cases, it must be assumed, as already mentioned, that there was local lymphatic spread (KLEINSASSER and MAJDID 1969). Only one patient had a recurrence in the hypopharynx: this was a carcinoma with infiltration of the cricoid lamina.

Among the **subglottic carcinomas**, two developed recurrences in the tracheostoma, one of which resulted from incomplete resection of the primary tumour, as shown histologically. This tumour had grown so far in the direction of the trachea, however, that complete resection was no longer possible.

The **oropharyngeal carcinomas** of the base of the tongue and the valleculae were resected completely in only two cases residual tumour tissue being detected in the lateral part of the base of the tongue. We did not see any recurrences.

The **hypopharyngeal carcinomas** could be resected completely with one exception: the residual tumour tissue in this case was found in the upper oesophagus. Recurrences occurred twice on the upper edge of the tracheostoma, twice in the tonsils and once in the retrolingual region. In the last-named case local lymphatic dissemination could be involved.

6.2.4 Management of Regional Metastasis

When the preepiglottic, paraglottic and lower subglottic spaces are affected, the prognosis of the patients is worsened less by limitations on surgical removal of the primary tumour than by the associated tendency towards metastasis into the regional lymph nodes.

All patients with primary subglottic, supraglottic, hypopharyngeal and oropharyngeal carcinomas, as well as glottic T3 and T4 carcinomas, at the Frankfurt University ENT Clinic are subjected to **elective neck dissection** even without lymph node metastasis being suspected. On the basis of our histological findings on the incidence and location of lymph node metastasis in relation to the site of the primary tumour, we consider **bilateral neck dissection** to be necessary in case of proven unilateral lymph node metastasis in the following carcinomas:

1. Carcinomas with subglottic-tracheal spreading
2. Supraglottic carcinomas with ventral spreading
3. Hypopharyngeal carcinomas
4. Caudal oropharyngeal carcinomas

In 1979 we reported on an increased frequency of regional recurrences in the submandibular region and the lower parotid pole in patients with supraglottic carcinomas (MEYER-BREITING and VON ILBERG 1979). We made similar observations with other carcinomas when the paraglottic space was infiltrated as well as with caudal oropharyngeal carcinomas. Since 1977, in all these cases this region has been resected in addition, and this has led to a convincing decrease in regional recurrences in this area. Lymph node metastasis in the submandibular region has not occurred, and metastasis to the lower section of the parotid gland has been observed only in three patients with hypopharyngeal carcinomas.

BOCCA (1981) described **functional neck dissection** and proposed that this technique is universally applicable. We do not agree, and apply it only to elective neck dissection and in cases without involvement of the upper jugular lymph node group. This is based on the histological observation that in isolated cases, small lymph nodes with tumour metastasis are found in the sternocleidomastoid muscle at the site where the accessory nerve enters the muscle. Therefore, when the upper jugular lymph node is affected, performance of **radical neck dissection** with the sacrifice of this nerve is in our experience mandatory. Contralateral neck dissection can, as a rule, be performed 6 weeks after the primary neck dissection without significant problems. In isolated cases, **simultaneous bilateral neck dissection** with unilateral preservation of the internal jugular vein may prove necessary when there is histological proof of bilateral lymph node involvement. We have had no adverse experience with this procedure.

6.3 Radiation Therapy

6.3.1 The Biology of Irradiated Tumours

In order to facilitate the understanding of the morphological changes in squamous cell carcinomas, described in more detail below, we shall deal first with the basic effects of radiation on living tissue (see Sect. 7.3).

The exact site at which radiation induces cell damage or death has still not been ascertained. Most probable is damage to the nucleus, more exactly to the DNA of which it is known that molecular changes can lead to mutation and/or to cell death (STREFFER 1969, ALTMANN et al. 1970). Investigations by HOWARD and PELC (1953) showed that all cells undergo generation cycles with phases of different length; these are, in part, of critical importance for synthesis of DNA (Fig. 6.6). In detail in proliferating cells the sequence of events is as follows:

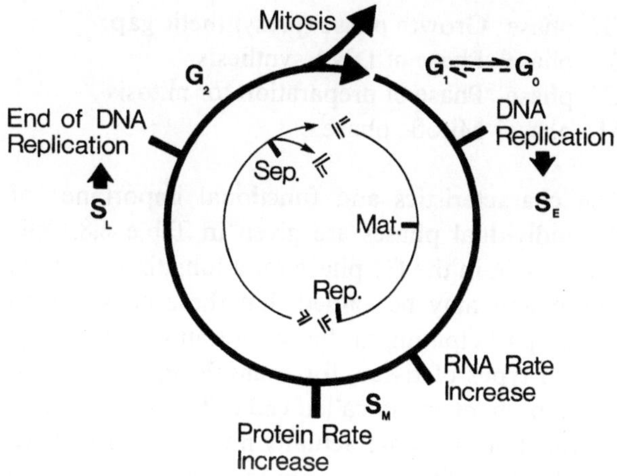

Fig. 6.6. Cell proliferation cycle (HOWARD and PELC 1953)

Table 6.8. Characteristics and properties of the stages of the cell cycle (According to KOLLMORGEN and BEDFORD 1973)

G_1 phase
- Cells which lose proliferative ability (muscle, nerve) leave the cell cycle in G_1 and enter G_0.
  - Enzymes necessary for DNA synthesis (kinase, polymerase, synthetase, desaminase) are synthesized. All species of RNA are made.
  - In renewing tissues, the rate of renewal is partially regulated by retention of cells in G_1.
  - Mammalian cells in embryogenesis, as well as some protozoa, slime molds and bacteria, have no G_1.
  - Histone acetylation and phosphorylation are probably initiated.
  - Synthesis of regular proteins which initiate DNA synthesis probably occurs.

S phase
- Synthesis of chromosomal DNA occurs.
- Maturation of daughter centrioles occurs.
  - Centriole reproduction begins.
  - Histone synthesis und other protein synthesis necessary to maintain DNA synthesis occurs.
  - Rate of RNA synthesis is about the same as during G_1 and G_2.

G_2 phase
- Centrioles separate into two pairs.
  - Proteins required for mitosis are synthesized.
  - RNA required to direct protein synthesis necessary for mitosis is synthesized.

M phase
- RNA synthesis ceases.
  - Protein synthesis decreases.
  - Condensation and segregation of DNA along with associated RNA and proteins occurs.

G1 phase	Growth phase (presynthetic gap)
S phase	Phase of DNA synthesis
G2 phase	Phase of preparation for mitosis
M phase	Mitotic phase

The characteristics and functional importance of the individual phases are given in Table 6.8. Cells can remain in the G1 phase for a long time, and the impression may be gained that these cells are no longer participating in the proliferation process. In certain types of tissue, for example squamous epithelium, there are so-called **end cells** with a particular function; they are actually no longer capable of proliferating. Other cells are in a resting condition from which they can again be mobilized for proliferation; these are said to be in the G0 phase. Determinations of the cell cycle times can be made using various methods which have been reported in more detail by SCHULTZE (1968). The length of the S, G2 and M phases is considered to be relatively constant (TUBIANA 1970). The length of the G1 phase, or rather the persistence of cells in the G0 phase, is dependent mainly, in non-neoplastic cells, on the rapidity with which cell death has to be compensated for by cell proliferation. For the volume of a given tissue there are two primary factors of significance: growth fraction and cell loss. Tumour tissue is no longer subjected to functional regulation of growth, and the "growth fraction" as a rule is larger than the cell loss. The ratio of growth fraction to cell loss is not constant, however, but dependent upon a series of other factors which in part are associated with the growth of the tumour itself (TUBIANA 1970). STEEL (1968) and DENEKAMP (1970) showed that with an increase in tumour cell loss, the doubling time of the tumour volume is prolonged. High rates of cell loss have been observed especially in carcinomas (FOWLER et al. 1971). Figure 6.7 shows an infiltrating squamous cell carcinoma marked by an antiproliferation antibody (Ki67). Only a small layer of cells is pink-stained (black in Fig. 6.7) representing the proliferating i.e. growth-fraction. They mostly surround the other, nonproliferating (colourless) cells characterized by a higher degree of differentiation of squamous epithelium (LÖRZ and MEYER-BREITING 1987). Besides the extent of differentiation of the carcinoma, nutritional factors, in particular oxygen supply, determine the tumour's rate of cell loss. HERMENS and BARENDSEN (1969) and SHIRAKAWA et al. (1970) demonstrated a decrease in the labelling index from the periphery of the tumour to its centre. This means that in deficient nutritional conditions, increasing numbers of cells are taken from the growth fraction and are transferred to the G0 phase. If the oxygen concentration in the centre of the tumour decreases further, cell death can ensue. Conversely, with an improvement in the nutritional situation the G0 cells again enter the proliferative G1 phase. On this basis it is possible to explain the direct oxygen dependence of the radiosensitivity of malignant tumours shown by HOLDHUSEN (1921) and GRAY et al. (1953). We shall only mention here the importance of the reoxygenation phenomenon (THOMLINSON 1968) and the variable radiosensitivity of tumours.

According to the rule of BERGONIÉ and TRIBONDEAU (1906) tumours with a low degree of differentiation and rapid growth exhibit high radiosensitivity; thus the proliferation and the generation cycle of tumour cells must be of particular importance as regards the effect of radiation. The effect of radiation is strongest if synchronized cells in the G2 and late S phases are irradiated (SINCLAIR 1968, THOMPSON and SUIT 1969). Even if cells in the other two phases are irradiated, there is a protraction of the S and G2 phases, i.e. the period in which the doubling of the DNA helix and the preparation for mitosis occur (ALTMANN et al. 1970). In general, G1 cells are to a large extent radioresistant. The radiosensitivity constantly increases at the transition from the G1 to the S phase, and declines again at the end of the S phase. During the G2 phase radiosensitivity is again increased, reaching a peak in the mitotic phase. Cells in G0 are regarded as especially radioresistant. Basically, however, these cells should be viewed as cells with a remarkably long growth phase which corresponds to the G1 phase. The data obtained up till now on the radiosensitivity of cells in the G0/G1 phase are, however, contradictory (Streffer 1980).

6.3.2 Histological Changes in Irradiated Carcinomas

An understandable wish of the oncological practitioner is that the pathologist should be able to recognize the radioresistance or radiosensitivity of a malignant neoplasm. Changes caused by radiation occur in the individual cell, but by a variety of factors certain patterns of alterations may result throughout the tumour; in particular, the success of radiation depends on the nutritional condition of the tumour. If valid, the rule established by

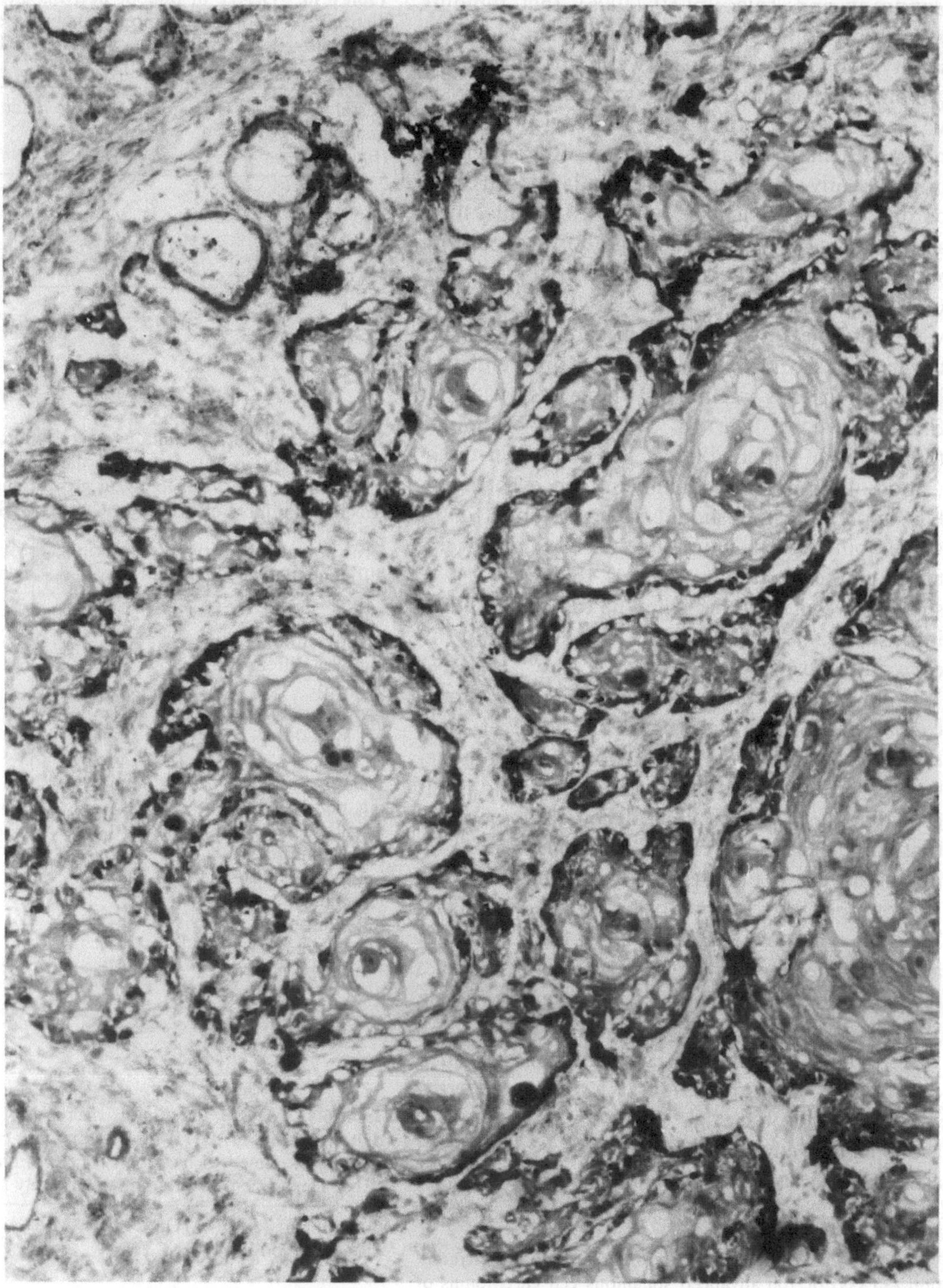

Fig. 6.7. Infiltrating squamous cell carcinoma marked by an antiproliferation antibody (Ki67). Only a small layer of cells is pink-stained *(black)* representing the proliferating, i.e. growth fraction of the tumour. These mostly surround the other non-proliferating colourless cells characterized by a higher degree of differentiation of squamous epithelium (LÖRZ and MEYER-BREITING 1988)

Bergonié and Tribondeau (1906), that tumours with a lower differentiation exhibit higher radiosensitivity, should provide an answer to the question of tumour irradiation response. According to Hansemann (1890), the proliferative activity of a malignant epithelial neoplasm increases with a decrease in the relative number of differentiated cells. According to Bergonié and Tribondeau's rule, then, a squamous cell carcinoma of grade IV should respond better to irradiation than one of grade I or II. Olofsson and van Nostrand (1973), however, were not able to establish such a relationship between radiosensitivity and degree of differentiation in squamous cell carcinomas; this agrees with our findings (Meyer-Breiting 1981b). In addition to the degree of differentiation, the peripheral dissociation of a tumour apparently influences its vascular supply, and this should have relevance for its vulnerability to irradiation in terms of a "periphery-basis gradient" (see page 131). Tables 6.9–6.12 show, however, that this is not the case; in addition, intrinsic factors of the tumour must exert an influence on radiosensitivity.

From our first studies of glottic and supraglottic carcinomas (Meyer-Breiting 1977), however, there appeared to be a certain correlation between the response of squamous cell carcinomas and their growth pattern. It has been a general experience that papillary and "verrucous" squamous cell carcinomas have low radiosensitivity (Ackerman 1948, Kraus and Perez-Mesa 1966, Biller et al. 1971, Demian et al. 1973, Elliot et al. 1973, Ryan et al. 1977). This agrees with our observations; only a few authors are of the opposite opinion (Rider 1976, Schwade et al. 1976).

Reports of anaplastic transformations of such carcinomas with irradiation (Kraus and Perez-Mesa 1966, Fonts et al. 1969, Biller et al. 1971) are to be viewed with caution. We also saw isolated anaplastic areas in nonirradiated carcinomas dis-

Table 6.9. Pattern of tumour necrosis after low-dose irradiation (30 Gy) of 100 advanced squamous cell carcinomas of the larynx related to Broders grading (ENT Department of Frankfurt University Hospital)

Histological grading (Broders)	Periphery eliminated	Periphery rarified	Mixed pattern	Diffused spotted
I	5	3	2	2
II	35	13	15	8
III	–	2	4	7
IV	–	–	2	3

Table 6.10. Degree of tumour necrosis after low-dose irradiation (30 Gy) of 100 advanced squamous cell carcinomas of the larynx related to Broders grading (ENT Department of Frankfurt University Hospital)

Histological grading (Broders)	High grade	Middle grade	Low grade or no reaction
I	8	2	2
II	48	18	5
III	1	5	7
IV	–	2	3

Table 6.11. Pattern of tumour necrosis after low-dose irradiation (30 Gy) of 100 advanced squamous cell carcinomas of the larynx related to histological growth and differentiation (ENT Department of Frankfurt University Hospital)

Growth and differentiation	Periphery eliminated	Periphery rarified	Mixed pattern	Diffuse spotted
Papillary	–	1	4	4
Lightly infiltrating, well differentiated	38	12	8	1
Densely infiltrating, well differentiated	1	3	5	3
Densely infiltrating, poorly differentiated	–	1	2	4
Lightly infiltrating, poorly differentiated	1	1	2	5
Solid and/or anaplastic	–	–	2	3

Table 6.12. Degree of tumour necrosis after low-dose irradiation (30 Gy) of 100 advanced squamous cell carcinomas of the larynx related to histological growth and differentiation (ENT Department of Frankfurt University Hospital)

Growth and differentiation	High grade	Middle grade	Low grade or no reaction
Papillary	1	5	3
Lightly infiltrating, well differentiated	52	7	–
Densely infiltrating, well differentiated	3	7	2
Densely infiltrating, poorly differentiated	1	3	3
Lightly infiltrating, poorly differentiated	–	3	6
Solid and/or anaplastic	–	2	3

playing this growth pattern. Since these carcinomas have a high degree of differentiation and a low tendency to proliferate, BERGONIÉ and TRIBONDEAU's rule seems to be in accordance with these observations.

However, this lack of responsiveness does not apply to well-differentiated squamous cell carcinomas (grade I and some grade II) with a nonverrucous or nonpapillary growth pattern. On the contrary, these show the most pronounced regression following irradiation. As can be seen from Fig. 6.8 a,c, the central, differentiating cells are the first to be eradicated in the peripheral extensions of carcinomas of this grade, showing cloudy swelling, hyalinization, eosinophilic necrosis and pronounced keratinization. Essentially this process is a devitalization of the tumour by keratinization, apparently induced by radiation (GLÜCKSMANN 1946, HALL and FRIEDMANN 1948, MICHAELS 1975, BURKHARDT 1980). This process, which occurs spontaneously in well-differentiated squamous cell carcinomas too, is also termed radiation keratogenesis (CROSSLAND 1962). But it is difficult to decide, in individual cases, to what extent such alterations have been induced by radiation and to what extent they are spontaneous. A narrow rim of small cells with a high nucleocytoplasmic ratio and nuclear hyperchromatism primarily remains vital. Being next to the stroma, these cells are most probably only secondarily affected by radiation. Especially in these squamous cell carcinomas with a high degree of differentiation and keratinization, multinuclear giant cells, often in clusters, are observed (GLÜCKSMANN 1959, GOLDMAN et al. 1969, BURKHARDT 1980). LELBACH (1955) considered these the lethal form of irradiated tumour cells. GOLDMAN et al. (1964, 1966, 1972), in contrast, interpreted them as foreign body giant cells. BURKHARDT et al. (1976) and BURKHARDT and GEBBERS (1977) were able to demonstrate, both enzyme-histochemically and by electron microscopy, their formation from monocytes and mononuclear phagocytes and their functional specialization for degradation of keratin lamellae. BURKHARDT et al. (1976) were not able to demonstrate on the ultrastructural level any structures whatsoever which were reminiscent of desmosomes, tonofilaments or other cell structures considered to be characteristic of epithelial cells. In the less differentiated squamous cell carcinomas, giant cells are seldom observed.

Changes caused by intrinsic properties of the carcinoma must be differentiated from radiation-induced alterations. In **differentiated tumours**, carcinoma cell groups in the centre may spontaneously undergo the ordinary maturation of squamous epithelium. Correspondingly, some of the cells keratinize and die. These changes caused by inversion (VON ALBERTINI 1974) can be recognized easily by their central position. Crucial in such cases is whether the "tumour matrix", i.e. the stem cell compartment, likewise matures. This does not usually occur spontaneously, but can happen in well-differentiated tumours (but not in papillary squamous cell carcinomas) after irradiation. There is often a typical pattern of radiation response: in the outermost tumour periphery there are concentric areas of granulation tissue of varying age containing multinuclear giant cells. In the centre of such zones eosinophilic cell detritus and horn lamellae can usually still be seen (Fig. 6.8 a). Towards the actual tumour centre, i.e. the tumour basis, the cytological changes described above are pronounced. Generally the nuclear atypia and the mitotic activity appear to be lower than in nonirradiated carcinomas of the same differentiation.

The behaviour of squamous cell carcinomas of grade II is very variable and to a certain extent dependent on the growth pattern. Carcinomas with **compact growth pattern** at the time of diagnosis are usually already in an advanced stage, completely filling one or two of the above-mentioned endolaryngeal spaces and in contact with the skeletomembraneous borders. They show a nonhomogeneous pattern of radiation response, which probably arises for several reasons. One of the most important is probably the tendency of advanced squamous cell carcinomas of the larynx towards "self-strangulation". It is conceivable that restricted growth, confinement for a certain time to a limited space, results in compression of supply vessels and thus impairment of nutrition. As a consequence, such poorly supplied regions may exhibit necrotic areas. The surviving cells remain in the G0 phase and are thus largely removed from the effect of the radiation. This tendency to self-strangulation is a phenomenon reflecting the anatomical peculiarity of the larynx and cannot be readily applied to other regions. A further explanation for the variable response pattern is that larger and more advanced squamous cell carcinomas also show considerable variations of growth pattern and degree of differentiation. It is noteworthy that in these carcinomas with solid growth, there persists a narrow peripheral rim of small cells with scanty cytoplasm and

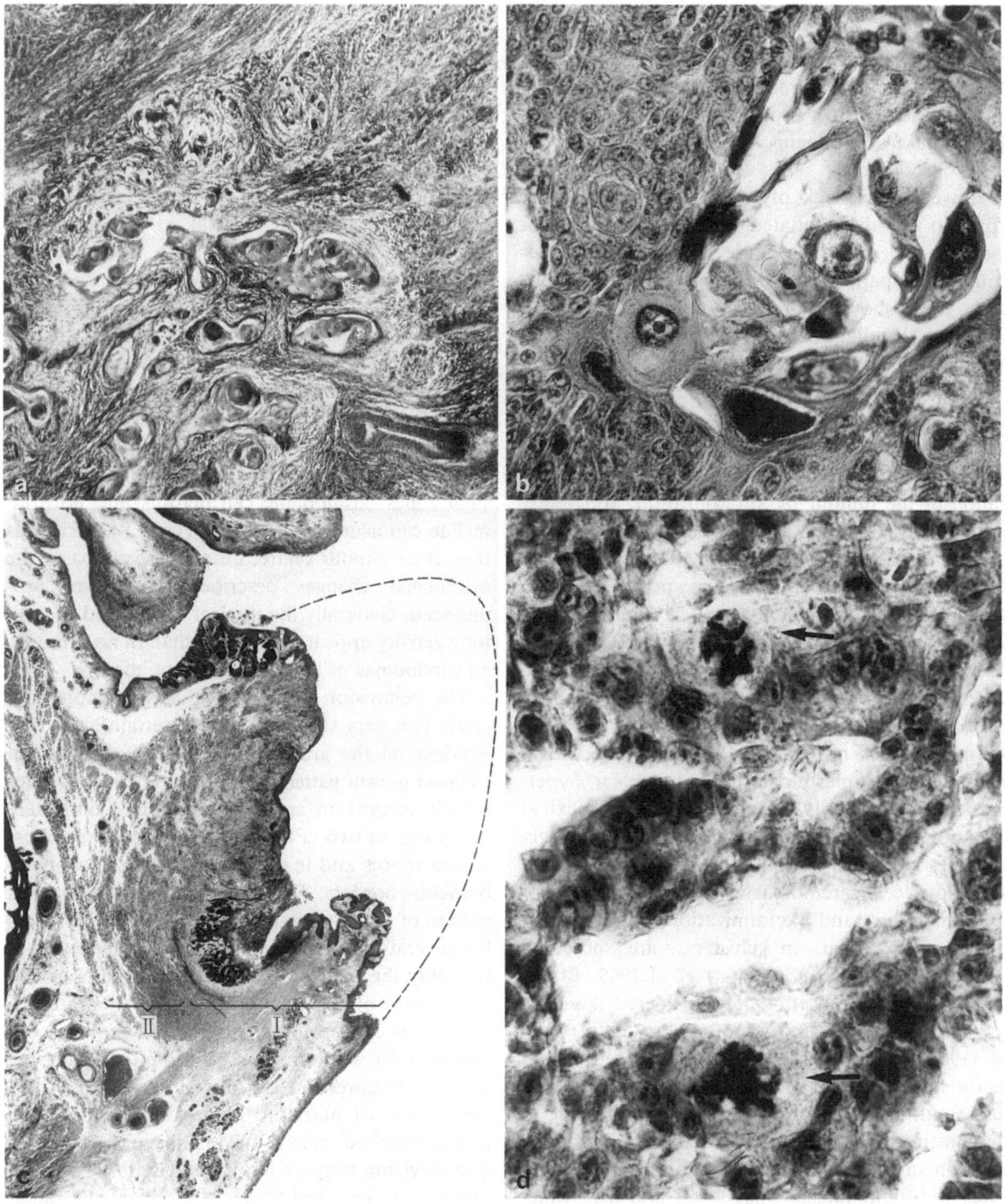

Fig. 6.8 a–d. Histomorphological alterations in preoperatively irradiated (30 Gy) squamous cell carcinomas of the larynx. **a** Peripheral extensions of a well-differentiated carcinoma. In these extensions the central, differentiating cells are the first to be eradicated showing cloudy swelling, hyalinization, eosinophilic necrosis and pronounced keratinization. HE, ×125. **b** Radiation-induced cellular changes in a poorly differentiated carcinoma. Enlarged cells with cytoplasm and nuclei achieving 3–6 times their original volume are numerous. Some nuclei lose their sharp boundary to the cytoplasm and kariolysis ensues. Structural changes in the chromatin can be seen in the nuclei of such cells: a shapeless mass of chromatin finally clumps together. HE, ×500. **c** Survey of a preoperatively irradiated glottic carcinoma, (30 Gy). *Area I* shows within the *broken line* the former shape of the glottic region, destroyed by carcinoma and irradiation. In this area residues of the tumour can be found. *Area II* consists of granulation tissue with multinuclear giant cells and debris of necrotic cells. Coronal section. HE, ×10. **d** Radiation-induced cellular changes in a poorly differentiated carcinoma. Mitotic figures. The chromosomes exhibit severed chromatin pieces which are connected only by narrow bridges or lie isolated in the cytoplasm. In giant nuclei, the mitotic figures are often multistranded or clumped together. HE, ×500

intensely staining nuclei; the nuclei exhibit a polar orientation to the stroma. The entire centre of the tumour mass, however, is necrotic.

In **dissociated carcinomas**, it is noticeable that there is no complete necrosis of the tumour cells in the peripheral extensions. Epidermoid stratification may be found but maturation and keratinization are rare. Cells of the basal, parabasal and intermediary cellular layer predominate and show only slight changes when irradiated. The dominant cell type is of average size, with large, intensely staining nuclei. This is the same type of cells surviving in the periphery of the carcinomas of compact growth pattern. We saw such cells most often in carcinomas which had been primarily irradiated with 60 Gy without success.

The same variable response pattern can be observed in **less differentiated and anaplastic carcinomas (grade III and IV)** which have reached a size necessitating laryngectomy. Owing to its poor vascular supply, the tumour is forced to maintain its growth fraction at a low level until more favourable nutritional conditions prevail. This can, for example, be accomplished by penetration of the tumour towards the prelaryngeal region and access to a better vascular supply, in which case marked proliferation may ensue again.

In **poorly differentiated carcinomas**, growing in solid formations or loosely disseminated in lymphatic clefts, diffuse foci with degenerative nuclear and cytoplasmic changes are found. Maturation as described for more differentiated carcinomas is virtually never seen. Enlarged cells with cytoplasm and nuclei achieving 3-6 times their original volume are numerous (Fig. 6.8 b). With time, the nucleus loses its sharp boundary to the cytoplasm and kariolysis ensues. Further, structural changes in the chromatin can be seen in the nuclei of such cells: a shapeless mass of chromatin finally clumps together. In mitotic figures, the chromosomes often exhibit severed chromatin pieces which are connected to one another only by narrow bridges or lie isolated in the cytoplasm. In giant nuclei, the mitotic figures are often multistranded or clumped together (Fig. 6.8 d). There are always vacuoles of varying size to be seen in the nuclei. The cytoplasmic boundaries become less and less clear during swelling until cytolysis results. The cytoplasm loses its internal structure in the course of these changes and becomes increasingly eosinophilic.

The scope of histomorphological assessment of radiotherapeutic effects is limited. Discrimination between vital and necrotic cells can be achieved more exactly by means of autoradiography than normal histology, but most autoradiographic studies restrict themselves to small pieces of tissue or cell suspensions which can hardly be representative of an entire tumour. Following initial unsuccessful experiments, OLOFSSON and VAN NOSTRAND (1973) stopped trying to examine the whole larynx autoradiographically. Our own efforts with such investigations also foundered because of technical difficulties. Morphometric determination and comparison of vital and necrotic tumour areas is not very meaningful, for two reasons. First, the technical problem of depicting these areas as exactly as necessary in a large piece of tissue, such as the larynx, has not been solved. Secondly, it remains exceedingly speculative just which region within a granulation tissue was originally true tumour and which region was tumour stroma with a lymphoplasmacellular reaction. Reports of morphometric studies (SCHUMANN et al. 1980) should thus be evaluated with appropriate reservation.

6.3.3 Preoperative Irradiation

So far there is no general agreement regarding the combination of surgery and radiation. The radiotherapist expects the maximal effect of his treatment in a tumour tissue with an intact stroma and favourable nutritional conditions. This is undoubtedly not the case immediately after surgery. In the stage of wound healing roughly between the 4th and 10th postoperative days, in which the vascular supply of any residual tumour cells is most favourable, irradiation is out of question since it would impair the healing process to an inestimable extent. During the later course of wound healing, however, there ensues an intensive vascular depletion and scarring of the tissue (HEGEMANN 1967, ZOLLINGER 1969, COTTIER 1980), which also impairs the nutrition of the residual tumour cells and thus reduces the prospects of effective postoperative irradiation. These disadvantages are assumed to be overcome with preoperative irradiation which has the following concept and aims (LEICHER 1963, POWERS 1968, KROKOWSKI 1971, SCHERER 1980):

1. Delimitation and reduction of the tumour based on the assumption that cells in the tumour periphery have a relatively better nutritional situation and are more radiosensitive than the cells of the tumour basis or tumour "nucleus"

2. Prevention of local recurrences by elimination of peripheral tumour cells which have already gained access to the lymph tract in the vicinity of the primary tumour
3. Prevention of metastasis by damage to tumour cells which by subsequent surgical manipulation might possibly have been dispersed into the lymph or blood system in the vicinity of the tumour
4. Blockade of the lymph vessels

Just how much relevance these theoretical considerations have for clinical practice can be proven by morphological investigations of the surgical specimens or statistical analysis of postoperative follow-up. Morphologically it has to be shown, on the basis of the extent and pattern of radiation effects on tumour tissue, whether the described aims of the preoperative radiation have been attained. Most important would be confirmation of the assumption that the tumour periphery (tumour extensions) shows a higher vulnerability to radiation than the tumour centre, i.e. tumour basis. The difference in radiation vulnerability between the centre and the periphery of a tumour will be termed "periphery-basis gradient". The existence of such a gradient of any significance would be essential for the whole concept of preoperative irradiation as it is the foundation of three of the four arguments given above.

6.3.3.1 Histological Changes in Preoperatively Irradiated Carcinomas: The Periphery-Basis Gradient

Tables 6.9-6.12 show the mode of response of 100 squamous cell carcinomas which were preirradiated with 30 Gy (15x2 Gy in 20 days) and were surgically removed within 1 week following irradiation. In assessment of the periphery-basis gradient of radiation vulnerability, as a first step it was simply registered whether such a gradient was recognizable or not. In cases with a recognizable gradient a better radiation effect in the tumour periphery could be presumed, but wether or not this had therapeutic relevance was not yet, taken into account. Less than 50% of such preirradiated carcinomas showed a periphery-basis gradient in their radiation response, and even in those with such a pattern the effect was so slight that this could hardly be considered to have clinical relevance. Similar observations were made by BRYCE and RIDER (1971), OLOFSSON and VAN NOSTRAND (1973) and not least by one of the main advocates of preoperative irradiation of laryngeal carcinomas, namely GOLDMAN himself (GOLDMAN et al. 1972). This is even more noteworthy since GOLDMAN and colleagues had preirradiated with 55 Gy. BRYCE and RIDER (1971) found that of 32 preoperatively irradiated squamous cell carcinomas, 5 regressed completely. In 11 other, the radiation-induced tumour regression was incomplete and irregular, and in 14 only a minimal response could be seen. The expected pattern of radiation response with predominantly peripheral regression, assumed to be of clinical relevance, was found by these authors in only two cases. Of 54 squamous cell carcinomas of the larynx described by OLOFSSON and VAN NOSTRAND (1973), 14 exhibited complete regression, 19 reacted incompletely and a further 19 minimally to radiation. The authors were able to recognize a radiation response pattern with a periphery-basis gradient in only two cases. Among 26 tumours, GOLDMAN et al. (1972) found a complete response in nine and a variable incomplete reaction in 17 cases. These authors expressly pointed out that in all cases with incomplete response, small tumour extensions could be seen right up to the periphery, and these could not with certainty be considered lethally damaged.

In the Frankfurt study of larynges that had been surgically removed owing to failure of radiotherapy, it was as a rule found that the tumour had spread. Thus it could be presumed that the tumour must have regenerated multilaterally: in two of these 10 carcinomas, however, the renewed tumour growth apparently proceeded from only one site. It can be concluded that irradiation with a complete tumour dose in advanced squamous cell carcinomas of the larynx succeeds in tumour eradication only in isolated cases; in most cases, it fails. Contrary to the hopes of the advocates of preoperative irradiation, such failure is due to vitality of residual tumour tissue not only in the centre of the tumour, but also in the periphery. This agrees with the findings of SKOLNIK et al. (1970).

The histologically recognizable changes of squamous cell carcinomas after irradiation and their dependence on the grade of differentiation (Tables 6.9-6.10) have been discussed in detail in Sect. 6.3.2.

The so-called **verrucous carcinomas** (see Sect. 7.1.1.1) or **papillary highly differentiated carcinomas** do not respond very well to radiation, and preoperative irradiation in these tumours cannot be recommended for a number of additional reasons, such as risk of anaplasia and subsequent metastatic potential.

Well-differentiated carcinomas (grade II) with enhanced maturation and "radiation keratogenesis" as a rule, respond well to radiation and exhibit the most extensive changes in the centre. However, a peripheral rim of cells usually remains vital. Probably through selection, this less differentiated "subline" of carcinoma cells is responsible for recurrences, which ensue in the peripheral portion of the tumour.

Moderately differentiated carcinomas (grade III) of both the compact and the dissociated growth pattern tend to central necrosis and proliferation of an anaplastic carcinoma cell subline of the basal-parabasal or intermediary type in the periphery. In carcinomas of **compact growth** type the above-mentioned self-strangulation (see page 131) also has to be taken into consideration, which results in focal necrosis, variations in radiovulnerability of the affected cells and further contributes to a nonhomogeneous response pattern.

In our experience, all **poorly differentiated squamous cell carcinomas** (grade III and IV) tend to a pattern of focal but diffusely distributed radiation response. There is no periphery-basis gradient in these cases. This is true for solid and compactly-growing tumours of this degree of differentiation as well as for dissociated carcinomas with lymphatic spread. No patient with this histological pattern has achieved 3-year survival since radiosurgical combination therapy was started in our clinic. HUDSON and CAVANAUGH reported as early as 1965 on 20 patients with laryngeal carcinomas which had been irradiated with 55 Gy prior to extirpation of the larynx; in all cases of poorly differentiated carcinoma there was residual vital tumour tissue.

In view of the fact that in the Frankfurt University ENT Clinic also patients with early stages of carcinomas exhibited lymphangiosis carcinomatosa after preoperative irradiation, it can be concluded that preoperative irradiation with 30 Gy achieves no effective obliteration of the lymph vessels and thus no blocking of lymphatic metastasis.

6.3.3.2 Regions of Diminished Radiation Effect

In more than half the squamous cell carcinomas with prelaryngeal spread, we observed a marked response to radiation therapy of the endolaryngeal portion of the tumour, while the prelaryngeal tissue exhibited slight or no change whatsoever. This agrees with the clinical experience and the histological results of the investigation of other authors (BRIDGER 1970, KIRCHNER 1970, SOM and SILVER 1968). The customary cross-field irradiation (Fig. 6.9 a) could be responsible for this difference in response. It is easily possible that at times the single radiation fields are shifted too far dorsally, so that a "cold zone" arises here (INCH and MCCREDIE 1963). Accordingly, OLOFSSON et al. (1972) described a modified technique of irradiation (Fig. 6.9 b) with which they were able to obtain better results with primary radiation of tumours displaying prelaryngeal spread. These authors achieved a 5-year cure in more than 50% of the patients with squamous cell carcinomas of the anterior vocal fold commissure, whereas SOM and SILVER (1968) could cure only two of 18 patients and KIRCHNER (1970) five of 13 patients by primary irradiation. WANG

a
b
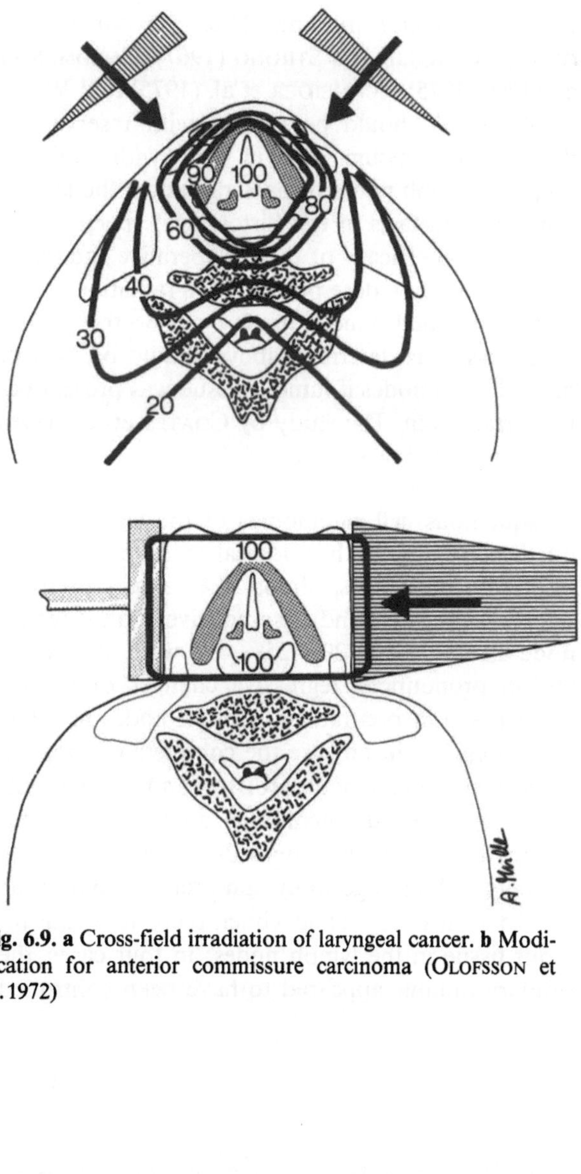

Fig. 6.9. a Cross-field irradiation of laryngeal cancer. **b** Modification for anterior commissure carcinoma (OLOFSSON et al. 1972)

and SCHULTZ (1963) reported a 5-year survival rate of 65% in a study of 34 patients. In 1975 KIRCHNER was able to report better results. Our histological observations relating to variable tissue response of tumours to radiation, however, agree with our disappointing treatment results. We achieved 5-year survival rates of less than 50% in patients with advanced squamous cell carcinomas of the glottic region; these results are worse than in prognostically less favourable supraglottic tumours.

6.3.3.3 Effect of Irradiation on Lymph Node Metastasis

With regard to the histological assessment of the effect of radiation on lymph node metastasis, it is unfortunate that so many authors make no discrimination between the clinical N1 and N2 stages of histologically-proven lymph node metastasis. Nonspecific lymphadenitis is common in tumour patients and this explains the frequent discrepancies between clinical N classification and the subsequent histological finding. Thus the conclusions drawn by CATLIN and STRONG (1967), GOLDMAN et al. (1969, 1975), SCHNEIDER et al. (1975) and WANG et al. (1975) should be viewed with reservation: these authors assume that in cases with clinically palpable lymph nodes prior to radiation, the lack of tumour metastasis in the histological specimens is proof of the efficacy of the preoperative radiation. At least with low-dose preoperative radiation (up to 30 Gy), residual tumour tissue or resorptive granulation tissue as described above should be present in the lymph nodes if tumour tissue was present before irradiation. The study by COATES et al. (1976) and our own investigations (MEYER-BREITING and VON ILBERG 1979) in preirradiated and nonirradiated squamous cell carcinomas of the larynx show, on the basis of the histological study of the neck dissection specimens, almost the same error rate, with false-negative and false-positive clinical lymph node assessment of 20%-25%. We were able to establish pronounced regressive changes of the tumour tissue in preirradiated lymph nodes in a few rare cases, but in no case the complete eradication of the metastatic tumour. HUDSON and CAVANAUGH (1965) in the study mentioned above, carried out prophylactic or curative neck dissection in 18 of 20 patients with laryngectomy and preirradiation of 55 Gy. In 13 histological specimen there was vital tumour tissue in the lymph nodes; in four cases, the primary tumour appeared to have been controlled by surgery. Based on these findings and our own observations, it appears to us that in patients with suspected metastasis in the regional lymph nodes, preoperative irradiation with 30 Gy is not a suitable method of increasing the success of therapy.

6.3.4 Late Results After Preoperative Irradiation of Squamous Cell Carcinomas of the Larynx

6.3.4.1 Local Recurrences

Preoperative irradiation should lead to a significant decline in the number of local recurrences compared to surgery alone and to postoperative irradiation, if the assumption of a special effect of radiation on the peripheral tumour tissue were correct. In experimental investigation with carcinomas in rats and mice, INCH et al. (1963, 1970) actually were able to demonstrate a reduction in the rate of local recurrence by preoperative irradiation. Likewise, BELLI et al. (1970) showed that the shorter the time between irradiation and tumour excision, the more effective the radiation with regard to the prevention of local recurrences. Perusual of some publications with regard to the late results of preoperative high-dose (CONSTABLE et al. 1975, GOLDMAN et al. 1975, SNOW et al. 1980) or low-dose (BILLER et al. 1969, SKOLNIK et al. 1975, MEYER-BREITING 1978) radiotherapy reveals that the rate of local recurrences varies between 6% and 19% in endolaryngeal carcinomas. With hypopharyngeal carcinomas the rate of local recurrences is given as 17% with a preoperative irradiation of 50 Gy (CARPENTER et al. 1976) and as 7% with low-dose preirradiation (BILLER et al. 1969). The high variability of the percentage of local recurrences in these reports must be regarded as the expression of different clinical procedures. To compare different radiosurgical combination procedures, therefore it is, more appropriate to perform comparative studies in one and the same clinic, or randomized studies, as presented by MEYER-BREITING (1978), SCHULLER et al. (1979), SNOW et al. (1980) and GANZER et al. (1981). Neither SNOW et al. nor MEYER-BREITING were able to establish significant differences between pre- and postoperative irradiation in the rate of local recurrence. Only GANZER et al. report a clearly higher percentage of local recurrences in the group of postoperatively irradiated patients. It must be borne in mind, though, that in this comparative study virtually all sandwichirradiated patients had been treated at the Frankfurt University ENT Clinic, whereas more than half the postoperatively irradiated patients had been treated at the Düsseldorf University ENT Clinic (GANZER et al. 1981). Thus clinic-specific factors cannot be ruled out. CARPENTER and coworkers (1976), in their comparison of local recurrences, similarly report no significant difference in frequency of recurrence among high-dose preirradiation, postoperative irradiation and surgical treatment alone.

6.3.4.2 Regional Recurrences

The rate of recurrence in the regional lymphatic system reported by different authors is in the same range in preoperatively irradiated patients and in patients treated by other procedures (MEYER-BREITING 1978, SCHULLER et al. 1979, SNOW et al. 1980, GANZER et al. 1981). In between 8% and 14.7% of patients with endolaryngeal carcinomas there was residual tumour tissue after surgery which later became apparent clinically as lymph node metastasis. Figures for hypopharyngeal carcinomas lie between 15% and 25% (BILLER et al. 1969, CARPENTER et al. 1976, VANDENBROUCK et al. 1977). Only BYERS (1979) reports the amazingly low rate of 4% regional lymph node recurrence in 59 postoperatively irradiated hypopharyngeal carcinomas. The relatively high rate of 13% regional recurrence in preoperatively irradiated and 14.7% in postoperatively irradiated endolaryngeal carcinomas in our series resulted from a high percentage of unfavourable supraglottic carcinomas (MEYER-BREITING 1981), in which involvement of the submandibular and mandibular angle regions was most often found. With glottic carcinomas the location of the metastatic recurrences was preferably paratracheal, supraclavicular and mediastinal. In hypopharyngeal carcinomas, metastatic recurrences were found homolaterally on the base of the skull, the tonsils and the upper mediastinum as well as contralaterally. All clinical observations thus appear to contradict experimental findings of a decline in lymph node and distant metastasis even with low-dose preoperative irradiation (HOYE and SMITH 1961).

In this context the experiment carried out by LORENZ as early as 1957 on the mouse Ehrlich ascites tumour is worthy of attention: in these animals, LORENZ was able to detect vital tumour cells in the blood following whole-body irradiation with the full tumour dose.

6.3.4.3 Late Distant Metastasis

In patients with endolaryngeal carcinomas, accounts of the frequency of distant metastasis after surgical intervention vary between the relatively narrow limits of 3% and 13% (BILLER et al. 1969, GOLDMAN et al. 1975, SNOW et al. 1980, MEYER-BREITING 1981). Only BYERS (1979) reports a high number of distant metastases in patients with postoperatively irradiated hypopharyngeal carcinomas. Possibly he considers metastasis in the mediastinal area as distant. The variation in the frequency of distant metastasis in the literature (between 3% and 13% after preoperative irradiation and between 5% and 13% after postoperative irradiation) is mainly due to varying interpretation of manifestations of pulmonary tumour detected by X-ray. Some authors tend to interpret such findings as distant metastasis, whereas others consider them to be second bronchial carcinomas (see MEYER-BREITING 1981). The observation made by CARPENTER and coworkers (1976) is worthy of note: they found distant metastasis in 5% of the patients with preoperative irradiation (n = 15), in 13% of those with postoperative irradiation (n = 7) and in only 1% of those with surgical treatment alone (n = 5). MEYER-BREITING (1978) and SNOW et al. (1980) also failed to establish any significant differences between preoperative and postoperative irradiation in this context.

6.3.4.4 Survival Rates

The comparison of survival rates reported by various authors (BILLER et al. 1969, BRYCE 1972, CONSTABLE et al. 1975, GOLDMAN et al. 1975, SKOLNIK et al. 1975, CARPENTER et al. 1976, BYERS 1979, SCHULLER et al. 1979, SNOW et al. 1980, GANZER et al. 1981) is complicated considerably by different parameters used, such as radiation dose, period of observation, comparison of stages etc. But nonetheless, whilst still bearing in mind the differences in assessment, such a comparison can be made. BILLER et al. (1969) and BRYCE et al. (1972) presented their results prior to the establishment of the new TNM classification and staging by the UICC and AJCC; their results were compared on the basis of the American stages III and IV. Most authors preferred high-dose preoperative irradiation (CONSTABLE et al. 1975, GOLDMAN et al. 1975, SKOLNIK et al. 1975, CARPENTER et al. 1976, BYERS 1979, SCHULLER et al. 1979). This is presumably true for SNOW et al. (1980) too, although they did not specifically state it. Low dose preirradiation, including sandwich irradiation, was applied by BILLER et al. (1969), SKOLNIK et al. (1975) and VOSTEEN (MEYER-BREITING 1978, GANZER et al. 1981). With high-dose preoperative irradiation, the 3-year survival rate reported by SKOLNIK et al. was 35.1% (n=30), by BRYCE 52% (n=52), by CONSTABLE et al. 67% (n=69) and by GOLDMAN et al. 77% (n=64). SCHULLER and coworkers (1979) report a 65% and SNOW et al. (1980) a 53% crude survival rate for a 2-year period. It should be mentioned that some authors, such as GOLDMAN and CONSTABLE, and possibly BRYCE too, selected the preirradiated cases by discarding patients who did not prove to be radiosensitive during the course of treatment. Thus a falsely favourable impression could possibly be gained from these reports, perhaps leading to a mistaken preference for high-dose preirradiation, which is undoubtedly burdened by a high rate of complications. The number of patients discarded unfortunately cannot be deduced from these publications. A complete survey of all patients with advanced laryngeal carcinomas treated would certainly provide a more realistic picture.

The average survival rates in studies of low-dose preoperative irradiation differ only slightly. BILLER (1969) reported the highest rate, 67.3% (n=49) while MEYER-BREITING (1978) with 50.6% (n=77) and SKOLNIK et al. (1975) with 49.3% (n=62) obtained roughly equivalent results. The figure of 60.8% given by GANZER (1981) is based only on those patients who underwent complete sandwich irradiation.

If these results are compared directly with those of postoperative irradiation and with those of surgical treatment alone, as published in recent years (CARPENTER et al. 1976, MEYER-BREITING 1978, BYERS 1979, SCHULLER et al. 1979, SNOW et al. 1980, GANZER et al. 1981), no significant differences can be found. BYERS (1979), SCHULLER et al. (1979) and SNOW et al. (1980) restricted their reports to 2-year survival rates, which were between 51% and 80% for surgical treatment alone (BYERS n=53, SCHULLER n=81). The figures given by other authors are between 50% and 60%. Drawing on the large samples of KLEINSASSER and MADJD (1969) and ALAJMO et al. (1976) for an overall assessment, we must, in honesty, admit stagnation in the development of more effective radiological procedures for advanced laryngeal carcinoma. Both in hypopharyngeal and in endolaryngeal carcinomas, the combined radiosurgical procedures do not give better results as regards long-term cure. The increase of postoperative complications with preoperative irradiation cannot be denied and is conceded without exception by all authors. This fact must also be considered in therapeutic planning. SCHULLER et al. (1979) draws the conclusion that surgical treatment alone should be preferred. BYERS, in contrast to SCHULLER and coworkers, observed a higher rate of survival (64%; n=39) in patients with postoperative irradiation than in patients with surgical treatment alone (51%; n=53). Results better than those of SCHULLER et al. (1979), however were also achieved by CARPENTER et al. (1976), who treated hypopharyngeal carcinomas by surgery alone. KLEINSASSER (1980), considering these facts, believes it more important to examine the surgical specimens as carefully as possible and then to reoperate solely in those regions in which residual tumour tissue is found to extend into the resection margin. Our experience in the treatment of early vocal cord carcinomas is also in favour of such an approach (MEYER-BREITING and von ILBERG 1981). All patients in whom we had established, on the basis of the surgical specimen, that the tumour had not been completely removed were correspondingly immediately reoperated on and attained 5-year survival.

6.5 Changes Following Treatment with Cytostatic Agents

The action of most cytostatic agents is histologically characterized by marked destructive changes and anaplasia of the tumour. HAYES et al. (1964) were able to distinguish histologically three stages of tumour destruction following intra-arterial methotrexate perfusion:

1. Lysis of the intercellular bridges and cytoplasmic vacuolization
2. Nuclear swelling, nuclear pycnosis and nuclear vacuoles
3. Coagulation necrosis with only few vital tumour cells

GARAS et al. (1975) likewise observed predominantly a cellular degeneration following methotrexate perfusion, together with kariolysis, oedematous swelling and vacuolization of the cytoplasm.

Treatment with conventional cytostatic agents apparently conceals the risk of increasing anaplasia of

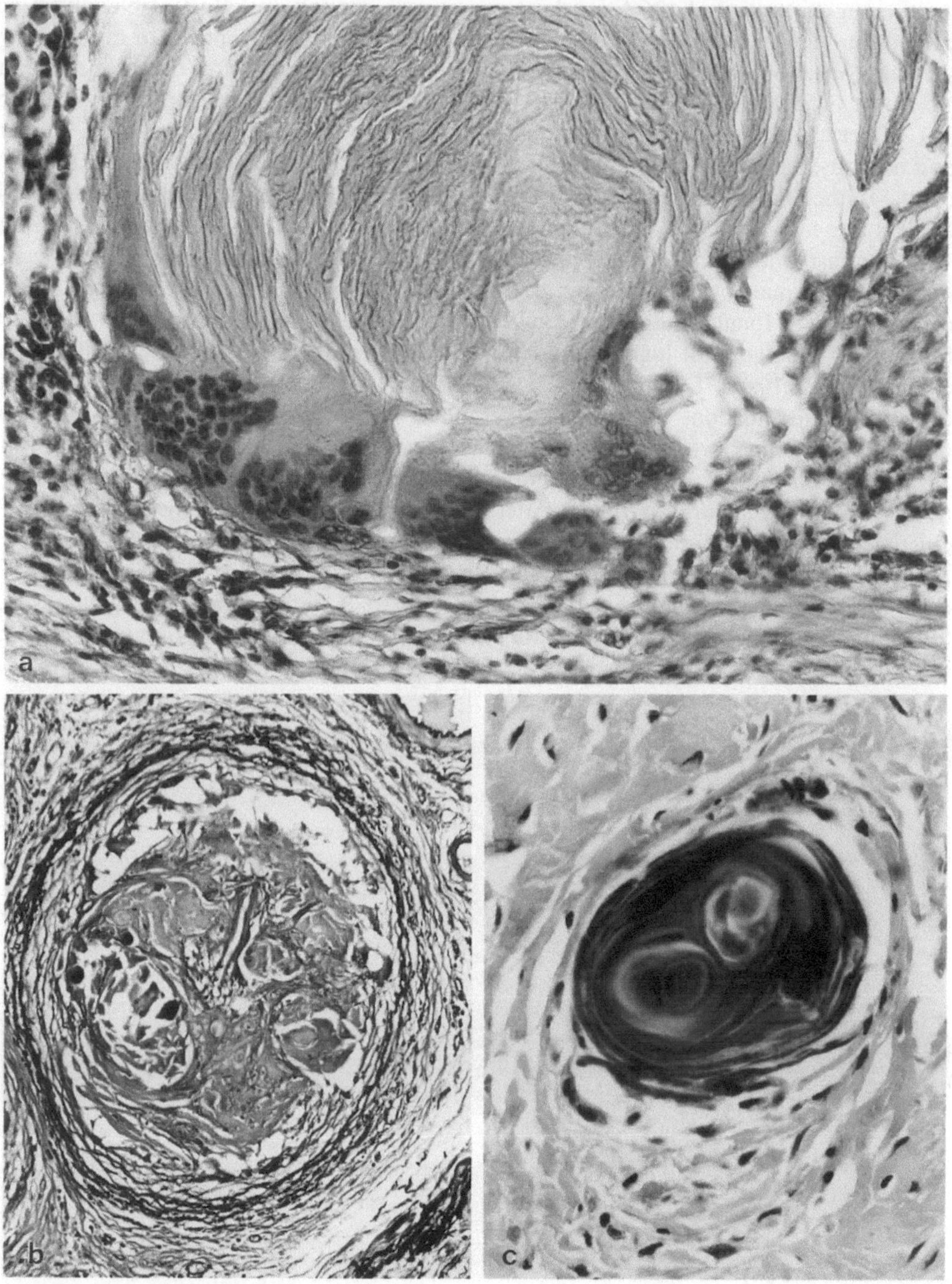

Fig. 6.10 a–c. Morphological changes of squamous cell carcinoma following bleomycin therapy. **a** Devitalized tumour area with keratinized cyst containing stacked horn lamellae and formation of multinuclear giant cells of foreign body type at the rim. Treatment with 225 mg bleomycin. ×600. **b** Completely keratinized former tumour cell nest with centrally stacked horn lamellae, a few giant cells and concentric fibrosis of the surrounding connective tissue. Treatment with 450 mg bleomycin. Van Gieson, ×120. **c** Keratinous pearl as a residue of a former tumour cell nest. Treatment with 435 mg bleomycin. Keratin stain, ×480

the tumour (SHKLAR et al. 1966). Furthermore, a co-carcinogenic influence could be demonstrated with several of these substances, for example methotrexate (SHKLAR et al. 1966, SHKLAR and SONIS 1975). This effect could play a role in recurrences or second tumours, particularly if multitopical disposition of the epithelium in the sense of "field cancerization" is present.

In contrast, with the use of the cytostatic agent bleomycin in squamous cell carcinomas, histological changes are found which correspond to those found after irradiation of highly differentiated carcinomas (Fig. 6.10a-c). Devitalization by means of increased differentiation, i.e. increased keratinization, is predominant (BURKHARDT and HÖLTJE 1975, BURKHARDT et al. 1976), while simple tumour necrosis is of only minor importance. After bleomycin therapy there is found a pronounced stromal reaction with the appearance of multinuclear giant cells; this reaction exceeds the extent of the changes following radiotherapy. This inflammatory reaction is apparently favoured by the lack of an immunosuppressive effect of bleomycin compared to other cytostatic agents or to radiotherapy. Squamous cell carcinomas after bleomycin monotherapy generally show a higher degree of differentiation than prior to the onset of therapy and an increase in the cellular stromal reaction (BURKHARDT 1980). Following irradiation a marked decline is noticeable in the cellular stromal reaction with diminished IgA- and IgG-containing plasma cells, while no significant change in the Ig-producing plasma cells or the Ig classes synthesized could be detected after bleomycin therapy (LÖNING and BURKHARDT 1979).

Since the beginning of the 1980s, cis-platinum has been introduced to treat head and neck tumours, usually in combination with bleomycin. Histologically the changes elicited by cis-platinum are comparable to those induced by methotrexate. Increased keratinization, such as seen with bleomycin, is not found.

Chemotherapy of squamous cell carcinomas of the head and neck region today is restricted to combination therapy, chiefly with bleomycin and cis-

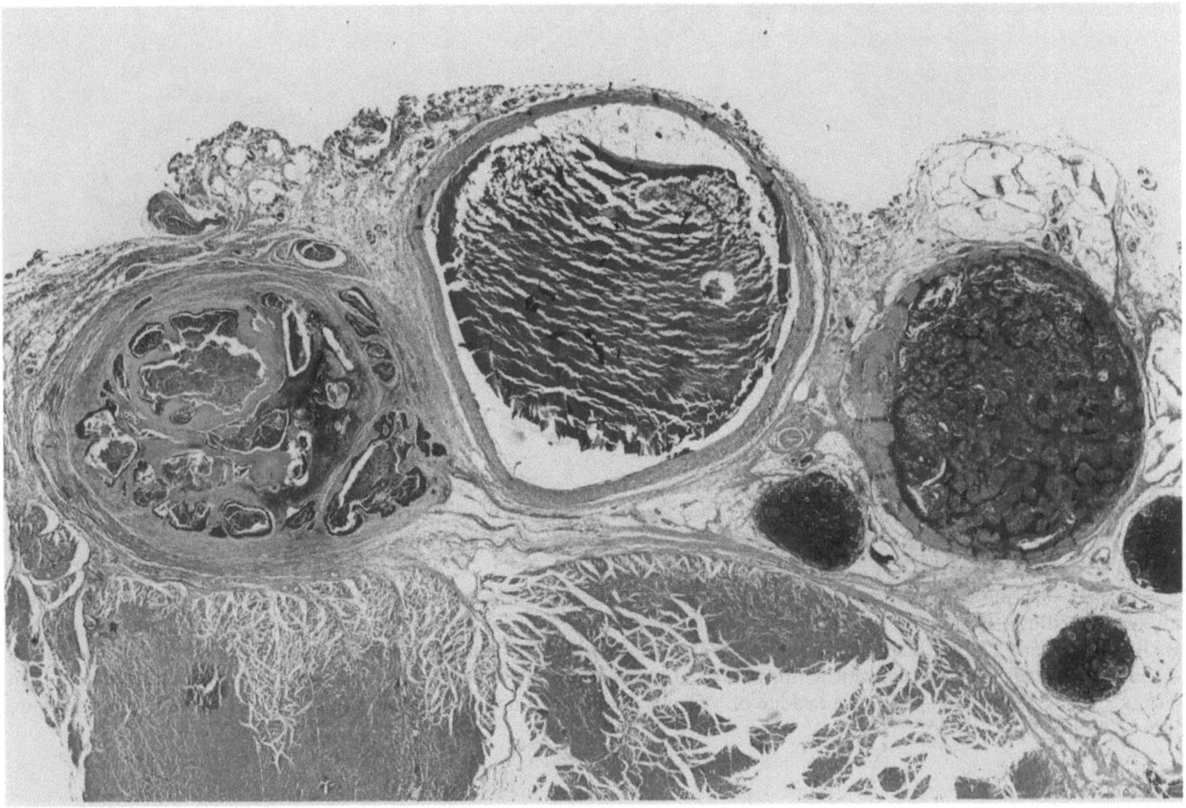

Fig. 6.11. Cervical node metastases preoperatively treated by a cytotoxic combination of cis-platinum, bleomycin and methotrexate. Next to the internal jugular vein there are two lymph nodes, both involved by a poorly differentiated squamous cell carcinoma. One of them shows a marked regression of the tumour, whereas in the other no convincing changes can be found. Horizontal section through a neck dissection block. HE, ×5

platinum. The use of these agents extends from preoperative treatment to therapy of nonoperable growths with or without radiation. The hope that a nonoperable tumour could be rendered operable by chemotherapy was not fulfilled, just as was the case with preoperative irradiation. Both these hopes were based on the assumption that squamous cell carcinomas have uniform behaviour, but actually, the larger a tumour is, the more different structures and patterns of behaviour are found. Correspondingly, some parts of a carcinoma may respond well to this therapy while in others there is no reaction. Figure 6.11 shows a metastasis in the jugular lymph nodes treated with bleomycin and cis-platinum preoperatively; different patterns of reaction can be clearly seen.

7 Unusual Malignant Tumours

7.1 Unusual Forms of Carcinoma

7.1.1 Special Forms of Squamous Cell Carcinoma

7.1.1.1 Verrucous Carcinoma

Verrucous carcinoma was first described as a separate entity by ACKERMAN (1948) and is also termed ACKERMAN tumour. ACKERMAN described 31 such tumours that had arisen in the oral cavity. All were in elderly patients with poor oral hygiene and badly fitting dental prostheses who often chewed plug tobacco.

Subsequently, these tumours were also described in other organs lined with squamous epithelium, such as the genito-anal area, nose, pharynx, oesophagus and middle ear. The most common site is still the oral cavity (1982: 283 case descriptions, McDONALD et al. 1982), the next most common, the larynx (1983: 150 case descriptions, KLEINSASSER 1983). Case reports of laryngeal verrucous carcinoma may be found, for example, in GOETHALS et al. (1963), KRAUS and PEREZ-MESA (1966), BILLER et al. (1971), DEMIAN et al. (1973), ELLIOT et al. (1973), BAK and ERDÖS (1975), FISHER (1976), FERLITO et al. (1976), RIDER (1976), VAN NOSTRAND and OLOFSSON (1972) and MAW et al. (1982).

Reports regarding the frequency of verrucous carcinomas in terms of percentage of total malignant laryngeal tumours are very variable: 1%-2% (BILLER and BERGMAN 1976), 1.4% (VAN NOSTRAND and OLOFSSON 1972), 3.8% (FERLITO 1985) and 11.2% (FISHER 1976, from a group of 276 patients; the cases classified as verrucous carcinomas included five with metastasis).

In the larynx too, the verrucous carcinoma, like other squamous cell carcinomas, arises mainly in older patients (fifth to sixth decade). Males predominate (male to female ratio approximately 3:1), but the proportion of women is larger than in normal squamous cell carcinomas. The symptoms resemble those of other carcinomas but growth is slower and metastasis usually absent. The preferred location of verrucous carcinoma is in the upper laryngeal region (supraglottis), however, it can occur on the ventricular floor and the vocal fold. If left untreated, the tumour can lead to death by respiratory obstruction (HYAMS 1976).

Clinically and macroscopically, usually extensive, often multifocal warty tumours are found; these have a grey-white, deeply clefted surface and are friable. They must be distinguished from hyperplastic exophytic-papillomatous leukoplakias, papillomas and other papilloma-virus-induced lesions, such as condyloma acuminatum and verruca vulgaris (FECHNER and MILLS 1982). The general similarity to the latter lesions, together with other features supposedly characteristic of viral infection, like vacuolar nuclei, intranuclear inclusions, nuclear pyknosis and perinuclear halos, have raised the question of a viral (human papilloma virus, HPV) etiology of verrucous carcinoma. However, no viral particles have yet been observed on electron microscopy by us or other authors. In addition, immunohistochemical testing for HPV capsid antigens was consistently negative (10 cases). Recently, ABRAMSON et al. (1985), while also unable to demonstrate HPV antigens with immunoperoxidase, found HPV-16-related DNA sequences in five verrucous carcinomas and in the surrounding epithelium using a molecular DNA hybridization technique (see Sect. 2.3.1.5). It is not clear whether these sequences are integrated into the host genome. This certainly raises the question of participation of HPV infections in carcinogenesis (see Sect. 4.2), in particular the genesis of verrucous carcinoma, which is at present far from proven in humans. The fact that tobacco abuse is found in almost all patients with verrucous carcinomas and that these lesions can be produced in experiments by application of 4-nitroquinoline 1-oxide (FISKER and PHILIPSEN 1984) point rather to a predominantly chemical carcinogenesis. Enhanced epithelial matu-

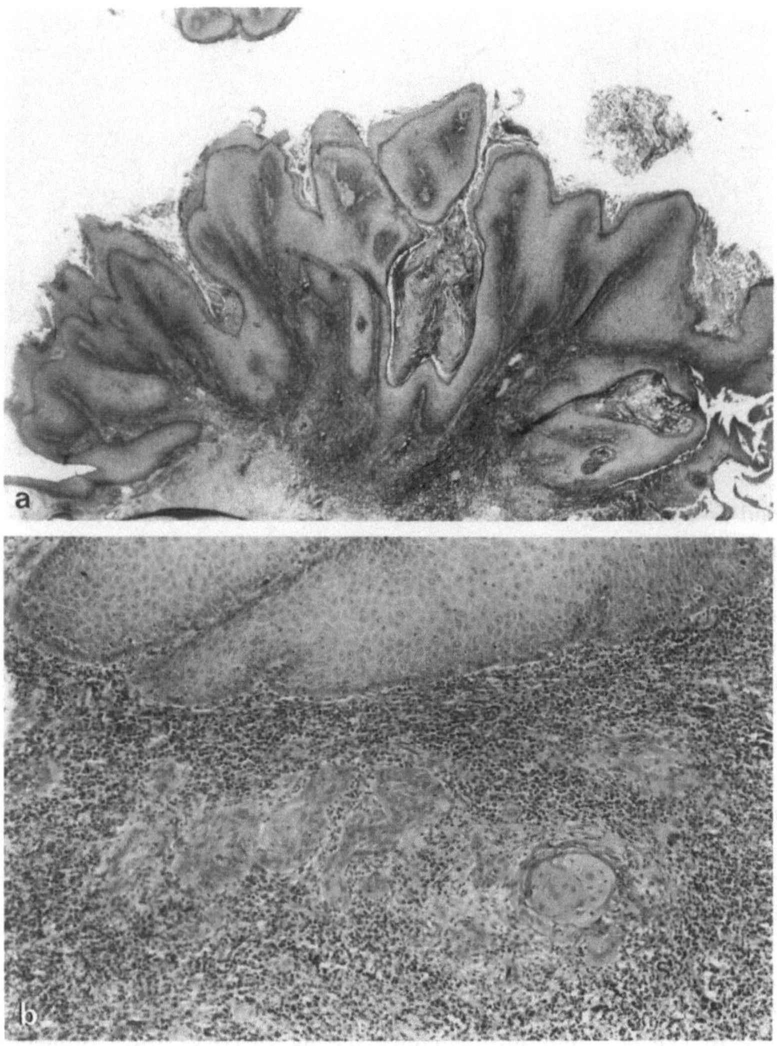

Fig. 7.1 a, b. Verrucous carcinoma: 68-year-old man with a tumour of the left vocal cord. **a** Overview of the wart-like tumour with a typical papillomatous hyperkeratotic surface. There are plump epithelial protrusions into depth with keratin plugs. Intense inflammatory infiltration. HE, ×20. **b** Higher magnification of the epithelial/mesenchymal interface of the same tumour. Beneath a well-delineated plump epithelial formation there is unequivocal dissociated invasive growth with a keratinous pearl at the right. HE, ×100

ration and hyperkeratosis could of course favour an opportunistic, persistent latent viral infection which might subsequently promote carcinogenesis. In view of these facts, Abramson et al. (1985) warn that irradiation further enhances the risk of DNA changes and malignant transformation.

Histologically the tumour is characterized by the following (Fig. 7.1 and 7.2):

1. The tumour surface protrudes like a wart and shows deep infoldings of the epithelium.
2. The tumour consists of an extraordinarily well-differentiated keratinizing squamous epithelium with few mitotic figures and without appreciable cellular atypia. There is a well-developed basal membrane.
3. The folds, which reach into the depth of the claviform or drop-shaped epithelial cones, contain pronounced keratin "plugs".
4. Tumour infiltration is on a broad "pushing" front supplanting the stroma, which exhibits an intense inflammatory reaction.
5. The usual dissociated infiltrative growth of squamous cell carcinoma should by definition be missing.
6. Metastasis should likewise not be present.

Verrucous carcinomas are generally regarded as distinct variants of differentiated squamous cell carcinomas with low-grade malignancy and no metastatic potential. Recently, however, the carcinomatous, i.e. true malignant, character of this lesion has been called into doubt. Shear and Pindborg (1980) distinguish, in lesions of the oral mucosa, between simple verrucous hyperplasia (exophytic growth above the level of the mucosa) and true verrucous carcinoma. Slootweg and Müller (1983), on the other hand, do not consider that this differ-

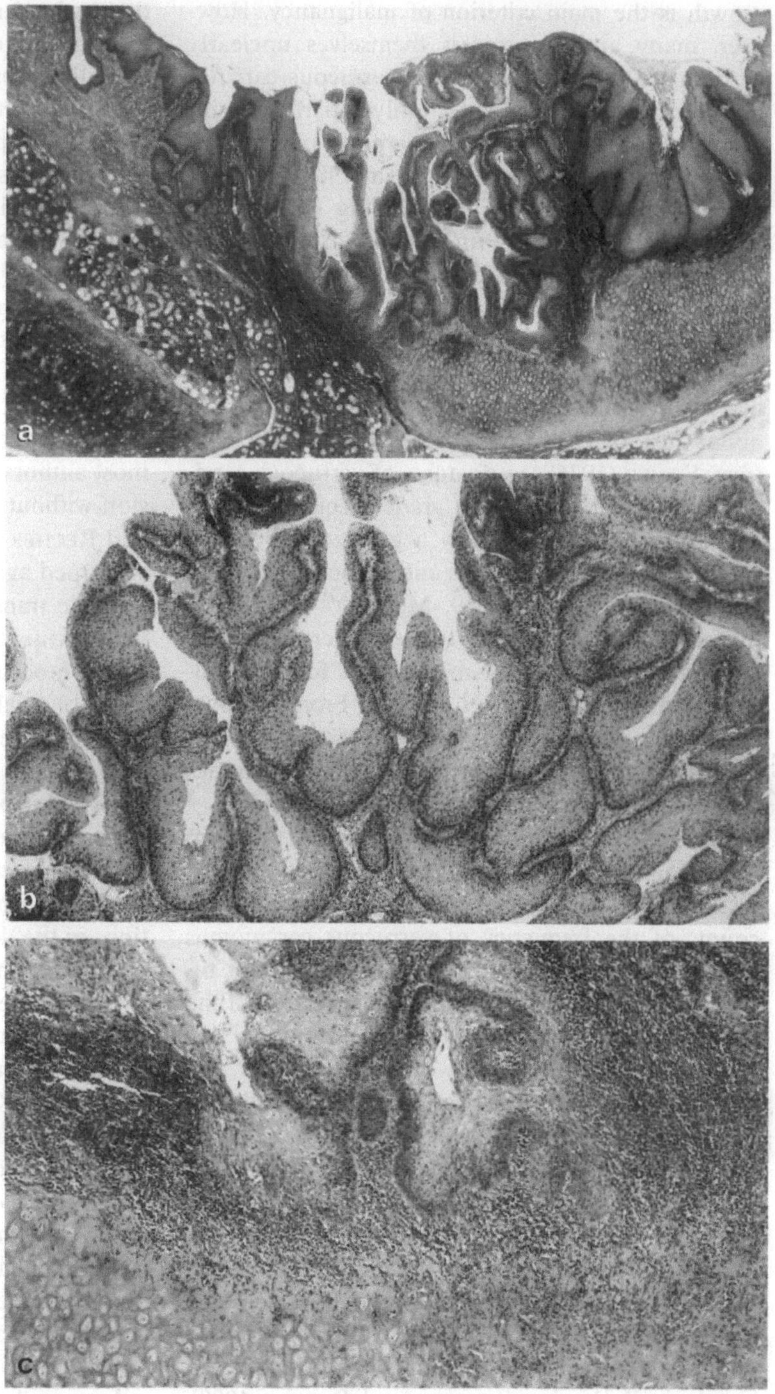

Fig. 7.2 a–c. Verrucous carcinoma: 64-year-old man with a tumour of the laryngeal epiglottic surface. **a** The hyperplastic epithelium at the right and left abruptly protrudes as a papillomatous tumor in the centre. The plump epithelium grows into depth on a broad, "pushing" front and has partially destroyed the cartilage of the epiglottis. HE, ×20. **b** The papillomatous epithelial formations on the top are well differentiated with orderly stratification and exhibit no marked dysplasia. Biopsy from this portion will not be representative of the lesion and will result in underestimation of the process. HE, ×35. **c** Tumour tissue in the depth is less well differentiated; however, also here no dissociated invasive growth is evident. There is a dense inflammatory reaction and the adjacent cartilage shows signs of dissolution. HE, ×60

entiation is possible in all cases. GLANZ and KLEINSASSER (1978) observed six "verrucous carcinomas" in the laryngeal region, of which only one clearly showed invasion; they concluded that most such tumours should not be termed carcinoma. They speak of verrucous acanthosis as a facultative precancerous lesion. MEYER-BREITING (1981b) is of a similar opinion: if dissociated infiltration is detected (Fig. 7.1), he views such carcinomas as papillary squamous cell carcinomas of grade I on the BRODERS scale.

The term carcinoma for a lesion which, according to the prevalent definition, is not supposed to grow invasively (ACKERMAN 1948, MASON 1972) is from the standpoint of the general pathologist highly unsatisfactory. Indeed, the feature of invasive growth is the main criterion of malignancy. However, many authors express themselves unclearly with regard to the ability of the verrucous carcinoma to invade - for example, "only superficially invasive" (SHAFER 1983); "free groups of invasive cells are unusual" (PRIOLEAU et al. 1980) - whilst others describe perineural spreading (MOHS and SAHL 1979, FISKER and PHILIPSEN 1984). The "coexistence of foci of less differentiated squamous carcinoma with verrucous lesions" is also pointed out (GOETHALS et al. 1963, KRAUS and PEREZ-MESA 1966, JACOBSON and SHEAR 1972, BATSAKIS et al. 1982, MEDINA et al. 1984) and is said to exist in about 20% of cases (MEDINA et al. 1984). In contrast, FISHER (1976) sees features of verrucous carcinoma in about half of the grade I squamous cell carcinomas and accordingly a grey zone between typical verrucous carcinoma and grade I carcinoma (see also FONTS et al. 1969, MICHAELS 1984). For this reason it is mandatory that each verrucous carcinoma be examined for microscopic foci of invasive carcinoma (MEDINA et al. 1984). From our own experience, such foci are found in more than half the cases; their presence in our opinion justifies classification as grade I squamous cell carcinoma.

Bearing these considerations in mind, the term "verrucous carcinoma" could be dropped (FRIEDMANN 1976, MICHAELS 1984). The differing accounts of the frequency of verrucous carcinomas with respect to the total number of malignant tumours of the larynx are simply the expression of the general uncertainty regarding the definition of this type of tumour. Thus many authors expressly emphasize that "verrucous carcinoma" is neither a purely clinical nor a histological diagnosis, but rather a term which should be applied only after synopsis of clinical and histological findings ("distinct clinico-pathological entity"; KRAUS and PEREZ-MESA 1966, BILLER and BERGMANN 1976, FISHER 1976, BAK and ERDÖS 1975, FERLITO and RECHER 1980, MCDONALD et al. 1982). The special feature of this tumour is that it appears clinically malignant but histologically benign (FERLITO and RECHER 1980). Verrucous and also papillary squamous cell carcinomas may accordingly raise considerable diagnostic problems for the clinician and the pathologist. If the biopsy specimen is not taken from the base of the tumour, the pathologist can as a rule only make the diagnosis "papillomatosis of the larynx". In our experience only biopsy material from the base of the tumour can provide the diagnosis of malignancy; this was the case in the majority of adult patients who came to us to be treated with the primary histological diagnosis "verrucous acanthosis" or "papillomatosis of the larynx". In diagnosing differentially between such lesions and squamous papillomas, morphometric studies may prove useful in some circumstances: according to MICHAELS (1984), the mean cell area is higher in verrucous carcinoma and there is a greater range of cell sizes.

Metastatic spread of verrucous or papillary squamous cell carcinomas was established in only one of more than 20 cases observed at the Frankfurt University ENT Clinic; in this tumour, however, there was an anaplastic focus in the depth.

With regard to therapy, there is controversy, but most authors recommend radical local tumour excision without neck dissection (FISHER 1976, FERLITO and RECHER 1980, MAW et al. 1982). Radiotherapy is warned against by a number of authors owing to possible transformation into anaplastic metastasizing carcinoma (SMITH et al. 1985). Such anaplasia can also occur spontaneously.

AIRD et al. (1954) described a further type of squamous cell carcinoma on the sole of the foot and termed it "carcinoma cuniculatum" (cuniculus = rabbit burrow). It is, like the verrucous carcinoma, a more "pushing" supplantive, endophytically growing tumour with a papillomatous surface and deep "burrow-like" crypts and sinus formations in the depth which are filled with keratin. Histologically this tumour is easily confused with a pseudoepitheliomatous epithelial hyperplasia. Carcinoma cuniculatum also resembles verrucous carcinoma in that the tumours are reminiscent of viral lesions (MCKEE et al. 1981); but testing for papilloma (HPV) antigens is negative (KAO et al. 1982). Such squamous cell carcinomas have since been observed in other regions of the body and in the oral cavity, but so far there has been no description of a tumour under this name in the larynx. Several lesions termed verrucous carcinomas have, however, fulfilled the criteria of carcinoma cuniculatum.

In accordance with its similarity to verrucous carcinoma, most authors today consider carcinoma cuniculatum as a special form of this tumour ("inverted verrucous carcinoma"; BROWNSTEIN and SHAPIRO 1976, SEEHAFTER et al. 1979, HEADINGTON 1978, PRILEAU et al. 1980, REICH 1982, KAO et al. 1982, RATZENHOFER 1982).

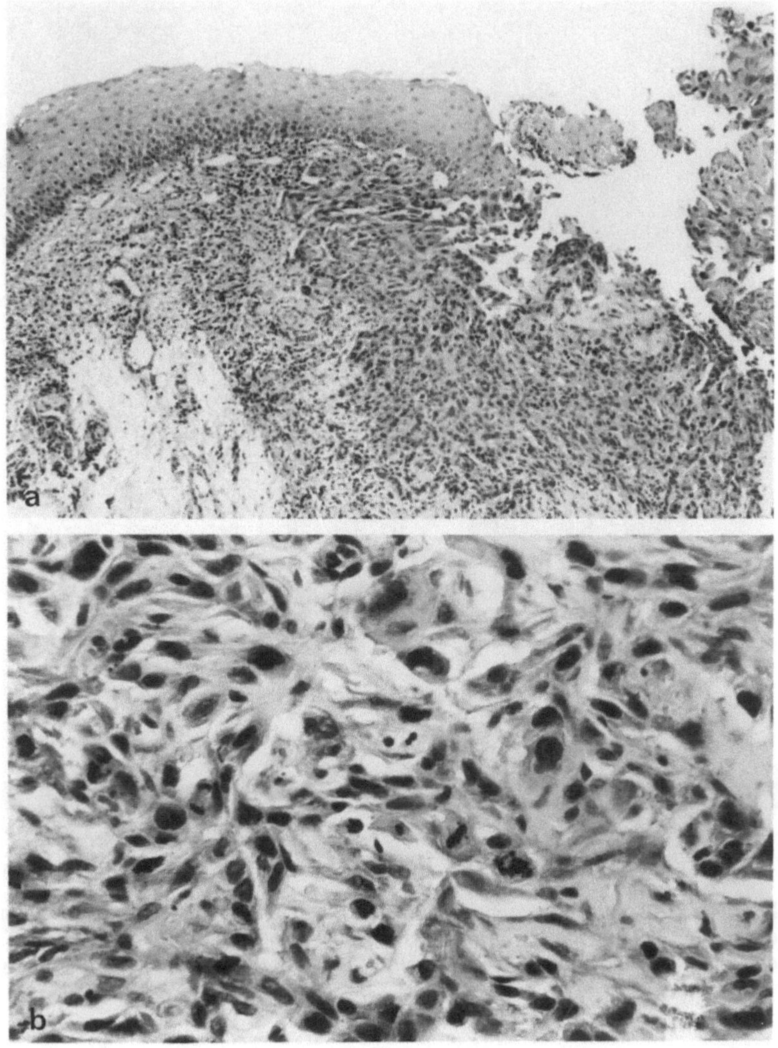

Fig. 7.3a, b. Spindle cell carcinoma: 45-year-old man, epiglottic fold. **a** The covering epithelium is destroyed at the right, and here an invasive, dissociated spindle cell tumour can be seen. HE, ×90. **b** The cells are highly pleomorphic with a predominance of spindle-shaped types. There are some atypical mitotic figures. Epithelial cohesion is not evident. HE, ×350

7.1.1.2 Spindle Cell Carcinoma and Carcinosarcoma

This probably heterogeneous group of neoplasms has been described under a number of names, including pseudosarcoma and sarcomatoid carcinoma. The tumours have been observed in the uterus, breast, bladder, stomach, oesophagus, oral cavity and pharynx. Up to 1% of all malignant neoplasms of the larynx contain a spindle cell fraction, sometimes in combination with better differentiated squamous cell carcinoma (MEYER-BREITING and ROSEMANN 1977).

These tumours are on average observed in somewhat older patients than the common squamous cell carcinomas - between 48 and 87 years of age with a peak at 68 (HYAMS 1975). There is a sexual predilection for men. The main location in the larynx is in the region of the vocal cord (up to 80%). Occurrence following irradiation is not uncommon (see Sect. 7.3; KLEINSASSER and GLANZ 1978, LASSER et al. 1979), and transformation of squamous cell carcinomas to spindle cell carcinomas is occasionally seen after treatment with cytostatic agents (BURKHARDT 1980). The prognosis depends largely on the depth of invasion (LEVENTON and EVANS 1981). Some authors report in general a better prognosis for this neoplasm than for common squamous cell carcinomas. According to recent communications, however, the prognosis for spindle cell carcinoma corresponds to that for poorly differentiated squamous cell carcinoma (HYAMS 1975, RECHER 1985). Thus the therapy does not differ from that for squamous cell carcinomas and is primarily surgical (GIORDANO et al. 1983).

Macroscopically, in about two-thirds of cases the

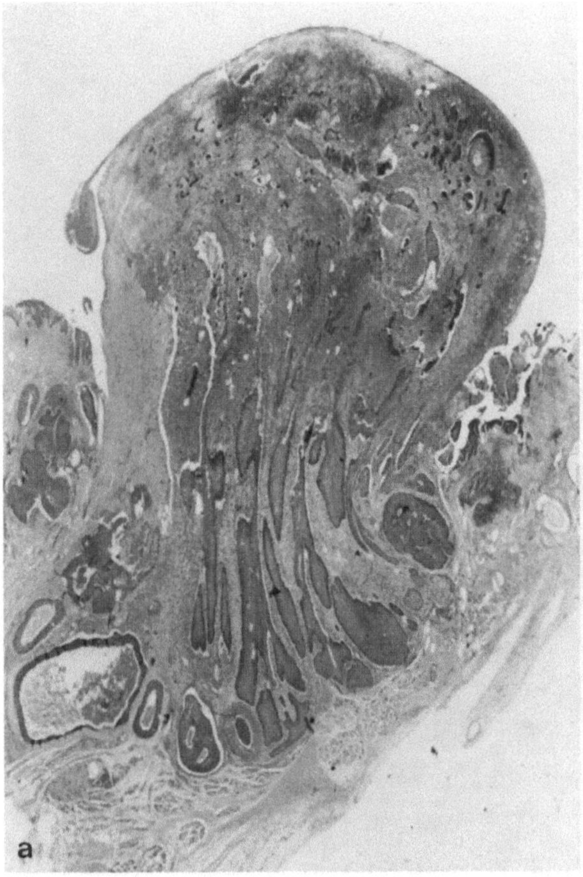

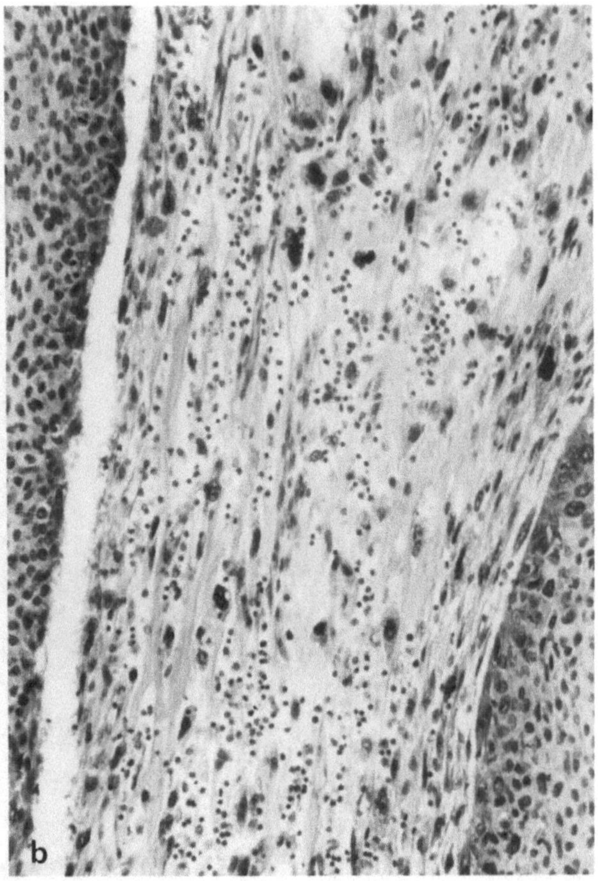

Fig. 7.4 a, b. Spindle cell carcinoma (so-called carcinosarcoma): 47-year-old man, vocal cord. **a** Polypous tumour with broad ulceration. Plump epithelial formations growing into depth can be seen. HE, ×25. **b** Between the cohesive, clearly epithelial components of the tumour a spindle cell tissue with cellular atypia and mitotic figures is established. HE, ×350

tumour exhibits a polypous exophytic, highly friable excrescence, and in one-third, primarily infiltrative growth.

Histologically the tumour has as a rule a biphasic structure. The marginal regions exhibit in most cases the morphological characteristics of a squamous cell carcinoma of grade II-IV. This fraction may, however, be quite unremarkable; occasionally there is only carcinoma in situ. Towards the centre of the tumour the epithelial surface becomes ulcerated, either in multiple small spots or over larger areas: spindle cells and sometimes also large, anaplastic cells can be found which are disseminated singly and occasionally form small groups. In the depth, the tumour cannot be distinguished by means of light microscopy from spindle cell sarcoma (fibrosarcoma, malignant fibrous histiocytoma, leiomyosarcoma, rhabdomyosarcoma and occasionally myxoliposarcoma). The spindle and anaplastic fractions have a high cellularity, exhibit numerous mitotic figures and sometimes contain scattered multinuclear giant cells. A dense reticulin and collagen fibre network can be demonstrated surrounding the single cells. Chondroid and osteoid foci and areas resembling malignant giant cell tumour are occasionally observed (Lasser et al. 1979, Lambert et al. 1980, Alguacil-Garcia et al. 1984). More rarely, the spindle cell component also resembles atypical granulation tissue.

In some tumours a transition zone is found between the squamous epithelial and the spindle cell fraction; in this zone, strands of squamous epithelium "stream in" between loosely distributed, spindle-shaped cells (Figs. 7.3, 7.4).

The infiltrative growth of the tumour may take the form of solid carcinomatous tissue or of diffusely disseminated immigration of spindle-cell elements. Both the clearly epithelial and the spindle cell fraction of the tumour have metastatic potential (Küpper and Blessing 1974, Randall et al. 1975,

LEVENTON and EVANS 1981). Metastasis exhibiting the structure of ordinary squamous cell carcinoma is not uncommon.

The histological diagnosis has to differentiate such neoplasms from the above-mentioned sarcomas and from benign vocal cord polyps with atypical granulation tissue (RANDALL et al. 1975). In lesions thought to be spindle cell sarcomas a clearly recognizable epithelial component should be looked for in serial sections in order to exclude spindle cell carcinoma (LEVENTON and EVANS 1981, ALGUACIL-GARCIA et al. 1984).

The numerous terms used for spindle cell carcinoma and carcinosarcoma reflect the controversy of its histogenesis and the uncertainty of its classification. The following interpretations have been given (review: BRODSKY 1984):

1. The spindle cell component corresponds only to an atypical stromal reaction (pseudosarcoma).
2. The lesion is a collision tumour (true carcinosarcoma).
3. Squamous cell and sarcomatous tumour elements differentiate from a common undifferentiated pluripotent cell (carcinosarcoma).
4. True mesenchymal metaplasia of the malignant epithelial cells occurs (carcinosarcoma).
5. Malignant transformation ensues in the stroma formed as a reaction to tumour growth, perhaps by the influence of the epithelial component (carcinosarcoma).
6. Both components are of an epithelial nature (spindle cell carcinoma).

Today it is generally considered that probably a heterogeneous group of tumours is involved and that different histogenesis is possible (LASSER et al. 1979, BRODSKY 1984, FECHNER 1984). The application of advanced methods has also led to inconsistent results. Electron microscopically, in some tumours features of fibroblasts and myofibroblasts could be discerned on the spindle cell elements (LASSER et al. 1979), but in most tumours structural elements of epithelial tissue, namely primitive desmosomes and tonofilaments, were detected (LICHTIGER et al. 1970, BATTIFORA 1976, LASSER et al. 1979, BURKHARDT 1980, KATHOLM et al. 1984). Similarly, in some tumours the immunohistological demonstration of cytokeratins and epithelial membrane antigen (EMA) in the spindle cell elements was positive, in others negative, in our experience and that of other authors (ALGUACIL-GARCIA et al. 1984). In most cases the tumour concerned is apparently a carcinoma with a pronounced spindle cell component, i.e. a spindle cell carcinoma (option 6 of those listed above; RANDALL et al. 1975, KLEINSASSER and GLANZ 1978, BURKHARDT 1980, KLEINSASSER 1983, KATHOLM 1984, MICHAELS 1984). It can be assumed that the tumour is a squamous cell carcinoma of deficient intercellular coherence. Since these tumours are primarily observed at sites of mechanical stress, where granulation polyps and other laryngeal polyps also arise, the deficient coherence and the bursting of the squamous epithelial surface possibly contribute to this peculiar morphological picture. The parallels between the vascular architecture of granulation polyps (see Chap. 8) and the surface of spindle cell carcinomas would also suggest such a relationship. A few of these tumours, however, may be true carcinosarcomas. Today transfection, i.e. transfer of genetic material, including oncogenes, from the carcinomatous cells to the stromal cells, is being discussed (option 5 above). Thus in every single case modern methods of cell typing (see Sect. 2.4) should be employed to define these tumours. Examples are given in Sect. 7.3.

Detailed accounts can be found in KLEINSASSER and GLANZ (1978) and BRODSKY (1984). Other accounts have been published by KAHLER (1908), ULLMANN (1920), RICII (1933), SCHWARZ (1936), FRANK (1940), WESSELY (1940), GRIEPENDROG (1955), WALTHER (1962), VERHEST and JORTAY (1968), MINCKLER et al. (1970), GALLE et al. (1971), KÜPPER and BLESSING (1974), RANDALL et al. (1975), SCHMIDT-BULER and RUPP (1975), RICHARDSON et al. (1978), RATZENHOFER (1979), LASSER et al. (1979), SRINIVASAN and TALVALKAR (1979), LAMBERT et al. (1980), BROICH (1981), LAGACE et al. (1981), LEUSZLER et al. (1981), LEVENTON and EVANS (1981), DESHOTELS et al. (1982), WOODS et al. (1982), ALGUACIL-GARCIA et al. (1984), KATHOLM et al. (1984) and RECHER (1985).

7.1.1.3 Transitional Cell Carcinoma

This type of carcinoma was first described in 1927 by QUICK and CUTLER. It is considered to originate from the transitions of the squamous epithelium to prismatic or respiratory epithelium in the region of the tonsils, the base of the tongue, the nasopharynx, the larynx and the excretory ducts of mucous glands (VON ALBERTINI 1974). VON ALBERTINI, in contrast to EWING (1928), is of the opinion that this

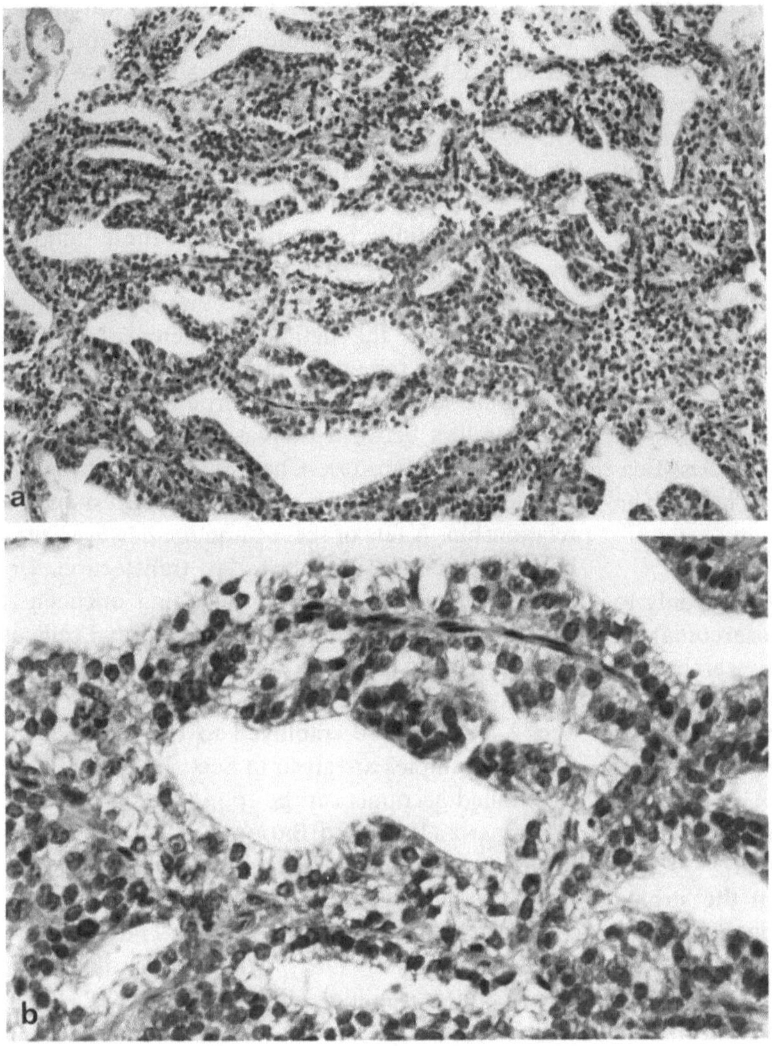

Fig. 7.5 a, b. Adenocarcinoma: 73-year-old woman, aryepiglottic fold. **a** Tubular, partly cystic tumour. HE, ×140. **b** Tubular and cribriform formation of mostly cylindrical tumour cells. Immunohistological testing for thyroglobulin was negative. HE, ×350

is not a uniform type of tumour but that different types of carcinomas are concerned which possess, as common characteristic, high radiosensitivity. Some carcinomas of this type may be undifferentiated squamous carcinomas (FERLITO 1976), others probably belong to the lymphoepithelial carcinomas.

7.1.1.4 Lymphoepithelial Carcinoma

Lymphoepithelial carcinoma (WHO: lymphoepithelioma, undifferentiated carcinoma of nasopharyngeal type) was described simultaneously in the 1920s by SCHMINCKE (1921) and REGAUD (1921). It is thought to develop from the lymphoepithelial tissue of Waldeyer's ring in the area of the embryonal branchial arches or branchial clefts. Since associations of epithelial and lymphatic tissue also occur in the piriform sinus and Morgagni's ventricle, occurrence of these tumours has been observed in these locations. Morphologically, as a rule, relatively anaplastic carcinomas are involved with loosely distributed nonkeratinizing cell complexes interspersed to a greater or lesser extent with lymphocytes. The lymphatic component possesses no real malignant character, so that it is justified to view this type of carcinoma as an anaplastic carcinoma which has arisen in an area of lymphoepithelial tissue. There is an association of nasopharyngeal lymphoepithelial carcinomas and Epstein-Barr virus (EBV) infection, but no such association has yet been established in laryngeal carcinomas of this type.

The particular feature of this carcinoma is early metastasis to the regional lymph nodes, at a time when the tumour is often not yet clinically appar-

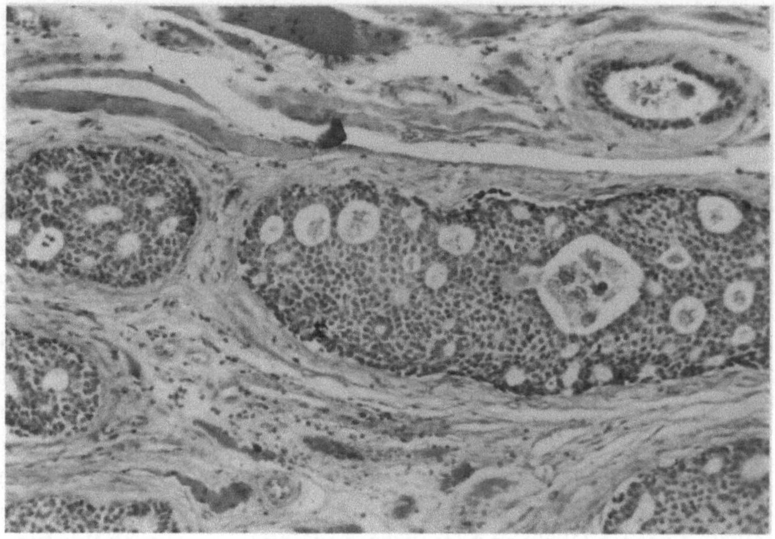

Fig. 7.6. Adenoid cystic carcinoma: 42-year-old male, submucosal subglottic tumor. Well-delineated solid tumour formations consisting of small relatively uniform cells containing typical round ("cylindrical") spaces. HE, ×140

ent; this is especially the case with tumours originating in the piriform sinus or Morgagni's ventricle. Like transitional cell carcinoma, lymphoepithelial carcinoma is highly radiosensitive but must be viewed as having an unfavourable prognosis owing to early and widespread metastasis (STANLEY et al. 1985).

Reports concerning lymphoepithelial carcinoma of the laryngohypopharyngeal regions can be found in DOCKERTY et al. (1968), FERLITO (1976), MICHEAU et al. (1976, 1979) and TOKER and PETERSON (1978). In our clinic we have seen a patient with lymphoepithelial carcinoma of the piriform sinus. Six reports from the literature and four additional cases have been compiled by STANLEY et al. (1985).

7.1.2 Carcinomas of the Adnexa of the Laryngeal Mucosa

Malignant tumours of the serous and mucous glands of the larynx amount to less than 1% of malignant laryngeal tumours (KLEINSASSER 1961, FERLITO 1976, MEYER-BREITING and ROSEMANN 1977, COHEN et al. 1985). All known types of salivary gland tumours, including those not mentioned here, can also occur in the laryngeal region. Adenocarcinomas and adenoid cystic carcinomas are most frequent. They occur more often following irradiation (SQUIRES et al. 1981).

In patients with adenocarcinomas of the larynx clinical examination must exclude distant metastasis from a primary tumour elsewhere and thyroid gland carcinoma which has penetrated into the endolarynx (SEBASTIAN and KLEINSASSER 1985).

7.1.2.1 Adenocarcinoma

The frequency of adenocarcinomas is 0.1%–1% of all carcinomas of the larynx. They comprise about two-thirds of all glandular laryngeal carcinomas (FECHNER 1976).

The age of the patients affected does not differ from that of patients with squamous cell carcinoma of the larynx, and there is a similar predilection for men (TOOMEY 1967, CADY et al. 1968). The main site is the supraglottic region, in particular the region of the ventricle and the vestibular ligament. A case of a papillary adenocarcinoma of the vocal cord was reported by MERTENS et al. (1986) and considered to be the first such observation.

Most adenocarcinomas metastasize early into the regional lymph nodes. CADY et al. (1968) reported that in half the patients with clinical N0 stage tumours postoperative histological examination detected regional metastasis. The prognosis of these patients is as a rule very unfavourable, since besides regional metastatic spread, distant metastasis also ensues at an early stage (COHEN et al. 1985); according to CADY et al. (1968) distant metastases appear within 2 years.

Morphologically adenocarcinomas display the following characteristics (Fig. 7.5):

1. Macroscopically they push forward a usually smooth, intact mucosal surface.
2. Histologically, well-differentiated, papillary, ductular and glandular structures or solid and cribriform cell formations can be observed.
3. Cytologically, cuboid or polygonal cells of vari-

able pleomorphism with or without mucus production are found.

Besides the well-differentiated adenocarcinomas, primary anaplastic giant cell adenocarcinomas of the larynx have been observed (FERLITO 1976). Differentiation from anaplastic squamous cell carcinomas may be difficult. These tumours correspond to the giant cell carcinomas of the lung (FERLITO et al. 1985 a). By immunohistological means it is usually possible to identify thyroid gland carcinomas which have broken into the larynx by demonstration of thyroglobulin.

Reports of laryngeal adenocarcinomas can be found in WHICKER et al. (1974), FECHNER (1976), CRISSMAN and ROSENBLATT (1978), MALLONEE et al. (1979), FERLITO (1980) and HOMMERICH (1985).

7.1.2.2 Adenoid Cystic Carcinoma

Adenoid cystic carcinomas (obsolete synonym: cylindroma) occur even more rarely than adenocarcinomas in the larynx. OLOFSSON and VAN NOSTRAND (1977), and FLEISCHER et al. (1978), surveyed 60 cases reported in the world literature and added four and five respectively of their own. Patients with adenoid cystic carcinomas of the larynx are usually younger than those with squamous cell carcinomas, according to FECHNER (1976) between 30 and 70 years of age with a slight predilection for the female sex. The most common location is the subglottic region, followed by the supraglottic. Of the 64 cases compiled by OLOFSSON and VAN NOSTRAND (1977), 27 were subglottic, 16 supraglottic and only three glottic. The remainder were so extensive that several regions were affected. Metastasis to the lymph nodes is encountered, but far more, these tumours tend towards perineural growth and penetration of vessels. Therefore clinical problems arise regarding the assessment of local extension and the decision on surgical removal of these tumours. Adenoid cystic carcinomas generally tend to local recurrences which repeatedly necessitate subsequent resection until the patients finally succumb to the underlying disease. Possibly due to the slow development of the tumour, local recurrences can often appear 5 years or more following initial surgical removal. Courses of up to 16 years are not unusual with this type of tumour. A tendency to distant metastasis further limits the chances of cure (STILLWAGON et al. 1985). Adenoid cystic carcinomas are considered in general to be radioresistant, and for this reason radical surgical procedure is recommended (FLEISCHER et al. 1978). Morphologically, adenoid cystic carcinomas have a typical architecture and are characterized by (Fig. 7.6):

1. The absence of a capsule.
2. Trabecular, tubular and sometimes also solid, well demarcated cell formations surround cell-free spaces of varying size with hyaline material, giving them a cribriform appearance. The stroma may be slightly myxoid.
3. Relatively uniform, small cells with little basophilic cytoplasm and small dark nuclei, occasion-

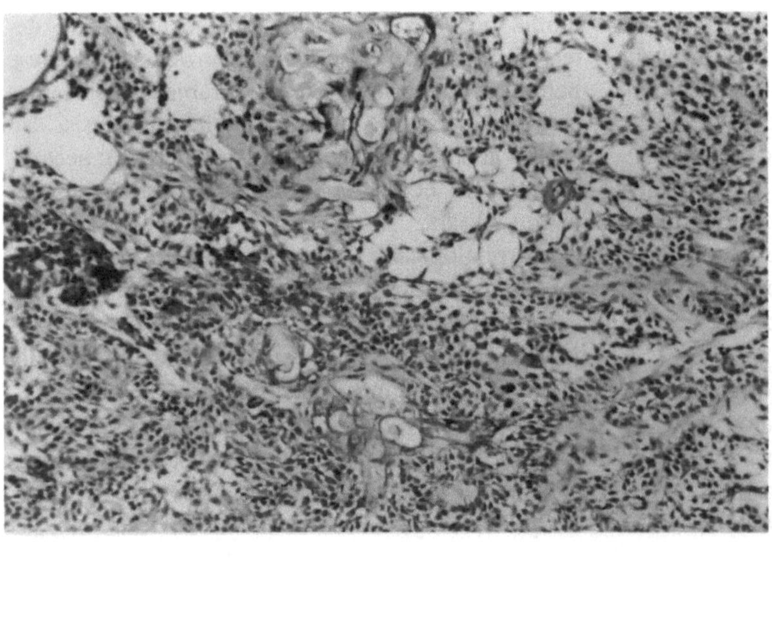

Fig. 7.7. Mucoepidermoid carcinoma: 63-year-old man, vestibular fold. Solid tumour with areas of keratinization and cyst formation containing mucus. HE, ×120

ally with a vesicular nucleolus. They resemble the basal cells of the skin and mucosae and are probably related to myoepithelial cells.

7.1.2.3 Mucoepidermoid Carcinoma

Mucoepidermoid carcinoma (WHO: mucoepidermoid tumour) is observed very rarely in the larynx (CADY et al. 1968, GERUGHTY et al. 1968, THOMAS 1971, MEYER-BREITING and ROSEMANN 1977). DAMIANI et al. (1981) found 32 case reports of mucoepidermoid or adenosquamous carcinomas of the larynx and hypopharynx in the literature and added a further 21 cases from the tumour register of the Armed Forces Institute of Pathology gathered between 1945 and 1979.

The age of the patients is lower than that of those with squamous cell carcinoma of the larynx (25–76 years of age); the male sex is quite clearly preferred (FERLITO et al. 1981, TOM et al. 1981, DAMIANI et al. 1981). Since glands exist in all laryngeal regions, mucoepidermoid carcinomas can arise in any area. The supraglottis is most often affected, the vocal cord only exceptionally (GATTIE and ERKMAN-BALIS 1980). We observed a 65-year-old man with a mucoepidermoid carcinoma in the supraglottis under the mucosa of the vestibular ligament.

The therapy of choice is surgical removal. Mucoepidermoid carcinomas are considered radioresistant. The overall 5-year survival rate of the cases reported by DAMIANI et al. (1981) was 77%. The low-grade mucoepidermoid carcinomas displayed better survival rates than did the adenosquamous and high-grade tumours. However, it must be noted that these tumours behave in an unpredictable manner (BINDER et al. 1980).

The histological picture of mucoepidermoid carcinoma offers, as a result of its composition from solid, epidermoid, glandular and ductular components, unusual variability. The characteristics of mucoepidermoid carcinoma are essentially as follows (Fig. 7.7):

1. The cellular component of the tumour consist of basaloid cells, mature squamous epithelia, intermediary cells and mucus-secreting cells.
2. These primarily solid or epidermoid formations contain focal mucus-forming cells or microcysts filled with mucus.

A mucus stain (PAS, alcian blue) is useful for the histological diagnosis. If true glandular structures occur then the tumour is termed adenosquamous carcinoma, which, for example, arises more frequently in the lung. In addition there is a glycogen-rich clear cell variant of mucoepidermoid carcinoma (SEO et al. 1980), which must be distinguished from metastasis of a renal cell carcinoma by mucus staining.

7.1.3 Other Forms of Carcinoma

Besides the forms of carcinoma described, other malignant epithelial tumours occur albeit very rarely in the laryngeal region. To this group belong, as already mentioned, other rare salivary gland tumours, for example acinus cell carcinomas and salivary duct carcinomas (CRISSMAN and ROSENBLATT 1978, FERLITO et al. 1981, SQUIRES et al. 1981). Giant cell carcinomas, well known in the lung, have also been described in the larynx (FERLITO et al. 1985 a).

The so-called neuroendocrine carcinomas ("apudomas") may arise in the region of the larynx, as may the potentially malignant carcinoid tumours (MARKEL et al. 1980, TAMAI et al. 1981, PALADUGU et al. 1982, CEFIS et al. 1983, NONOMURA et al. 1983, MILLS and JOHNS 1984) and the related small cell carcinomas which occur primarily in the bronchial region similar in embryological origin to the larynx. For these neoplasms we have only a few single reports, so that no well-founded presentation of the biological behaviour of these tumours in the larynx is possible.

Most of the 19 cases of laryngeal **carcinoid tumours** compiled from the literature by BLOK et al. (1985) showed malignant behaviour. Half of these tumours were initially misdiagnosed as undifferentiated carcinoma or adenocarcinoma. The histological features of carcinoid tumours include "nesting" and trabecular growth pattern. The cytoplasm is often markedly swollen, granular, and eosinophilic, giving the cells the features of oncocytes or oncocytoid cells (STANLEY et al. 1986). Argyrophil and argentaffin stains may be positive. A dual endocrine and exocrine (mucos) differentiation has been observed (PALADUGU et al. 1982, CEFIS et al. 1983). Dense core granules can be found by electron microscopy; demonstration of NSE (neurone-specific enolase) is as a rule positive (MYEROWITZ et al. 1978). Case reports have been given by CAPPER et al. (1981), CEFIS et al. (1983), NONOMURA et al. (1983) and MILLS and JOHNS (1984).

GNEPP et al. (1983) compiled 43 cases of **small cell (oat cell) carcinomas** in the laryngeal region from the literature. As to be expected, the reports agree in describing particularly aggressive behaviour in these tumours (MYEROWITZ et al. 1978, THOMPSON et al. 1982). Histologically these tumours are identical to bronchial small cell carcinoma.

Combined small cell carcinomas - with squamous cell or adenocarcinomatous components - have also been observed (FERLITO et al. 1985b). The typical small cell is positive for cytokeratins, NSE and calcitonin in immunohistological examinations and contains neurosecretory granules (WEIDAUER et al. 1985). A variety of paraneoplastic syndromes may be associated with this tumour (MEDINA et al. 1984). Combined radiotherapy and chemotherapy, as for small cell bronchial carcinomas, is recommended.

7.1.4 Metastatic Cancer

Metastasis to the larynx is rare (GLANZ and KLEINSASSER 1978, ABEMAYOR et al. 1983). It can be blood-borne or ensue by lymphatic spread. FRIEDMANN and OSBORN (1965) report that among 72 patients with metastasis in the "head and neck" region the larynx was affected in 15 cases. BATSAKIS et al. (1985) reviewed 83 well-documented examples of metastasis to the intrinsic larynx, including 11 cases they were able to observe themselves. The primary tumours included renal cell ("hypernephroid") carcinoma (16.9% of all metastatic tumours to the larynx), bronchial carcinoma (9.6%), breast carcinoma (9.6%), prostate carcinoma (6%) and gastrointestinal carcinoma (2.4%). The rest were metastases of malignant melanomas (30%) and sarcomas.

The symptoms of metastasis to the soft tissues of the larynx are usually the same as with primary laryngeal cancer. No site of preference is evident, but the glottic area is seldom affected; multiple locations can be involved. Metastasis to ossified cartilage of the larynx may be unaccompanied by clinical symptoms. Prognosis is generally poor and depends on the underlying tumour disease. The occurrence of unusual malignant tumours in the larynx should always prompt a search for a primary lesion elsewhere.

7.2 Nonepithelial Malignant Tumours

7.2.1 Malignant Mesenchymal Tumours (Sarcomas)

Sarcomas of the larynx are exceedingly rare (KRATZ and RITTERHOFFER 1961, FRIEDMANN 1976, KRAJINA 1976, DRAETTA et al. 1980, GORENSTEIN et al. 1980, WILHELM et al. 1980). Accounts vary from 0.2% (from 4818 malignant laryngeal tumours (HACIHANEFIOGLU and ÖZTÜRK 1983) and 0.32% (KRAJINA 1976) to about 1% (FRIEDMANN 1976, MEYER-BREITING and ROSEMANN 1977). The most common form of sarcoma, according to older statistics, is fibrosarcoma (KRATZ and RITTERHOFFER 1961), the frequency of this lesion has been overestimated, however, owing to inadequate diagnostic possibilities (FERLITO et al. 1983, MICHAELS 1984). In the extensive collective statistical study carried out by KRAJINA (1976), there is, in addition to this type of sarcoma (three cases from 6067 neoplasms), a higher percentage of spindle cell sarcomas which could possibly have been more readily characterized using modern diagnostic methods (for example immunohistochemistry; Sect. 2.4).

The frequency of the individual types of sarcoma is more accurately described in the recent statistical studies carried out by GORENSTEIN et al. (1980) and FERLITO et al. (1983). The former, among about 3100 malignant laryngeal tumours encountered over an observation period of 25 years, diagnosed 17 sarcomas: seven chondrosarcomas, six fibrosarcomas, three rhabdomyosarcomas and one osteosarcoma. FERLITO et al. (1983), among 2874 tumours observed over a period of 17 years, found 25 sarcomas: seven fibrous histiocytomas, eight malignant lymphomas and plasmocytomas, three chondrosarcomas, two haemiangiopericytomas and one case each of angiosarcoma, leiomyosarcoma, liposarcoma, rhabdomyosarcoma and synovial sarcoma. The frequency of rhabdomyosarcomas can be deduced only with difficulty from older publications, since more particular experience regarding the diagnosis of this highly pleomorphic neoplasm has been gained only relatively recently. Some tumours reported as spindle cell sarcomas and immature fibrosarcomas, especially in small children, were in all probability embryonal rhabdomyosarcomas. CACHIN and SCHWAB (1978) even described a preponderance of rhabdomyosarcomas among the sarcomas of the head and neck region in children.

For this reason, FRIEDMANN'S (1976) demand should be followed, namely that in diagnosing sarcomas, all available histological means, including immunohistochemistry and electron microscopy, should be employed. Only through such efforts can comparative statistics for these tumours be compiled and consistent and comparable conclusions reached. When dealing with spindle cell neoplasms the possibility should always be borne in mind that the tumour could be a spindle cell carcinoma (Sect. 7.1.1.2). MICHAELS (1984) emphasizes that a "pedunculated lesion with a malignant fibroblastic histological appearance growing in the region of the anterior vocal cord is most likely to be a spindle cell carcinoma", whereby even focal osteoid formation can be present.

In the following the sarcomas that occur in the larynx will be dealt with in order of their presently known frequency.

7.2.1.1 Fibrosarcoma and Malignant Fibrous Histiocytoma

BATSAKIS and FOX (1970) report the frequency of fibrosarcoma to be 1%-2% of all malignant neoplasms of the larynx: according to KRATZ and RITTERHOFFER (1961), it comprises more than 50% of all laryngeal sarcomas. From the results gained by advanced methods of histological examination, however, these numbers should be regarded with some scepticism (FERLITO et al. 1983). In the Frankfurt University ENT Clinic we found, among 850 malignant neoplasms of the larynx, only one well-differentiated fibrosarcoma, compared to eight

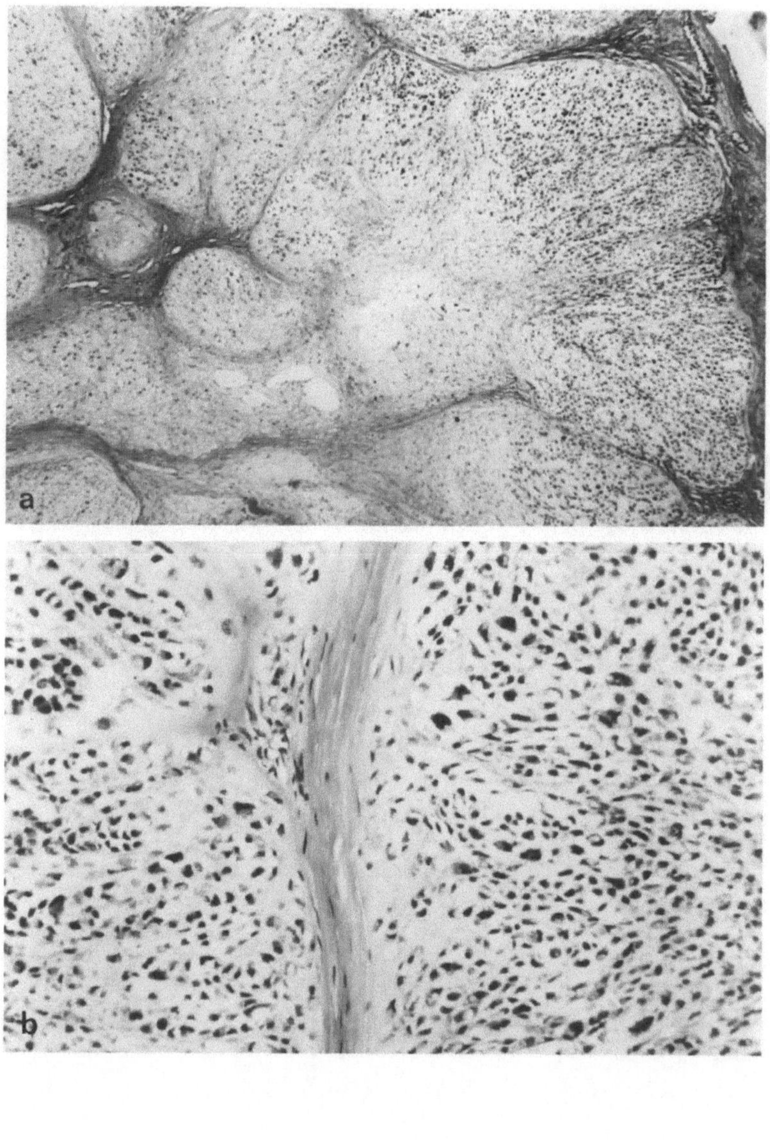

Fig. 7.8a, b. Chondrosarcoma: 55-year-old woman, subglottic region. **a** Lobulated tumour mass with formation of cartilage and high cellularity, especially in the periphery. HE, ×25. **b** The high cellularity with nuclear pleomorphism is evident at high magnification. HE, ×220

mesenchymal malignant tumours. According to the publications cited below, patients in every age group can be affected by fibrosarcoma. There is no certain sexual predilection, but in most surveys men predominate.

Fibrosarcoma of the larynx is found most often in the vocal fold and in the supraglottic region, but occasionally also at the transition to the trachea, as in one of our cases, an 11-year-old girl.

Macroscopically, laryngeal fibrosarcoma is often polypous. If the site of origin is fairly deep in the tissue, the mucosal surface is pushed forward from a broad base into the lumen.

Histologically these tumours are derived from the fibroblasts and resemble fibromas but exhibit cellular atypia and mitotic figures. In general, fibrosarcomas are divided into poorly and well-differentiated forms depending on the proportion of fibre-forming and/or anaplastic cellular elements (BATSAKIS and FOX, 1970). PERILLI and BAGNARIOL (1969), in contrast, divided fibrosarcomas into four grades of differentiation.

The more common, well-differentiated fibrosarcomas hardly metastasize at all, but tend to recur locally (40%, GORENSTEIN et al. 1980), whereas poorly-differentiated types form distant metastasis, in particular in the lung (25%). Consequently, partial laryngectomy is recommended (if possible) in the former instance and radical laryngectomy in the latter.

The first report of a fibrosarcoma in the larynx and upper tracheal region was by KAHLER (1908). Thereafter followed numerous further observations (CITELLI 1912, HART and MAYER 1928, FIGI 1933, RIGBY and HOLLINGER 1943, BROUGHTON and BARNES et al. 1948, COAKLEY and SALE 1948, HOL-

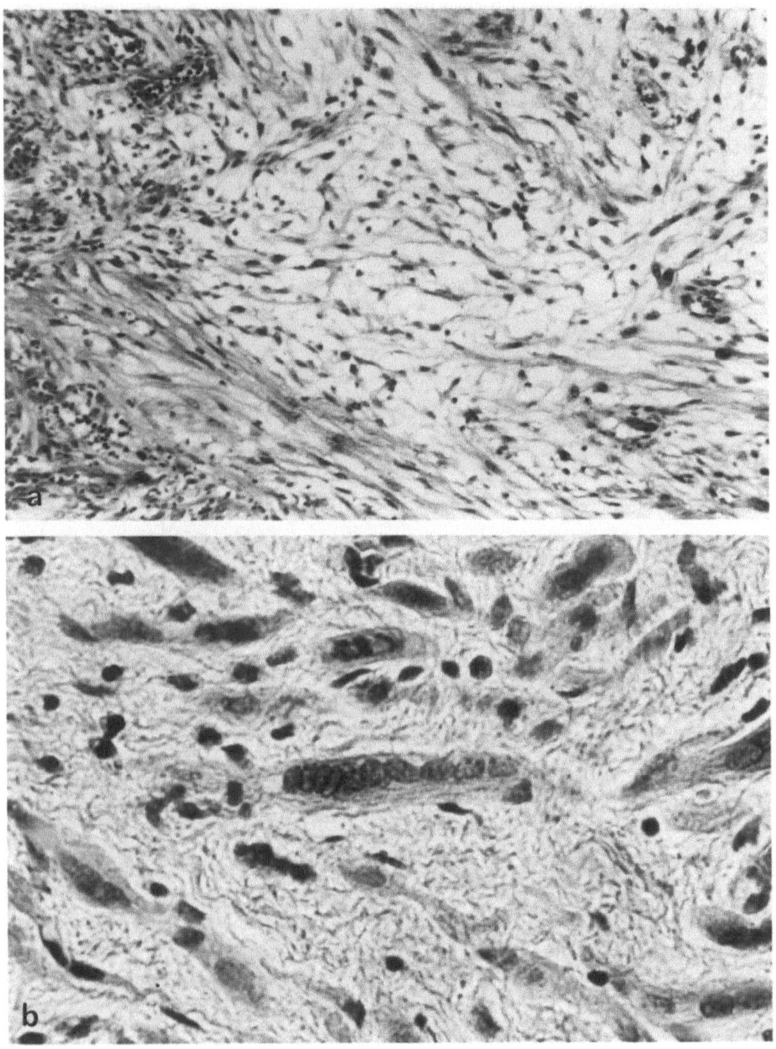

Fig. 7.9 a, b. Rhabdomyosarcoma: 11-year-old boy, polypous tumour of the vocal cord. **a** Loosely textured spindle cell tumour tissue. HE, ×60. **b** At high magnification the scattered tumour cells exhibit marked nuclear pleomorphism and elongated cytoplasm, with cross-striation occasionally discernible. HE, ×600

LINGER et al. 1950, MILLER 1950, LACHMANN 1951, DIEHL 1953, DWYER 1953, VYXLONZEL 1956, GIRAUD 1957, JOHNSTON 1957, HALL 1958, KRATZ and RITTERHOFFER 1961, FLANAGAN et al. 1965, CALVET et al. 1968, PERILLI and BAGNARIOL 1969, FRIEDMANN 1976, KRAJINA 1976, DONALDSON 1978, DRAETTA et al. 1980, GORENSTEIN et al. 1980).

FERLITO (1978) and FERLITO et al. (1983 a and b) pointed out that under the term "fibrosarcoma" are subsumed, in part, the so-called **malignant fibrous histiocytomas** and xanthomas (see Sect. 3.3.1.1). In more recent papers this term has been increasingly applied to the tumours of the fibrohistiocytic spectrum, wherein fibrous, pleomorphic, giant cell, angiomatoid, myxoid and xanthomatous forms can be distinguished. A storiform growth pattern of spindle cells is thought to be characteristic of this neoplasm.

FERLITO et al. (1983 b) compiled 17 case reports from the literature and added their own observations. The pleomorphic subtype was found in six patients, the fibrous and giant cell subtypes in four patients each. The tumours have an unpredictable clinical behaviour and exhibit a tendency toward recurrence and - depending on the grade of anaplasia - metastatic spread (four cases). Recent case reports were published by RAMADAS et al. (1984), VOLMER (1985) and GODOY et al. (1986).

7.2.1.2 Chondrosarcoma

The most common site of chondrosarcomas is the dorsal part of the cricoid cartilage (75%). From here the tumour can extend to the oesophageal inlet and sometimes result in dysphagia prior to dyspnoea. Older patients and men are affected most frequent-

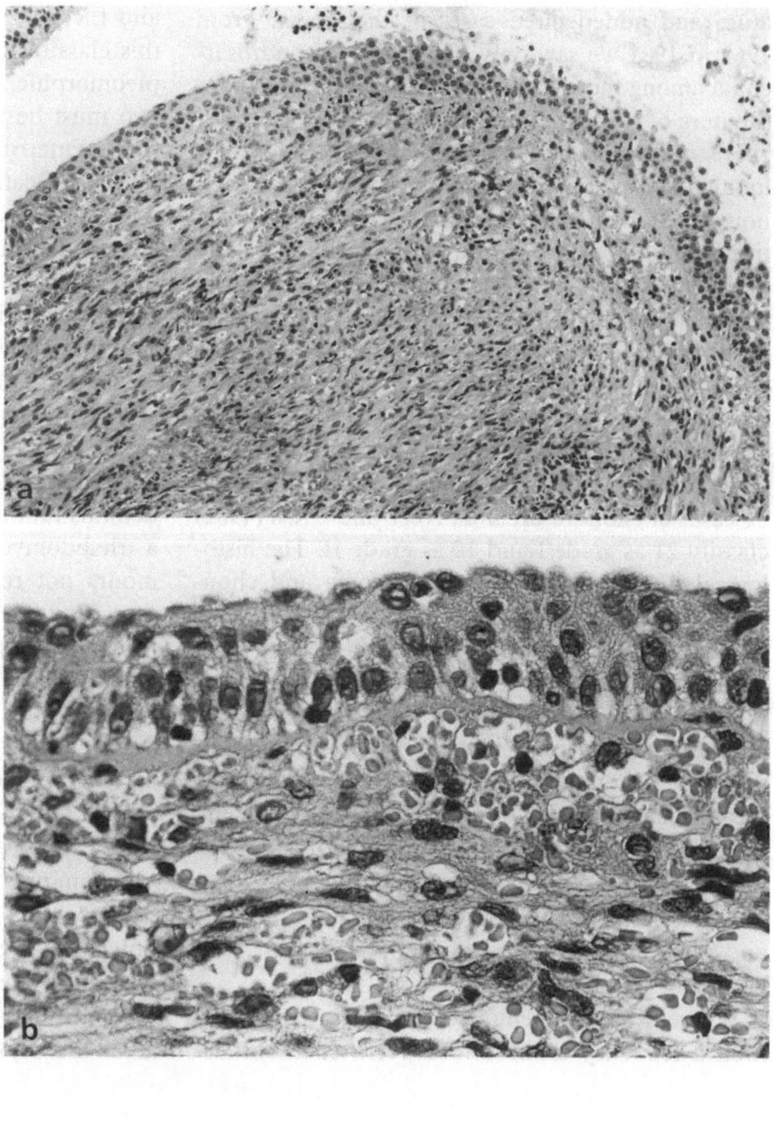

Fig. 7.10 a, b. Kaposi's sarcoma: 54-year-old man with acquired immunodeficiency syndrome (AIDS). Multiple blue-red tumorous lesions in the trachea and subglottis. **a** Protrusion of the intact epithelium by an atypical spindle cell tissue with abundant cleft formation containing erythrocytes. HE, ×150. **b** The spindle cells exhibit nuclear atypia, between them there are spaces without clear endothelial lining, filled with erythrocytes. The majority of the spindle cells give a positive reaction for factor-VIII-associated antigen. HE, ×350

ly. Tumour growth is slow. The X-ray picture is relatively typical and exhibits tumour nodules of varying radiodensity with irregular spots of calcification. Macroscopically these hard, often globular tumours push the intact mucosa forward into the lumen of the larynx.

One of the first to report such neoplasms in the larynx was NEW (1935). Two years later AUBRY and LEROUX-ROBERT (1937) likewise reported on chondrosarcoma in the larynx. These initial descriptions were followed by further, at first isolated but later more frequent, reports (LINK 1949, UNGERECHT 1951, SIROTA and HURWITZ 1952, HUIZENGA and BALOGH 1970, BUSUTTIL and FORBES 1978, COYAS et al. 1978, WEBER et al. 1978, HELLQUIST et al. 1979, OESTBERG et al. 1979, CANTRELL et al. 1980, EIBLING and ROSNAGLE 1980, GORENSTEIN et al. 1980, MOHR and HUSSAIN 1981, FISH et al. 1982, NEEL and UNNI 1982). FERLITO et al. (1984) compiled 149 cases of chondrosarcomas of the larynx reported in the literature and added three cases of their own. From 1962 to 1981 we saw only one case of chondrosarcoma among more than 850 patients with malignant tumours of the larynx (Tab. 5.1).

Histologically chondrosarcomas are composed of lobulated, usually hyaline, in part myxoid, cartilaginous tissue of variable maturity, with thin connective tissue septae (Fig. 7.8a). The coarse, usually dark, chromatin-rich nuclei of the tumour cells are remarkable, irregular large cells can be binuclear, multinuclear giant cells are not uncommon (Fig. 7.8b). Well-differentiated forms can be distinguished from poorly differentiated forms. HUIZENGA and BALOGH (1970) found a 3:1 ratio of differentiated to undifferentiated chondrosarcomas. Of 31 cases of chondrosarcoma, NEEL and UNNI (1982) classify 21 as grade I and 10 as grade II. The histological distinction between chondroma and chondrosarcomas has been defined by LICHTENSTEIN and JAFFE (1943) and is discussed in Sect. 3.4.1. In our experience, there is a danger of occasionally underestimating differentiated chondrosarcomas as chondromas, especially if the biopsy material is insufficient. Photometric investigations, in particular measurement of the DNA and, to a lesser extent, the nuclear size, can be of assistance in this distinction (HELLQUIST et al. 1979). The differential diagnosis of chondrosarcoma comprises chondroblastic and myxoid osteosarcoma and, in cases with abundant spindle cells, spindle cell sarcoma.

Whereas the differentiated chondrosarcomas exhibit a tendency towards local recurrence but seldom metastasize, in less differentiated tumours blood-borne metastasis occurs, most often to the lung. This latter subtype behaves no less malignantly than the same tumours arising in skeletal bones (ESCHER et al. 1984). The choice of operative procedure thus depends on the degree of differentiation.

7.2.1.3 Rhabdomyosarcoma

Probably as a result of improved diagnostic methods (see Sect. 2.4) and better information, most published accounts of rhabdomyosarcomas in the larynx have appeared in the last few decades, particularly in recent years. DIEHN et al.(1984) found 28 case reports in the literature and added a further six observations.

In the histological classification of this morphologically very variable tumour, the system of HORN and ENTERLEIN (1958) has generally been adopted: this classifies rhabdomyosarcomas into embryonal, pleomorphic, alveolar and botryoid forms. The last two must be viewed as subtypes of the embryonal form. FRIEDMANN (1976), in contrast, recommends the classification proposed by ASHTON and MORGAN (1965), into embryonal rhabdomyosarcomas with and without cross-striation and alveolar rhabdomyosarcomas. Whereas the pleomorphic type is mostly seen in adults (KLEINSASSER and GLANZ 1979), the embryonal forms of rhabdomyosarcoma occur particularly in children. According to DITO and BATSAKIS (1962), of 170 patients with rhabdomyosarcomas in the head and neck region, 80% were under 12 years of age. Immunohistological demonstration of myoglobin gives an indication of a rhabdomyomatous nature in pleomorphic tumours not readily identified as rhabdomyosarcomas. Up to 1979, only four cases of the particularly rare pleomorphic (adult) rhabdomyosarcoma had been reported (FRANZ 1979). WILHELM et al. (1980) added a fifth.

Embryonal rhabdomyosarcomas of the larynx, as in other mucosal areas, not uncommonly present with a polyp-like protrusion into the laryngeal lumen, the so-called botryoid type. Cursory histological examination of these tumours often reveals only nonspecific alterations compatible with granulation polyp. Only close observation reveals that this polyp is interspersed with spindle-shaped cells having pleomorphic, in part bizarre, nuclei. Whereas large areas are myxoid, an increased density of cellular elements is sometimes found towards the surface (Fig. 7.9).

Alveolar rhabdomyosarcoma may, owing to its larger proportion of small cell elements with little cytoplasm, be confused with malignant lymphomas. Only the alveolar structure and the presence of a few large cells which have a pronounced, eosinophilic cytoplasm and occasionally detectable cross-striation point to its true origin. The phenomenon of cross-striation can be particularly well assessed following staining with phosphotungstic acid-haematein (PTAH, Mallory).

Rhabdomyosarcomas are generally highly malignant tumours with a tendency towards both local recurrence and early lymphatic and blood-borne metastatic spread. Besides surgical treatment these tumours respond to combined chemotherapy, which according to accounts by WILBUR et al. (1975) and TAN et al. (1975), is superior to combined surgery and radiotherapy.

Case reports of rhabdomyosarcomas can be found in PIAGET et al. (1943), PEARSON et al. (1956), HARRIS (1961), FRUGONI and FERLITO (1976), MEYER-BREITING and ROSEMANN (1977), IWASAWA (1978), WINTHER and LORENTZEN (1978), FRANZ (1979), SENJUKOW et al. (1979), STANKIEWICZ and PAPIEL (1979), KLEINSASSER and GLANZ (1979), BATSAKIS et al. (1980), DEGROOT et al. (1980), GORENSTEIN et al. (1980), WILHELM et al. (1980) and ABRAMOWSKY and WITT (1983).

7.2.1.4 Leiomyosarcoma

EGGSTON and WOLFF (1947) first mentioned two cases of this tumour in an endolaryngeal location. Further reports came from KAWABE (1967) and WOLFOWITZ and SCHMAMANN (1973). Owing to the small number of cases no statement can be made regarding preferred location, age and sexual predisposition.

The histological picture corresponds to that of leiomyomas but cellular atypia and mitotic figures are present. KLEINSASSER and GLANZ (1979) point out the difficulties of histological differential diagnosis between leiomyosarcoma and fibrosarcoma. Demonstration of desmin can support the diagnosis of leiomyosarcoma.

7.2.1.5 Angiosarcoma

Only scarce reports on angiosarcomas of the larynx are available (MEYER-BREITING and ROSEMANN 1977, FERLITO et al. 1985).

Malignant haemangioendotheliomas are usually haemorrhagic and cystic and often polypous. The endothelial cells are the malignant cell of these tumours. We observed a 65-year-old male patient with tumour formation in Morgagni's ventricle and spread to the piriform sinus. Histologically there was intense capillary proliferation as well as the development of lacunae of variable size; on their edges the otherwise single-layered, cytoplasm-rich endothelial cells formed aggregates of pleomorphic smaller cells with little cytoplasm, increased mitotic figures and deficient coherence; they were shed in great numbers into the lumina of the lacunae. Besides endothelial proliferation, haematopoietic elements and their precursors are not uncommonly found in this type of tumour. Immunohistochemical demonstration of factor VIII associated antigens helps to distinguish this tumour from other pleomorphic sarcomas. Malignant haemangioendotheliomas metastasize very early via the blood and have a particularly poor prognosis.

Haemangiopericytomas consist of blood vessels surrounded by spindle- to round-celled malignant cellular elements which are derived from pericytes. Such a tumour was observed by FERLITO (1978) in a 50-year-old man in the anterior region of the vocal cord.

MURRAI et al. (1962) reported on the laryngeal occurrence of a special form of the haemangiosarcoma, namely **Kaposi's sarcoma.** This tumour appears primarily on the skin and in recent years has been observed more often in immunosuppressed patients, such as those suffering from AIDS (acquired immunodeficiency syndrome). Affection of the larynx, mostly in the subglottic area, often together with the trachea, is almost always associated with involvement of the skin. There are further observations of laryngeal Kaposi sarcomas (MORITSCH et al. 1978, COYAS et al. 1983). Increasing occurrence is to be reckoned with.

Histologically Kaposi sarcoma involves the proliferation of endothelial and spindle cells (Fig. 7.10). Angioblastic zones with endothelium-lined cavities and areas with bundles of spindle cells are intermingled. In addition, round cell infiltrates and numerous microhaemorrhages are typical.

7.2.1.6 Malignant Lymphoma

Since lymphatic tissue is found in the larynx, in particular in the piriform sinus and in Morgagni's ventricle, malignant lymphoma can develop. In practice, however, both primary malignant lymphoma in the larynx and laryngeal involvement in generalized lymphoma are encountered extremely seldom (0.1% of malignant laryngeal tumours; HACIHANEFIOGLU and ÖZTÜRK 1983); thus the difficult problems of lymphoma classification need not be dealt with here (for further information see LENNERT 1981).

In the case of **plasmacellular proliferations** in the larynx, appropriate clinical diagnostic investigations must be performed to determine whether a solitary plasmocytoma (see Sect. 3.5.1) or a generalized process involving other regions of the body is presented. Paraproteinaemia indicates generalized plasmocytoma.

KRAJINA (1976) reported on lymphomas of apparently higher grades of malignancy observed in the larynx. SWERDLOW et al. (1984) compiled a survey of 18 cases of laryngeal non-Hodgkin lymphomas (17 from the literature plus one of their own). The patients were between 14 and 81 years of age and women were affected about twice as often as men. Only five of these cases could be classified as low grade malignant; the remainder were high grade malignant. Further subsequent classification of cases reported in the literature is unfortunately not possible if immunohistological examinations have not been performed. MICHAELS (1984) reported on a laryngeal Burkitt lymphoma in a 9-year-old boy.

An extreme rarity, described by HOOD et al. (1979), was a primary affection of the larynx by mycosis fungoides - a T-cell lymphoma usually originating in the skin - in an 80-year-old woman; only 3 years later did a pronounced skin affection appear. A similar case was described by KLEINSASSER (1983). Secondary involvement of the larynx occurs more often but is still rare (FERLITO and RECHER 1986).

So-called **reticulum cell sarcomas** (retothelial sarcomas) have been seen in the larynx and described by GRIMAUD and WERNER (1955), NORRIS and PEALE (1961), KRAJINA (1976), WATANABE (1978) and DRAETTA et al. (1980). Among 850 patients with malignant neoplasms of the larynx treated in Frankfurt University ENT Clinic, two cases were classified as reticulum cell sarcomas. Usually those affected are elderly. As long as the tumour is limited to the region, the prognosis, with radiotherapy, appears to be relatively favourable. In case of distant metastasis or general spread it becomes poor.

According to recent interpretation, the majority of the neoplasms earlier termed reticulum cell sarcomas belong to the immunoblastic group of malignant lymphomas. Distinction between the latter group of malignant lymphomas and the true histiocytic malignant neoplasias is possible only immunohistologically, by demonstration of immunoglobulins or of histiocytic features such as lysozyme, alpha-1-antitrypsin, vimentin and S-100 protein (see Sect. 2.4).

MEYER-BREITING (1975) found that only seven cases of **Hodgkins's disease** in the larynx had been reported in the literature and added one further case of his own. In two patients the disease originated primarily in the larynx, and in four there was simultaneous involvement of the laryngeal and cervical lymph nodes (CHATELLIER and GUERIN 1927, HALPHEN 1927, TANTURRI 1927, ZEIDLER 1929, COOKE 1931, REBOUL et al. 1956, LAUTZ 1958, DONAT 1959). As a rule, an unremarkable superficial distension of the soft parts of the larynx is described. Hoarseness and dyspnoea cause patients to seek medical care.

Malignant lymphoma (SWERDLOW et al. 1984) must be distinguished histologically from the rare pseudolymphomas. Immunohistochemical investigations are necessary in cases of unclear nature. Treatment of the lymphoreticular neoplasias is best placed in the hands of an oncologist.

7.2.1.7 Other Malignant Mesenchymal Neoplasms

Besides the tumour types described above, other malignant mesenchymal neoplasms can of course occur in the laryngeal region. However, these are all extremely rare and often have been described only in solitary case reports. With regard to the details of these tumours, reference will be made to the appropriate special publications.

Isolated observations have been made of **liposarcomas** in the laryngeal region (MILLER et al. 1975, VELEK et al. 1976, KRAUSEN et al. 1977, TOBEY et al. 1979, OTTE and KLEINSASSER 1981, GAYNOR et al. 1984, ALLSBROOK et al. 1985). The supraglottic region is apparently the preferred site. These tumour can be multiple (KRAUSEN et al. 1977) and tend to local recurrences. The prognosis depends on the histological type and on the degree of differentiation. Local excision and postoperative irradiation are recommended.

Reports of **alveolar soft part sarcomas** in the laryngeal region are only isolated (MICHAELS 1984).

The case of a questionable extraskeletal **Ewing sarcoma** in the larynx of a newly-born baby was described by ABRAMOWSKY and WITT (1983).

Neurofibrosarcomas are similarly mentioned only in a few isolated cases (GORENSTEIN et al. 1980); they must be distinguished from fibrosarcomas.

The malignant synovioma or **synovial sarcoma,** which normally derives from the synovial membrane or the bursae in the vicinity of joints, is occasionally seen in the larynx and the adjacent hypopharynx (GATTIE et al. 1975, MILLER et al. 1975, WILHELM et al. 1980, GEACHAN et al. 1983, KLEINSASSER 1983, MOHR and PIRSIG 1984). This tumour, which is usually composed biphasically of spindle cells and cleft spaces lined by thelial cell formations, must be distinguished in particular from fibrosarcoma (FERLITO et al. 1983, KLEINSASSER 1983).

Osteosarcomas occur exceedingly seldom in the laryngeal region (MORLEY et al. 1973, DAHM et al. 1978, GORENSTEIN et al. 1980, REMAGEN et al. 1983). REMAGEN et al. (1983) were able to find only five case reports in the literature and added one of their own. Only elderly patients were affected. The tumours are predominantly cell-rich and composed of spindle cells with reticular osteoid formation; giant cells and cartilage formation are common. HAAR et al. (1978) reported on a pronounced chondroblastic osteosarcoma of the larynx. Osteosarcoma must be distinguished primarily from chondrosarcoma, myositis ossificans and spindle cell sarcomas.

Giant cell tumours (osteoclastomas) are likewise rarely seen in the larynx (KLEINSASSER 1983). Histologically, benign and aggressive forms cannot be distinguished. In the larynx, giant cell tumours tend to behave rather aggressively (KLEINSASSER 1983).

Malignant mesenchymoma - mixed mesenchymal neoplasm - has also been described in the larynx (TOBEY et al. 1979).

7.2.2 Malignant Neuroectodermal Tumours

7.2.2.1 Malignant Melanoma

Primary malignant melanomas in mucosal surfaces, particular in the laryngeal region, are considered extremely rare. In each case it must be ensured that no primary tumour of another location - in particular the skin - is metastasizing to the larynx. Even in cases of melanoma confined to the larynx the question arises of whether a primary tumour in the region of the skin has possibly regressed, as has been postulated by several authors.

Primary laryngeal melanomas are thought to derive from melanocytes in the laryngeal mucosa, which were described, for example, by GOLDMANN et al. (1972) employing the Fontana silver stain. These results have been questioned, however, by MICHAELS (1984), who pointed out that the dendritic Langerhans cells are similar to melanocytes. It can be assumed that the occurrence of true melanocytes in the larynx is at least rare (BUSUTTIL 1976). Thus, lentigo (melanoplakia) of the larynx is extremely rare (GOLDMAN et al. 1972, TRAVIS and SUTHERLAND 1980) and there is only one report of a benign melanocytic tumour (compound naevus) in the larynx (SCHIMPF et al. 1969).

KIM and PARK (1982) compiled 27 cases of probable primary malignant melanoma of the larynx from the world literature, REUTER and WOODRUFF (1986) accepted 22 cases as true laryngeal melanomas. Affected were patients over 50, men more frequently than women (about 2:1). The location was chiefly supraglottic, and the symptoms were hoarseness and dysphagia. The tumours were as a rule nodular to polypoid and only some were of a dark brown/black colour. The rest were grey-white, i.e. no pigment could be seen macroscopically. Lymph node metastasis in the neck region was generally not present at the time of the initial diagnosis.

Histologically, only the nodular type of melanoma has been described so far. About half the cases were amelanotic. Junctional changes at the epithelial mesenchymal interface are considered an indication that the tumour concerned originated in the laryngeal mucosa (LORENTZ 1979).

The prognosis of laryngeal melanoma is extremely poor, since rapid and pronounced distant metastatic spread usually ensues. The survival times are on the order of a few months to, at the most, a few years. Laryngectomy and neck dissection are recommended as treatment.

We observed a male patient aged 55 with a tumour in the region of the aryepiglottic fold which was certainly malignant, but could not be classified at first; it was surgically removed. Four years later a local recurrence appeared, and after a further 14 months (following hemilaryngectomy and irradiation), metastasis appeared in the cervical lymph nodes. The histological examination now showed a tumour resembling malignant melanoma and the

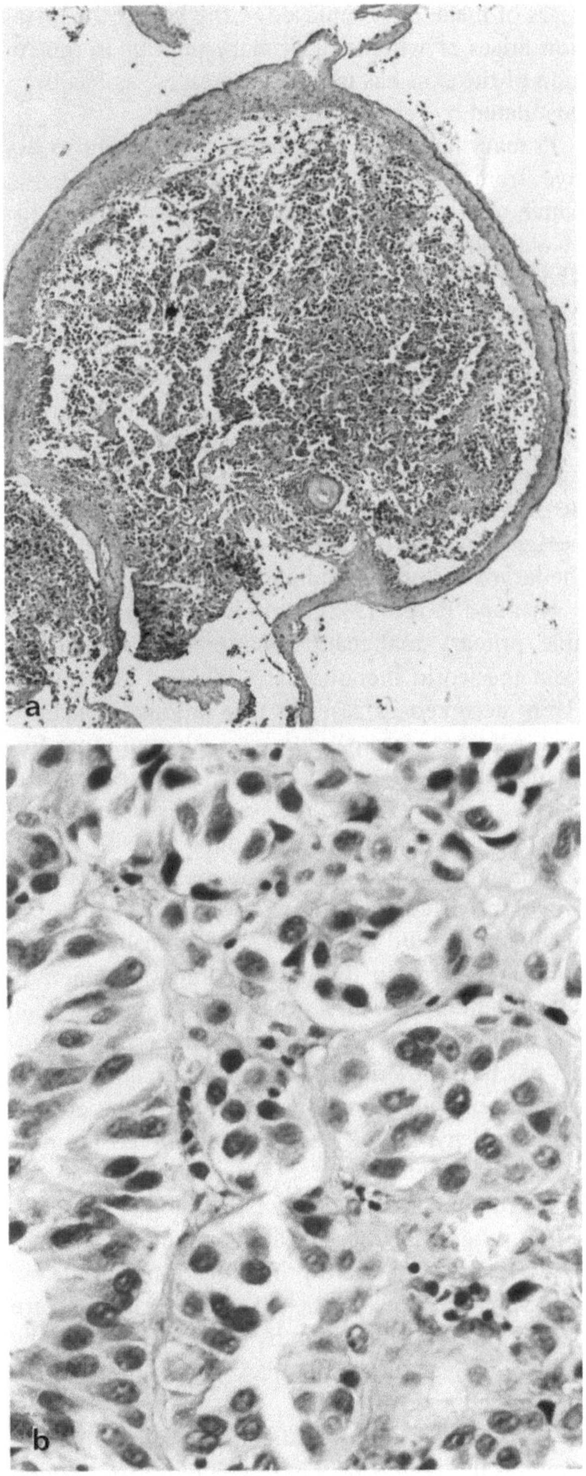

Fig. 7.11a, b. Malignant melanoma: 55-year-old man, aryepiglottic fold. a Polypous cellular tumour with intact epithelial covering. HE, ×35. b The tumour cells show "nesting" typical of melanocytic tumours, but no epithelial cohesion. Marked nuclear pleomorphism of the round to spindle-shaped tumour cells. HE, ×350

Fontana-Masson stain and the immunological test for the S-100 protein were positive. A competitive primary tumour could not be established during the entire course of the tumour disease.

Metastases from malignant melanomas are also rare, but are the most common of the metastases which occur in the larynx. Ferlito and Caruso (1984) documented 23 metastatic malignant melanomas among 81 metastatic tumours in the larynx described in the literature (28%). Metastasis was exclusively in the soft parts, and again men were affected more frequently than women.

7.2.2.2 Chemodectomas (Paragangliomas)

The possibility that chemodectomas (paragangliomas) of the larynx may be malignant has already been discussed in Sect. 3.3.2.3. The histological picture does not generally offer any help in establishing malignancy (Spagnolo and Paradinas 1985).

7.3 Radiogenic Tumours

It is undisputed today that irradiation of living tissue, including therapeutic application, can induce malignant neoplasms. There are basically three types of radiation damage (Gössner 1972):

1. Dystrophy (degeneration, necrosis)
2. Dysplasia
3. Neoplasia

All three changes cause considerable difficulties in the assessment of biopsy or surgical specimens of preirradiated tissue. Depending on the dose, there ensues, to a greater or lesser extent, epithelial metaplasia of the laryngeal mucosa. In regions of preexisting squamous epithelium, epithelial hyperplasia is found with a pronounced tendency to keratinization. Both are associated with epithelial dysplasia of variable extent. Also the subepithelial connective tissue shows, under certain circumstances, considerable cellular atypia and often inflammatory changes. Cellular atypia of the connective tissue cells is often difficult to distinguish from malignant mesenchymal tumours or carcinomatous extensions with markedly dissociated growth pattern, especially in small biopsy specimens.

An early report on the appearance of laryngeal

carcinoma following irradiation was made by VON EICKEN (1934). Malignant neoplasms after irradiation can originate from the laryngeal epithelium or from the soft tissue of the larynx (GAHLIB et al. 1969, BAKER and WEISSMANN 1971, LAWSON and SOM 1975, GLANZ and KLEINSASSER 1976, TAYLOW 1977, DONALDSON 1978). Proof usually cannot be obtained in these cases whether tumour recurrence, spontaneous new tumour disease or so-called radiogenic tumour is involved, because in general the risk factors which led to carcinomatous disease in the first place have continued to exert their effect, and in carcinoma patients often larger mucosal areas tend to malignant transformation (so-called multitopical or multicentric tumour growth or field cancerization, see Sect. 4.5): thus, even in nonirradiated patients treated for malignant neoplasms, carcinomas can be more frequently observed in the same and in related organs.

The radiogenic second neoplasms in the laryngeal region are, in the vast majority of cases, squamous cell carcinomas. From the true radiogenic second tumours must be distinguished the changes of the histological picture of squamous cell carcinomas observed following irradiation (see Sect. 6.3.2). Occasionally the transformation of a keratinizing squamous cell carcinoma into spindle cell carcinoma or carcinosarcoma (see Sect. 7.1.1.2) is seen, as in the case of a 51-year-old patient of ours in whom, 1 year after irradiation of a moderately differentiated, keratinizing squamous cell carcinoma with 64.6 Gy, a recurrence in the form of a pleomorphic, spindle cell carcinoma was found.

The relationship between irradiation and oncogenesis is relatively clear if the primary radiotherapy was performed for a non-neoplastic disease or a benign tumour. In the laryngeal area radiation has been applied for thyrotoxicosis, tubercular lymphadenitis, lupus vulgaris, thymic hyperplasia and juvenile laryngeal papillomatosis. Radiotherapy of these disorders is generally rejected today owing to the risk of tumour induction. GOOLDEN reported first in 1951, and in more detail in 1957, on the development of malignant neoplasms in the laryngopharyngeal region following radiotherapy for thyrotoxicosis and tubercular lymphadenitis. He found 24 cases in the literature, and added 18 of his own, in which, during an interval of 10-35 years (average 25 years) following radiotherapy, a malignant neoplasm appeared in the laryngopharyngeal region; of these, five were carcinomas clearly located in the laryngeal region. The malignant tumours were in the vast majority of cases squamous cell carcinomas and two were fibrosarcomas. Patients were aged 40-50 years and were thus without exception younger than the average patient presenting carcinoma in the laryngopharyngeal region. A large proportion of the patients in this account were women; this can be explained, however, by the high frequency of thyrotoxicosis in women.

Spontaneous malignant transformation of juvenile laryngeal papillomas is extremely rare: almost always there has been preceeding irradiation (WALSH and BEAMER 1950, KLEINSASSER 1958, GALLOWAY et al. 1960, KLEINSASSER and GLANZ 1979). In the Mayo Clinic series, the frequency of carcinoma following irradiation of juvenile papillomas was 14% (MAJORS et al. 1964). The carcinomas appear between 3 and 44 years after irradiation (average 20 years).

GOOLDEN (1951, 1957) established the following criteria for the recognition of a relationship between radiotherapy and tumour development:

1. Appearance following radiotherapy of a primary benign disease
2. A long latency period between radiotherapy and tumour disease
3. Development of the tumour in the region with the highest radiation dose, recognizable by distinct radiogenic skin changes in this area (hyperpigmentation, atrophy or necrosis)
4. Histological proof of a malignant tumour, i.e. first and foremost the exclusion of radiogenic necrosis
5. Unusual characteristics of the tumour disease with regard to sex, age, location or histology

Much more complicated is the assessment of a second neoplasm following radiotherapy of a malignant tumour. In order to accept and recognize a correlation between the irradiation and the development of the second tumour in such cases, it has been postulated that the two tumours should be histologically distinct from one another. This condition would be fulfilled, for example, in patients in whom a malignant mesenchymal tumour develops after irradiation of a carcinoma (see below), which has been reported repeatedly. RASINGER and ULRICH (1983) described the appearance of a differentiated adenocarcinoma 2 years after irradiation (25 Gy) of a moderately differentiated squamous cell carcinoma. COACKLEY (1985) observed a primary oat cell carcinoma of the larynx 11 years after successful radiotherapy (cobalt) for squamous cell carcinoma of the vocal cord. The occurrence of a squamous cell carcinoma in the larynx in a 20-year-old female nonsmoker who 3 years previously had received radiation therapy and chemotherapy for a rhabdomyosarcoma of the paranasal sinus was documented by AMENDOLA et al. (1985). In two patients treated for Hodgkins disease by irradiation, squamous cell carcinomas of the laryngopharyngeal area and the tongue developed 12 and 22 years later (WALLNER et al. 1985). Thus a radiogenic etiology can be considered as probable if tumour manifestation is unusual in the patient concerned or if tumours unusual in the respective organ are involved (GOOLDEN'S point 5 above).

The observations by GOOLDEN (1951, 1957), as well as numerous observations on different organ systems, have shown, however, that the radiogenic neoplasms are generally histologically of the same or similar type as arises spontaneously in the corresponding organ system. Thus, in bone there is a propensity for the development of osteosarcomas (ARLEN et al. 1972), and in the laryngeal region for squamous cell carcinomas, which are indeed the most common tumours arising spontaneously (see Sect. 5.1). A few authors consider tumour tissue in the depth as recurrence, while a second carcinoma is acknowledged if there is a connection with the surface epithelium. But this can, of course, be a secondary association.

In any one particular case, therefore, absolute proof can never be obtained as to whether the carcinoma in question is a radiogenic second carcinoma, a recurrence, or has developed spontaneously (metachronic carcinogenesis). BAKER and WEISSMANN (1971), on reviewing the clinical course of a large number of patients, found that simple tumour recurrences - i.e. residual tumours - generally appear within the first few years after treatment. In seven patients, however, they observed neoplasms which arose between 5 and 25 years after radiotherapy. They state that in all these cases the tumour appeared to be an independent second neoplasm. Nonetheless, they noted that at least in one patient who continued to smoke after radiotherapy, preexisting risk factors continued to exert an influence. Relatively arbitrarily, BAKER and WEISSMANN (1971), like other authors (GLANZ and KLEINSASSER 1976, LUND et al. 1982), postulated a tumour-free interval of 5 years after irradiation of the first tumour for the recognition of the second tumour as radiogenic.

Three patients at the Frankfurt University ENT Clinic between 1975 and 1985 had tumour growth detected between 6 and 9 years after conservative surgery with no radiotherapy whatsoever. This proves that either late recurrence or spontaneous metachronic carcinogenesis does occur.

Although it is not possible in an individual patient, statistically a clear relationship can be shown to exist between irradiation and the development of second tumours. VAN DISHOECK (1968) found that in 8% of the carcinomas in the head and neck region, this area had been irradiated 15-20 years previously for different diseases. More recently, GLANZ and KLEINSASSER (1976) have discussed the problem of late recurrences of laryngeal carcinomas providing an extensive review of the literature on the subject. Among 1086 patients with laryngeal carcinomas observed by these authors over a period of 23 years, there were 32 cases of carcinoma which appeared 5-18 years (average 9.9 years) after treatment. Three of these patients had been treated solely by surgery, the other 29 either by surgery and postoperative irradiation or by irradiation alone. GLANZ and KLEINSASSER (1976) conclude that these carcinomas in all probability resulted from radiation; according to their observation, the probability of developing a new carcinoma rises from year to year. Like BAKER and WEISSMANN (1971) they draw the conclusion that radiotherapy should be avoided in younger patients. Similar experience was reported by LAWSON and SOM (1975), who described 18 patients (5.6%) with development of carcinomas 5-21 years after irradiation. LUND et al. (1982) found that of 266 patients irradiated for laryngeal carcinoma, 10 (3.7%) developed a second carcinoma within 5-17 years later (average 11.8 years). All 10 carcinomas were located in the radiation field and five were in the area of the maximum dose (100%) whilst three were located peripherally in the marginal zone (50%-80% of the dose). LUND et al. (1982) also consider it highly probable that radiation plays an etiological role in the development of second carcinomas.

In contrast to these observations are the findings of KOGELNIK (1977): he followed up 1057 carcinoma patients who were either irradiated (720 cases) or treated by surgery only (337 cases). All had a recurrence-free interval of at least 5 years. Between 8 and 25 years after initial treatment, 78 (10.8%) irradiated patients and 36 (10.6%) operated patients developed a second tumour in a different location. In 39 (5.4%) of the irradiated patients these tumours were located in the field of radiation and in 20

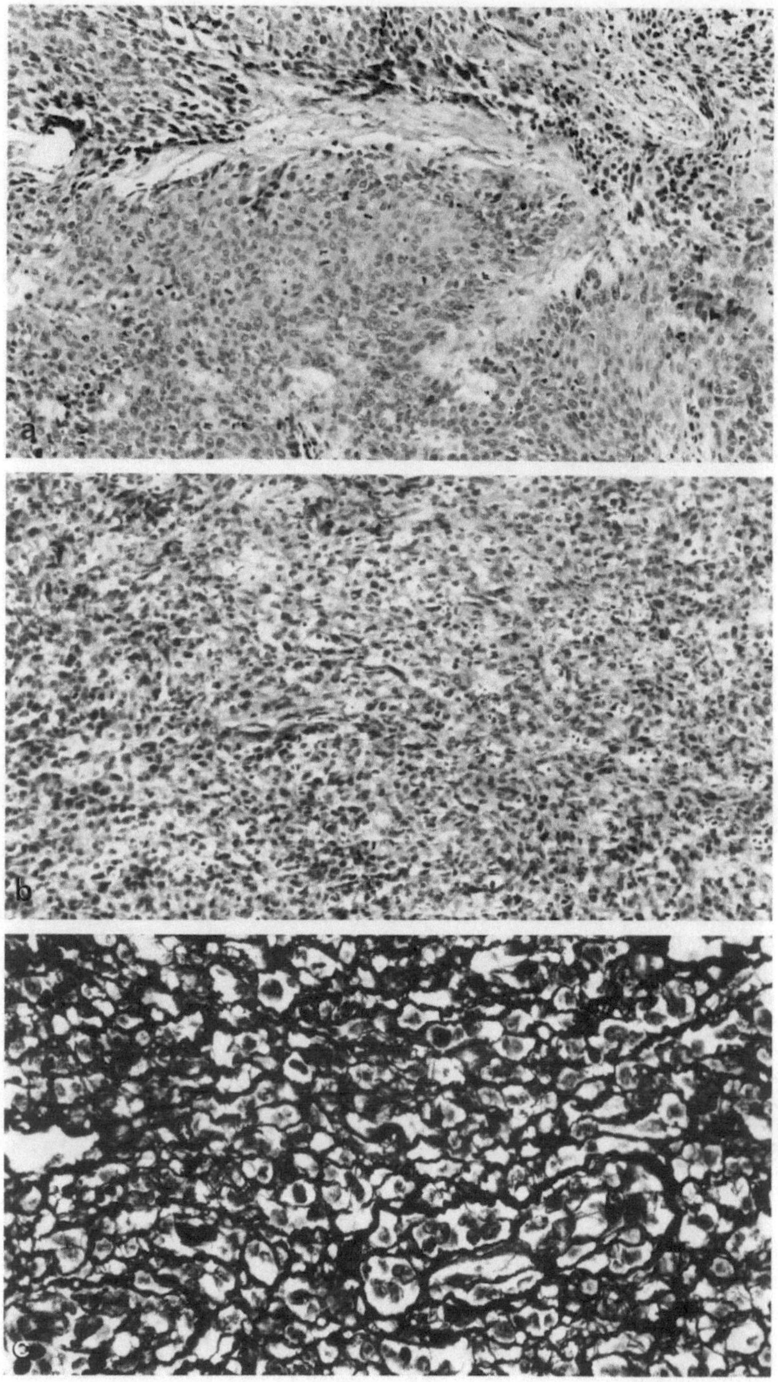

Fig. 7.12a–c. Radiogenic tumour: 46-year-old man, glottis. **a** Moderately differentiated squamous cell carcinoma with only scarce keratinization and high mitotic rate before radiation. HE, ×140. **b** Pleomorphic and spindle cell tumour tissue without epidermoid stratification or keratinization 1½ years after irradiation (54.25 Gy). HE, ×140. **c** Dense reticulin fibre network around the tumor cells, not compatible with an epithelial tumour. Silver stain, ×350

(5.9%) of the operated patients in the immediate vicinity of the operation field. These figures reveal no statistically significant difference between the two groups of patients. Second tumours in the vicinity of the primary tumour were, within the first 5 years, even more common in the patients subjected to surgery than in the irradiated patients – possibly because the precancerous mucosal fields were eradicated by the radiation.

Since at least with early vocal cord carcinomas, radiotherapy and surgery produce comparable rates of cure, the relation of mutilation and quality of life must be weighed against the safety of therapy and chances of survival in each individual patient (VAN

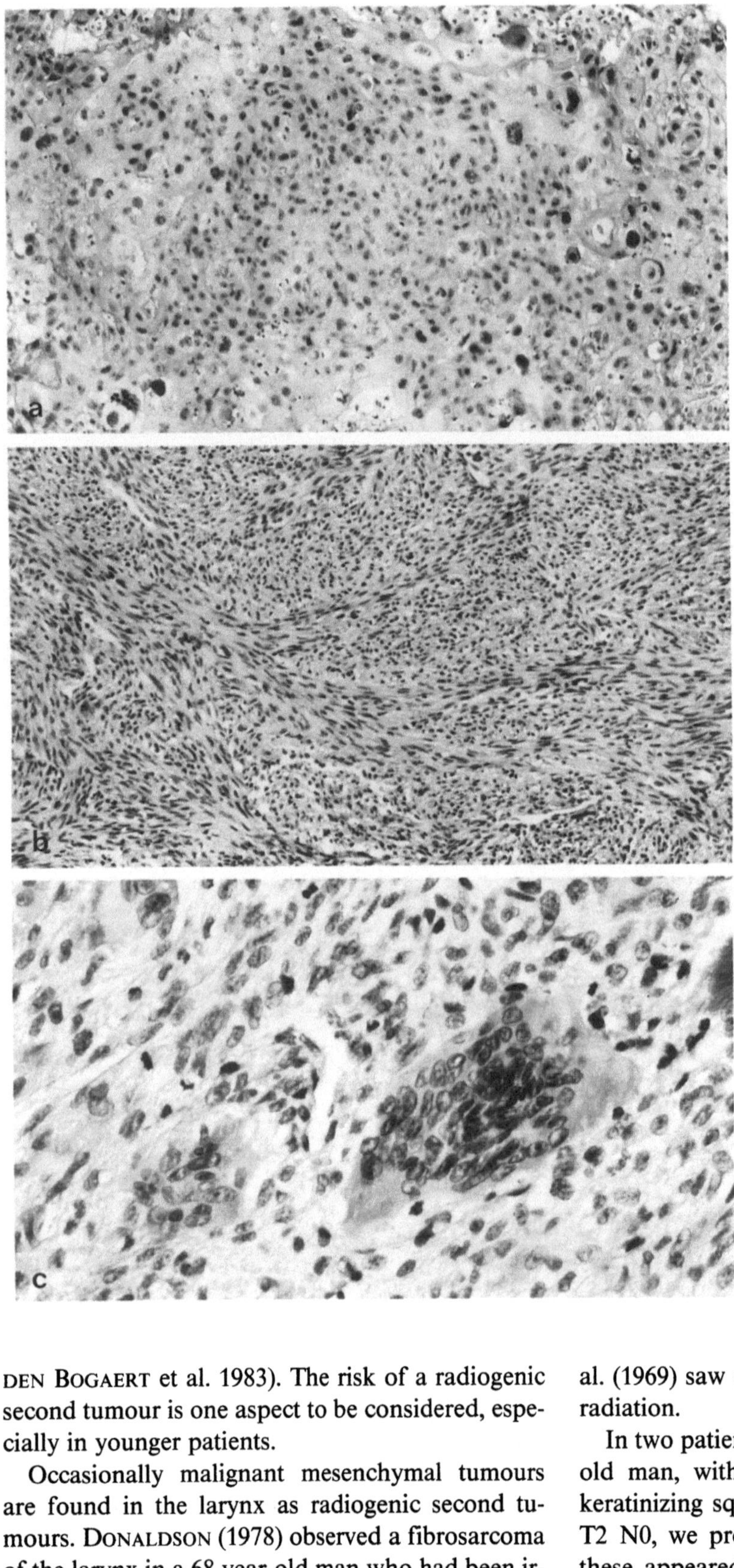

Fig. 7.13a–c. Radiogenic tumour: 64-year-old man, glottis. **a** Poorly differentiated squamous cell carcinoma with focal keratinization before radiation. HE, ×140. **b** Spindle cell tumour with formation of interlacing bundles 2½ years after radiation (65.8 Gy). HE, ×110. **c** Area of the tumour with formation of multinuclear giant cells. Note high mitotic rate. HE, ×350

DEN BOGAERT et al. 1983). The risk of a radiogenic second tumour is one aspect to be considered, especially in younger patients.

Occasionally malignant mesenchymal tumours are found in the larynx as radiogenic second tumours. DONALDSON (1978) observed a fibrosarcoma of the larynx in a 68 year-old man who had been irradiated 11 years previously with 56 Gy. GAHLIB et al. (1969) saw a laryngeal chondrosarcoma after irradiation.

In two patients, a 46-year-old man and a 64-year-old man, with primary moderately differentiated keratinizing squamous cell carcinomas, both grade T2 N0, we proved the development of sarcomas; these appeared 1½ and 2½ years after irradiation with 54.5 and 65.8 Gy respectively. We found spin-

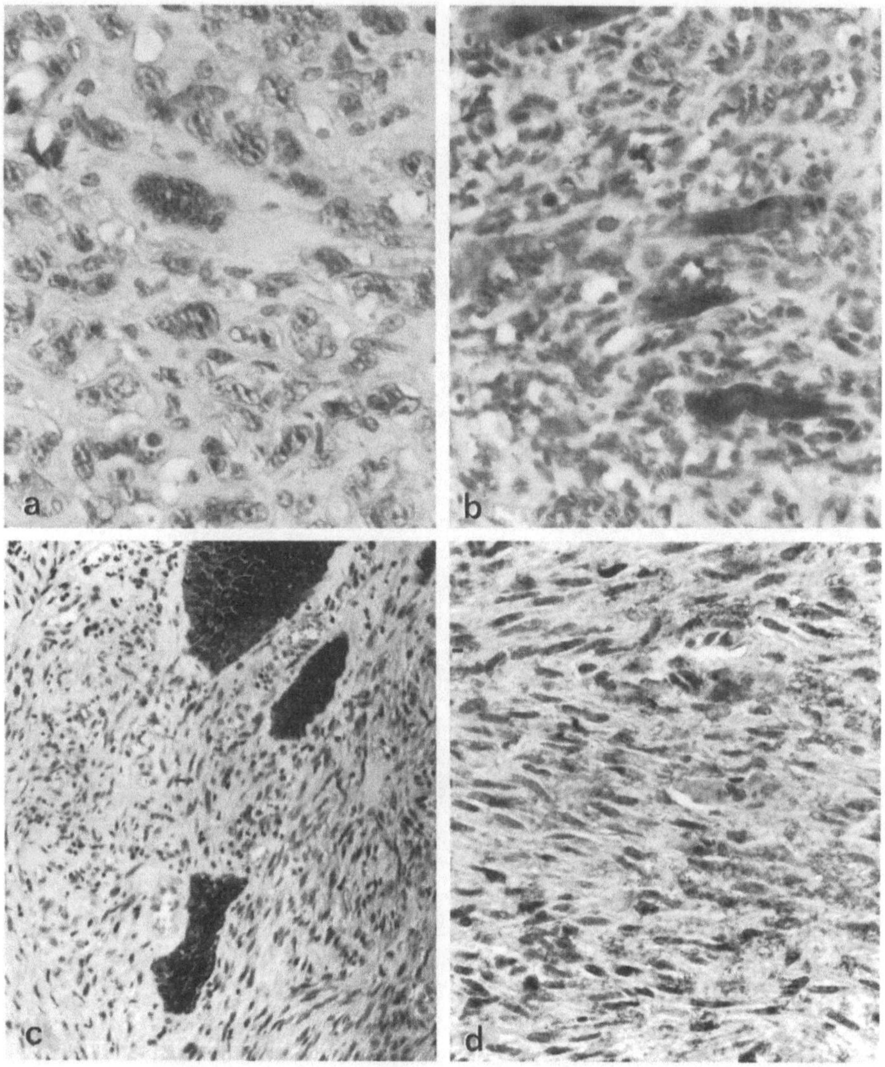

Fig. 7.14a–d. Immunohistological findings in radiogenic tumours. **a, b** Same case as Fig. 7.12. **a** Tumour tissue with highly pleomorphic cells; no reaction products for cytokeratins. ×350. **b** Demonstration of myoglobin in skeletal muscle fibres infiltrated by the tumour (brown in original slide; PAP method). Tumour cells show no reaction. ×220. **c, d** Same case as Fig. 7.13. **c** Positive reaction with cytokeratin antibodies in epithelium infiltrated by the tumour (brown in original slide; PAP method). No reaction in tumour cells. ×140. **d** Demonstration of desmin: there is a faint granular reaction product in the cytoplasm of the tumour cells (brown in original slide; PAP method). ×350

dle cell, partly pleomorphic, fibre-rich sarcomas, which in one case contained multinuclear giant cells (Fig. 7.12 and 7.13). Immunohistological examination (Fig. 7.14) excluded recurrences of spindle cell carcinoma in both cases (cytokeratin test negative) and supported the diagnosis of leiomyosarcoma. Desmin could be demonstrated in the tumour cells, while tests for myoglobin and S-100 protein were negative.

Owing to the relatively short time which had elapsed between irradiation and development of a second neoplasm in these patients, doubts may be raised as to whether these sarcomas can be considered as radiogenic tumours. The different histogenesis of the first and second neoplasms makes it appear possible that in both cases the tumours concerned are in fact radiogenic in origin. This view is also supported by the fact that such malignant mesenchymal tumours are exceedingly rare in the larynx (see Sect. 7.2.1).

8 Pseudotumours of the Larynx

As already defined in Chap. 3, pseudotumours, just like neoplasms, are tissue overgrowths. However, in contrast to true neoplasms, pseudotumours usually regress after elimination of the inflammatory or mechanical-functional causes, i.e. they are reversible in the broadest sense. Pseudotumours at an early stage exhibit the same signs and symptoms as true neoplasms of the larynx. Knowledge of them is therefore of practical significance for every practising laryngologist, pathologist and oncologist. For this reason the most important pseudotumours are briefly covered in this chapter.

We distinguish between four types: (1) inflammatory pseudotumours; (2) laryngeal cysts and laryngoceles; (3) metabolically induced pseudotumours; (4) endolaryngeal thyroid tissue. Over a period of 20 years, FRIEDMANN (1976) observed 1286 pseudotumours of the larynx of which 1122 were vocal cord polyps, 18 intubation granulomas, 14 contact granulomas, 44 tubercular lesions, 13 amyloid tumours, 72 retention cysts and three other lesions.

8.1 Inflammatory Pseudotumours

This group of tumours develops in nonspecific laryngitis or results from local, circumscribed chronic inflammatory processes caused by epithelial defects or damage to the subepithelial vascular connective tissue. Accordingly the pathogenesis may be inflammatory, mechanical or constitutional. Often all three factors combine clinically pseudotumours, appear as polyps of the laryngeal mucosa. Polyps of this type occur particularly frequently in the region of the vocal cords, but also occasionally found on the anterior wall of the subglottis. For this reason it would be better to speak generally of **laryngeal polyps**. While polyps of the vocal cord are usually diagnosed early due to changes of the voice, polyps in other areas can grow to larger inflammatory pseudotumours. KEEN et al. (1986) reported such a tumour in the subglottis in an 11-year-old girl which led to progressive upper airway obstruction.

8.1.1 Vocal Cord Polyps

Vocal cord polyps arise as a rule unilaterally and solitarily. They are coloured pinky-red, blue-red or livid (in colour (Fig. 8.1).

According to BECKMANN (1982) inflammation is the most important factor in the pathogenesis of laryngeal polyps. Functional mechanical influences such as vocal abuse or "phonotrauma" can similarly induce them or favour their development in the presence of corresponding constitutional disposition (KAMBIC et al. 1981, KLEINSASSER 1982, NAGATA et al. 1983, MICHAELS 1984). Special features of the lymph drainage in Reinke's space likewise play a role. Polyps are observed most frequently in people of middle age, 3 times more often in men than in women (EPSTEIN et al. 1957, KLEINSASSER 1982). In some statistical analyses nonsmokers are

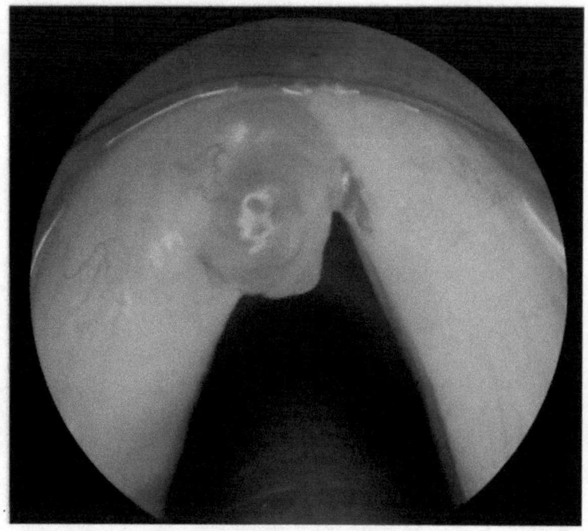

Fig. 8.1 Vocal cord polyp as seen laryngoscopically: 35-year-old man

affected just as often as smokers (KAMBIC et al. 1981, NAGATA et al. 1983), but in others smokers predominate (80%-90%; KLEINSASSER 1982). Seldom do vocal cord polyps attain such a size that they lead to airway obstruction (GILMAN et al. 1982).

FRENZEL et al. (1980) distinguished between the gelatinous or myxoid type and the telangiectatic polyp. The structure of the polyp is dependent partly on its age. The young polyp exhibits - apparently as a result of a disturbance in the permeability of the vessels by recurrent microtraumatization - oedematous swelling, haemorrhage and distinct distension, generally considered to be the fundamental initial change (FRENZEL et al. 1980, KAMBIC et al. 1981, KLEINSASSER 1977, 1982, GILMAN et al. 1982). The reaction of the vascular connective tissue can lead to an intensive proliferation of small vessels and to the formation of a telangiectatic polyp (FRENZEL et al. 1980, 1985), within which thrombi can develop. Fibrin exudation leads to fibrinoid swelling or necrosis and, at a further stage, to hyalinization and "amyloid" deposition (see Sect. 8.3.1; Fig. 8.2). A massive haemosiderosis can form subsequent to recurrent and pronounced haemorrhage (Fig. 8.3). Finally, fibrous transformation ensues with proliferation of fibroblasts and fibre formation in the polyp. For this reason it was considered a fibroma by some authors (KLUMPP 1938, RÖSSLE 1949, HOMMERICH 1952). Inflammatory changes can appear in these polyps either primarily or secondarily. The mucosal lining usually consists, especially in the oedematous phase, of normal squamous epithelium. This may exhibit hyperplasia, hyperkeratosis and even dysplasia (KAMBIC et al. 1981). Higher grade dysplasia is not found, however. SCHAUER et al. (1972) consistently found nonsuspect alterations (group I and II) in cytological smears. KAMBIC et al. (1981) did not see a single malignant transformation in 591 patients.

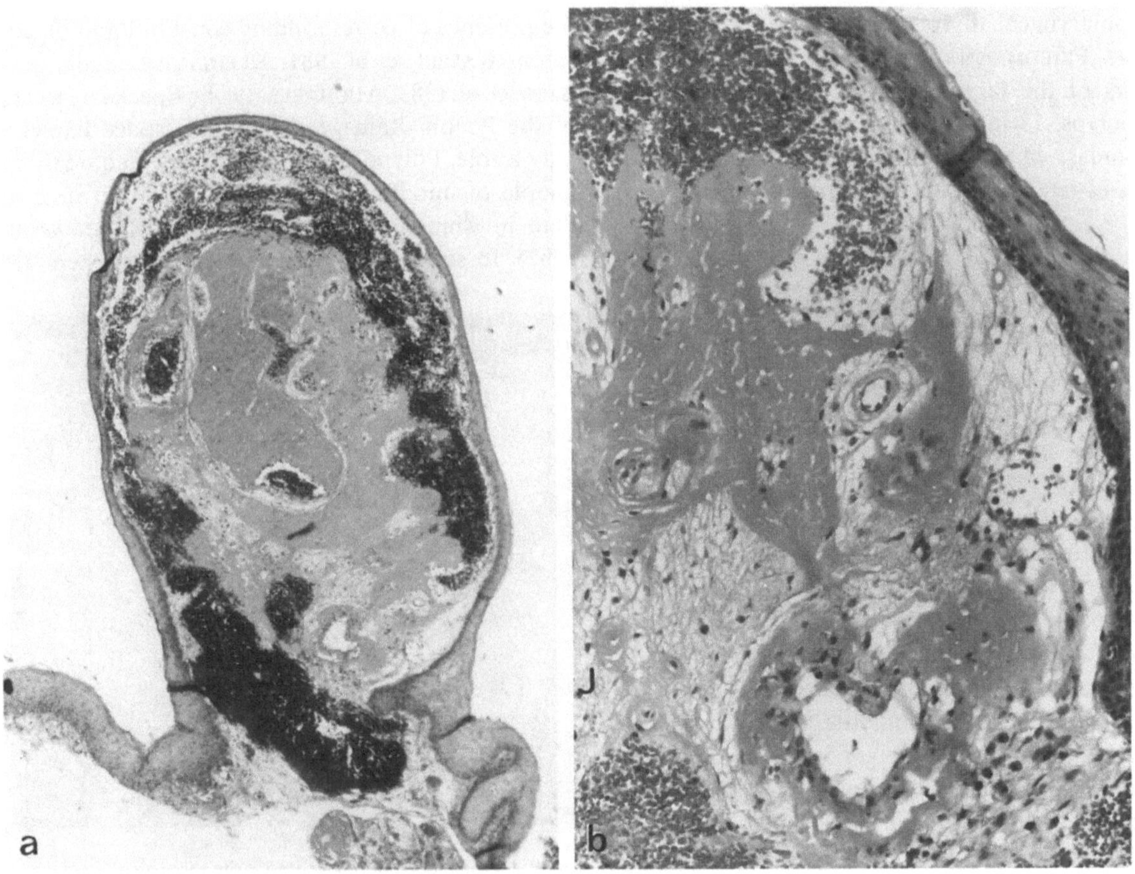

Fig. 8.2 a, b. Vocal cord polyp: 33-year-old man, glottis. **a** Polyp with fibrinoid stroma and haemorrhages covered by intact epithelium. HE, ×35. **b** Beneath the epithelium there is a loose myxoid stroma with deposition of fibrinoid hyaline masses. HE, ×90

8.1.2 Vocal Cord Nodules

HOFER (1928) defined vocal cord nodules as "small, maximally pin-head sized, sometimes round, sometimes coniform firm growth which perches, often bilaterally, on the free edge of the vocal cords, usually in the anterior part, has a smooth surface and corresponds in colour to that of the vocal cord upon which it rest". Histologically the changes found resemble those in vocal cord polyps. For this reason they are viewed by KÖHN (1969), KLEINSASSER (1977) and KAMBIC et al. (1981) as representing a special form of polyp which develops as a result of a localized disturbance in circulation and subepithelial oedema. But owing to the preference for women and children and the relatively constant location between the posterior and the medial third of the vocal fold, certain constitutional and functional factors must be postulated. Since vocal cord nodules occur predominantly in children with a tendency to screaming or forceful production of the voice, and in adults in occupations with heavy use of the voice, such as speakers, military instructors and mostly singers, the term screamer's or singer's nodules has come to be adopted. The comment made by BECKMANN (1982) that such nodule never develop in singers of the first class is a revealing indication that the underlying factor is nonphysiological straining of the voice.

8.1.3 Intubation Granulomas

Intubation granuloma is assumed to result from the pressure of the intubation catheter on the posterior section of the larynx. Here too constitutional factors must play a role, since women suffer markedly more often from intubation granulomas than men. In this context it appears superfluous to argue whether the damage is evoked by pressure of the tube on the apex of the vocal process (MATZKER 1953, BECKMANN 1982) or in some cases unsuitable,

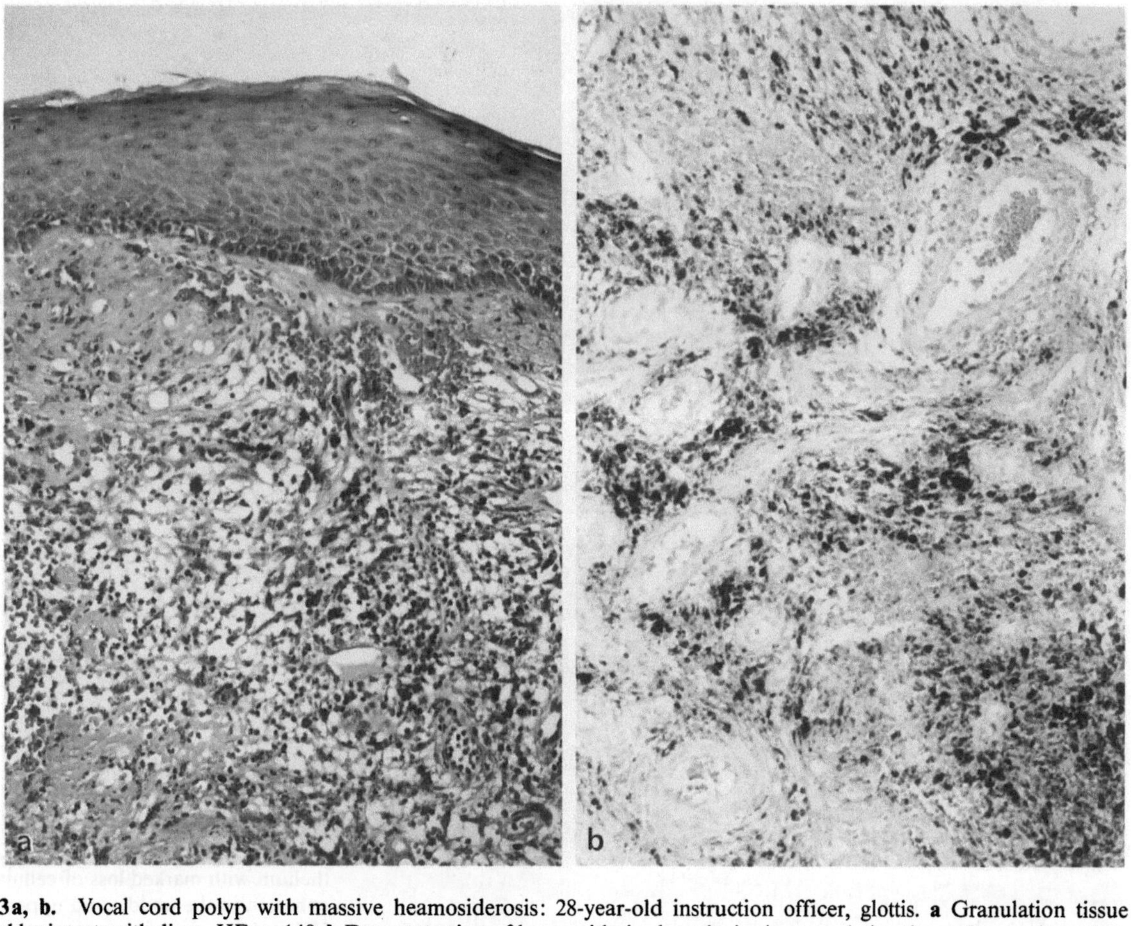

Fig. 8.3 a, b. Vocal cord polyp with massive heamosiderosis: 28-year-old instruction officer, glottis. **a** Granulation tissue covered by intact epithelium. HE, ×140. **b** Demonstration of haemosiderin deposits in the granulation tissue. Iron stain, ×140

forceful attempts at intubation. An epithelial defect at the level of the tip of the vocal process is the initial lesion. An ulcer, granulation tissue and finally granulomatous polyps develop. According to BAUER (1951) most of these changes regress at the latest by the 10th day after extubation. Should healing not take place, polypous granulations develop after several weeks which are composed of granulation tissue of the type of the teleangiectatic granuloma (pyogenic granuloma). These may be covered by thin squamous epithelium. As a rule, lymphocytic, plasmacellular and histiocytic infiltrations predominate while the occurrence of granulocytes depends on secondary bacterial infection. The vessels show a radial arrangement from the base to the periphery of the polyps, confluent in a cap-like network at the tip of the polyp.

After the first description of intubation granuloma by CLAUSEN (1932), the number of publications grew with the increased use of intubation, until nowadays it has become impossible to survey the literature.

8.1.4 Contact Hyperplasia

Contact hyperplasia (synonyms: contact ulcer, contact granuloma) of the vocal cords is caused by collisions of the vocal processes during strenuous phonation. Despite the designation "contact ulcer", ulceration usually does not occur. Men in the middle decades of life are those mainly affected. The cause is presumed to be multifactorial - constitutional influences and stress, especially of a mental nature, are considered to play a role.

Macroscopically, an annular mucosal thickening

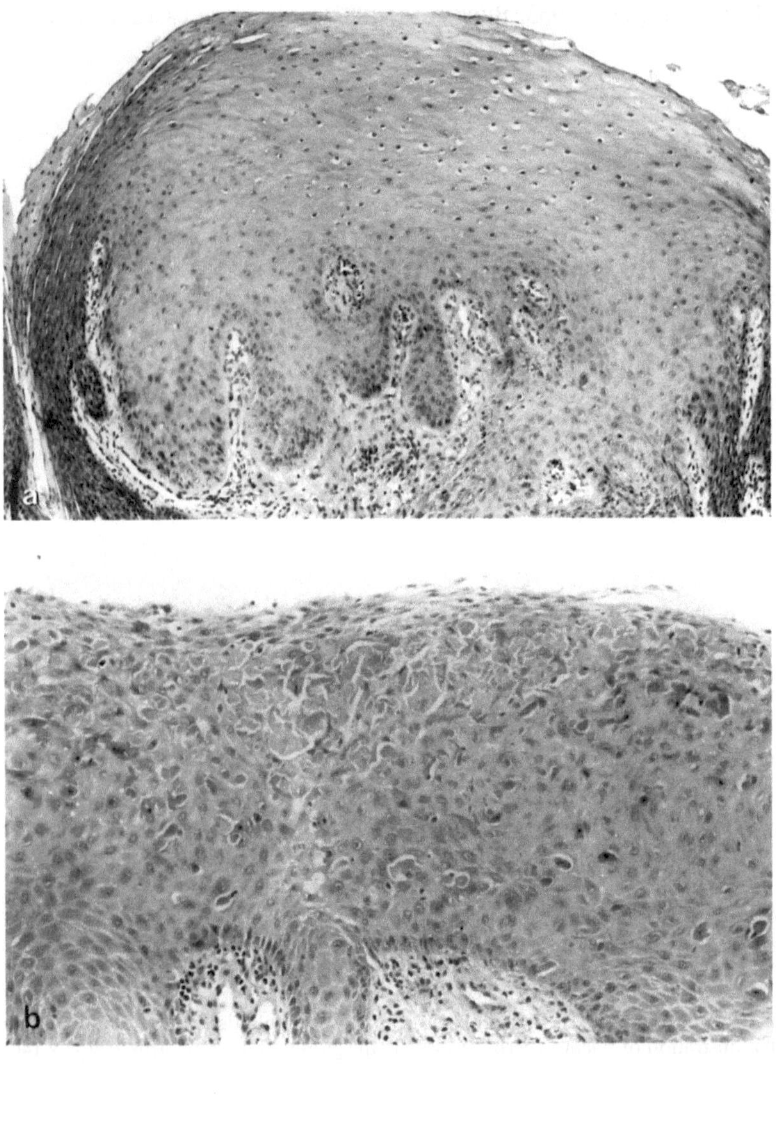

Fig. 8.4a, b. Contact hyperplasia: 45-year-old man, glottis. **a** Nodular thickening of epithelium with slight inflammation. HE, ×60. **b** Localized area of epithelium with marked loss of cellular cohesion in the middle and upper layers. HE, ×140.

on the inside of the vocal processes is formed, with a central depression resembling an ulcer. Histologically, the squamous epithelium is thickened but intact and shows slight inflammation (Fig. 8.4a). The hyperplastic epithelium exhibits marked loss of intercellular cohesion (Fig. 8.4b). Granulation tissue may be found in the subepithelial layer.

8.1.5 Infectious Laryngeal Tumours

A number of infectious lesions may lead to tumorous changes - often with granuloma formation - in the laryngeal region; only a few can be mentioned here.

Tubercular laryngeal tumours originate in broadly based or pedunculate fashion from the mucosa and appear partly smooth, like a fibroma, or verrucous to polypoid. The lesions may be solitary or multiple, sometimes occuring on the edge of a tuberculous ulcer. They originate usually in the posterior portion of the larynx, less frequently in the interarytenoid space, arytenoid cartilages, vocal cords, aryepiglottic folds, and epiglottis.

Corresponding with the decline in the incidence of tuberculosis reports of such changes are found chiefly in the older literature (AVELLIS 1891, TRAUTMANN 1902, MANASSE 1927, ZIEGELMANN 1932, GIANNI 1933, MALAN 1933, COPPO 1935). Recently, however, a renewed increase in laryngeal tuberculosis has been observed (PESCH 1976, LAHOVARY et al. 1986). GERTLER et al. (1985) in the department of otolaryngology in Cape Town, South Africa, observed nine patients with tuberculous laryngitis in only 1 year. Four had previously diagnosed pulmonary tuberculosis, in a further four pulmonary involvement was established.

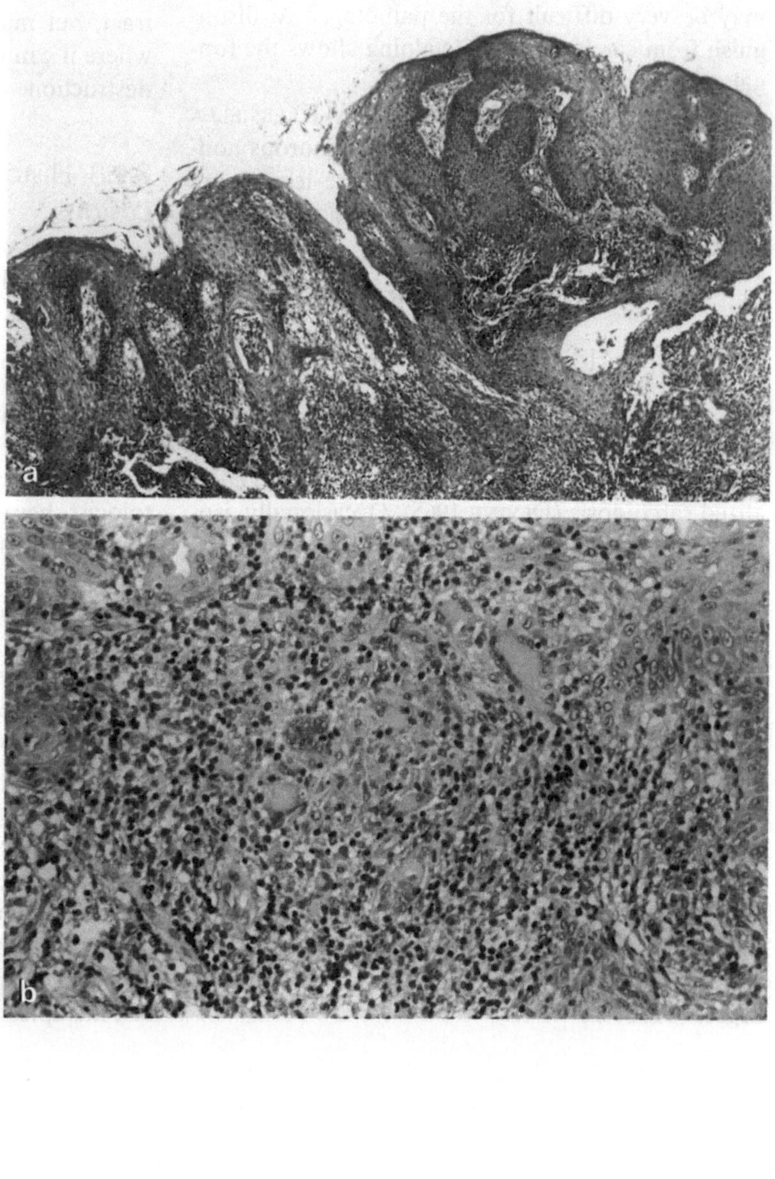

Fig. 8.5a, b. Tuberculous pseudotumour: 26-year-old woman, supraglottis. **a** Irregular papillomatous protrusions of the intensely inflamed mucosa. Pseudoepitheliomatous epithelial hyperplasia with formation of epithelial growth into depth. HE, ×56. **b** At higher magnification tuberculoid granulomas with epithelioid cells and multinuclear giant cells can be found. Demonstration of acid-fast rods by the Ziehl-Neelsen stain. HE, ×220.

We have observed two patients with laryngeal tuberculosis over the past 2 years; a 26-year-old woman and a 61-year-old woman. In both cases there was no affection of the lung and tuberculosis was not suspected. Clinically, as in most cases, suspicion of malignancy was pressing and motivated biopsy. Histologically, polypous protrusions of the epithelium were found with focal ulcerations, pseudoepitheliomatous hyperplasia, considerable chronic inflammation (Fig. 8.5 a) and typical tuberculoid granulomas with epithelioid cells and multinuclear Langhans giant cells. Some granulomas had central caseous necrosis. Acid-fast rods could be demonstrated using Ziehl-Neelsen staining, proving the tuberculous nature of the process (Fig. 8.5 b).

Similar lesions highly suspect of malignancy can be seen in **fungal infections**, such as histoplasmosis, blastomycosis (PAYNE et al. 1984) and aspergillosis (KHEIR et al. 1983). They are characterized by marked pseudoepitheliomatous hyperplasia which may be very difficult for the pathologist to distinguish from carcinoma. PAS staining allows the fungal colonies to be recognized.

The **scleroma** apparently caused by KLEBSIELLA rhinoscleromatis may similarly form tumorous nodules in the larynx. Histologically these lesions are characterized by large foamy histiocytic cells (Mikulicz cells).

8.1.6 Sarcoidosis

Sarcoidosis of the larynx, though not frequent, is not unusual. It occurs in 3%-5% of cases of generalized sarcoidosis (DEVINE 1965). Occasionally, isolated solitary sarcoid-like lesions can be observed in the larynx.

The main laryngeal location of sarcoidosis is the inlet; brownish nodules may be found in a reddened and slightly oedematous swollen mucosa and give rise to the suspicion of tuberculosis. Later a diffuse thickening may ensue, together with hardening of the laryngeal inlet. In some cases a circumscribed submucous tumour may form.

Histologically as well as clinically, the early stager of sarcoidosis resemble tuberculosis, the tubercles being composed of epithelioid cells and Langhans' cells. Only seldom is there very discrete central necrosis. In later stages fibrosis of variable degrees ensues.

8.1.7 Other Granulomas and Granulomatoses

Granulomas are nodular, under certain circumstances tumourlike, aggregations of inflammatory cells with a high content of mononuclear phagocytes (monocytes, histiocytes, macrophages, epithelioid cells) with or without the formation of multinuclear giant cells. The occurrence of granulomas caused by infections in the larynx has already been mentioned (see Sect. 8.1.5).

Rheumatic granulomas are seldom found in the laryngeal region (FRIEDMAN 1975).

In granulomatoses, besides true granulomas, abundant nonspecific granulation tissue, capillary proliferation, necroses, lymphocytic infiltration and angiitis may be found. The cause is not known in most cases but an immunologically mediated tissue damage is probable.

Wegener's granulomatosis affects primarily the nose, the paranasal sinuses and the respiratory tract, but may also occur in the laryngeal region, where it can cause deep ulcerous lesions and tissue destruction.

8.1.8 Histologically Pseudomalignant Lesions

Pseudoepitheliomatous epithelial hyperplasia (Fig. 8.6) is a proliferation of the epithelium which, at first sight, is reminiscent histologically of squamous cell carcinoma; it is found from time to time in the marginal area of ulcers, in vocal cord polyps, in infectious lesions and in granular cell tumours. Knowledge of this lesion is important to the histologist because of the serious consequences of false diagnosis. The characteristics of pseudoepitheliomatous hyperplasia which distinguish it from carcinoma are:

a) well-differentiated epithelium
b) few mitotic figures without atypia and
c) continuity of the cell complex with the surface.

In case of doubt the last-named has to be demonstrated by means of serial sections.

Necrotizing sialometaplasia is found in the region of seromucous glands subsequent to partial necrosis. Originating from the larger and smaller excretory ducts epithelial proliferation and squamous cell metaplasia, in part with epithelial dysplasia, en-

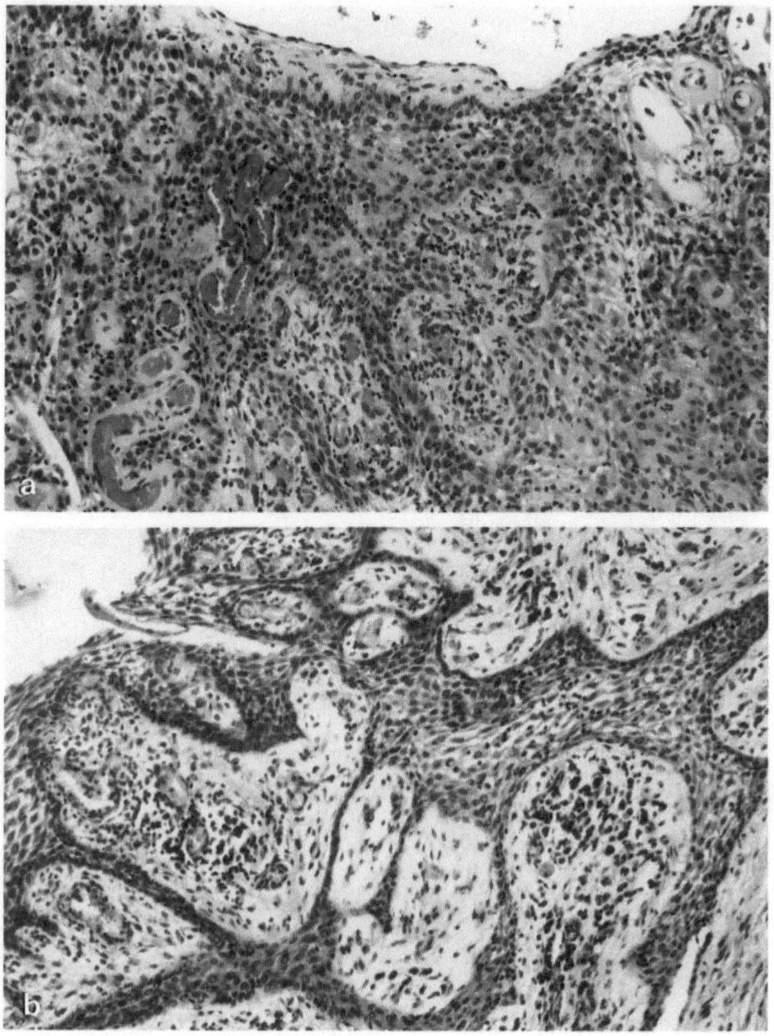

Fig. 8.6a, b. Pseudoepitheliomatous epithelial hyperplasia: 38-year-old woman with chronic laryngitis, supraglottis. **a** Intense inflammation of the mucosa with growth of epithelial formations into depth. HE, ×140. **b** Formation of reticular epithelial proliferations continuous with the surface epithelium. HE, ×140

sue. The picture can easily be confused with that of squamous cell carcinoma. The preferred lobular architecture is an indication of the benign nature of necrotizing sialometaplasia.

8.2 Laryngeal Cysts and Laryngoceles

8.2.1 Laryngeal Cysts

In as far as true malformations are the cause of cysts of the larynx, either dispersal of epithelium or failure of fusion of single lacunae to the later laryngeal saccule is involved. Dispersion of tissue from the third or fourth pharyngeal pouch can also lead to congenital cyst formation. Retention cysts, in contrast, are due to inflammatory or traumatic processes. Depending on their origin, cysts exhibit either cylindrical epithelial or squamous epithelial lining (Fig. 8.7). In the former, oncocytic transformation is often observed. It is necessary to distinguish these cysts from oncocytic cystadenomas.

Small intracordal epidermoid cysts are apparently not uncommon and lead to dysphonia (Monday et al. 1983, Bouchayer et al. 1985). Typical cases present as smooth white to yellow spheres shining through the mucosa. Inflammation is usually absent.

Cysts can occur in every part of the larynx but are observed chiefly in the supraglottic region.

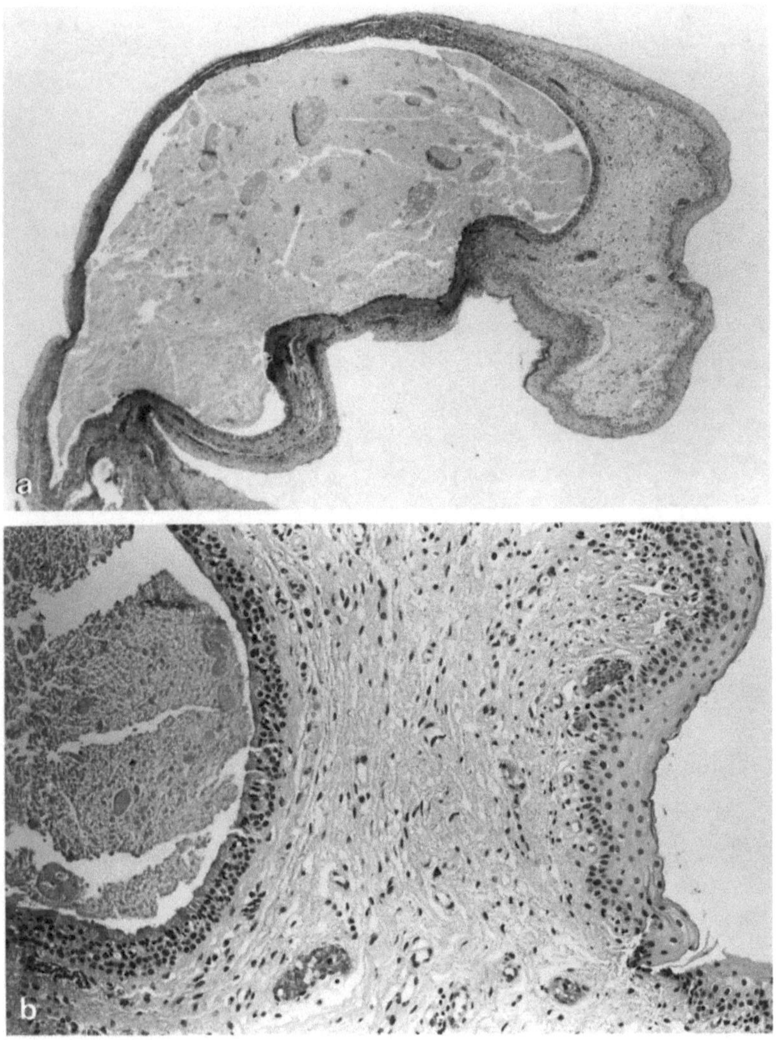

Fig. 8.7 a, b. Cyst of the vocal cord: 38-year-old woman with a nodule on the posterior portion of the right vocal cord for many years. **a** Large cyst with a protein containing fluid forming a polypous protrusion. HE, × 35. **b** The surface squamous epithelium **(right)** and the multilayered glandular epithelium of the cyst **(left)** at higher magnification. HE, × 150

8.2.2 Laryngoceles

The rare laryngoceles develop from structures of the laryngeal saccule, which only secondarily gains access to the laryngeal lumen. At an early stage of development the saccule is relatively much larger than the later Morgagni's ventricle. If involution fails to take place, it persists as the so-called primary laryngocele. In contrast to this, in patients so disposed secondary laryngocele formation can ensue as a result of certain external factors such as screaming, coughing, straining and in particular blowing (of instruments). Internal and external laryngoceles are distinguished on the basis of location and extension. The internal laryngocele remains within the laryngeal framework and causes, accordingly, endolaryngeal signs and symptoms such as hoarseness, aphonia and, in an advanced stage, dyspnoea and dysphagia. The external laryngocele expands outside the laryngeal framework through the lateral parts of the thyrohyoid membrane, which offers little resistance. As a result of this protrusion through a membrane, a valve-like mechanism leads to a continual distension of the laryngocele sac. External extension of a laryngocele thus must be viewed as acquired.

Histologically the lining of the laryngocele corresponds to that of Morgagni's ventricle. The mucosa shows typical respiratory epithelium which may, depending on the extensions, be flattened; lymphoid tissue may be present. More detailed descriptions of laryngoceles are given by MATZKER (1957) and TILLMANN and WUSTROW (1982).

The relationship between laryngocele and laryngeal carcinoma has been mentioned in Sect. 4.1.3.

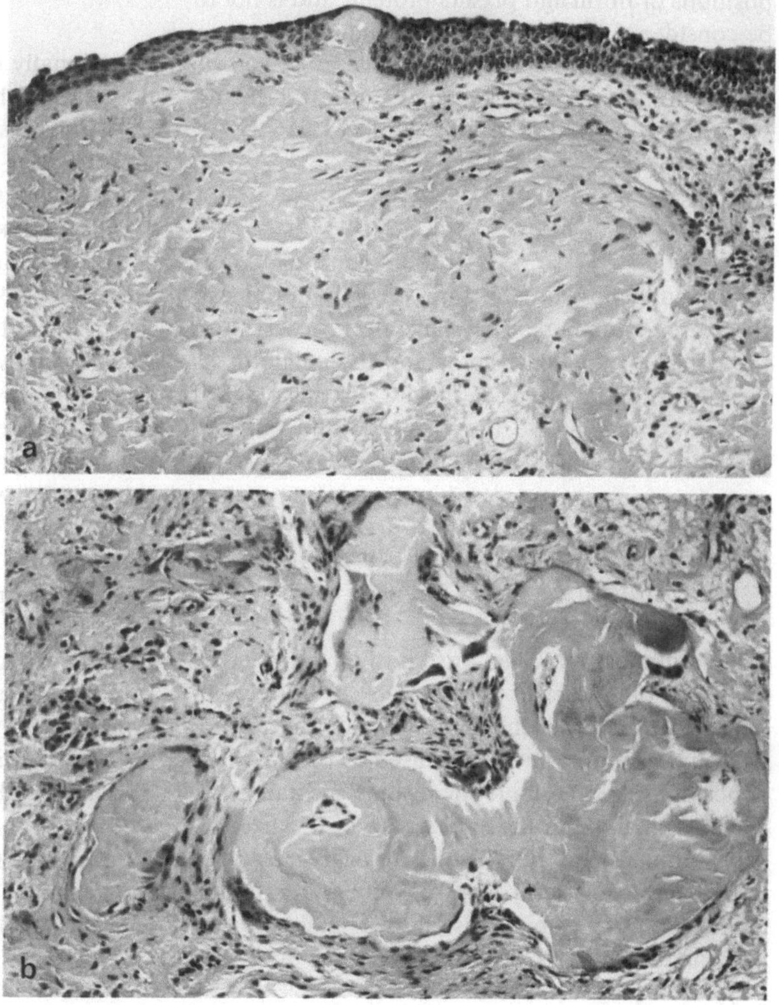

Fig. 8.8a, b. Amyloid tumour: 19-year-old woman, supraglottis. **a** Beneath the intact surface epithelium there is a homogeneous deposit of a hyaline material containing only few cells. Reactions for amyloid are positive. HE, ×140. **b** In the depth there are acellular deposits surrounded by granulation tissue and multinuclear giant cells of the foreign body type. Reactions for amyloid are positive. HE, ×140

8.3 Metabolically Induced Pseudotumours

8.3.1 Amyloid Tumours

Deposition of amyloid or amyloid-like material can appear in the form of a solitary lesion or as generalized amyloidosis. Three types can be distinguished in the larynx:

1. "Amyloid" deposition in vocal cord polyps
2. Circumscribed amyloid tumours
3. Diffuse subepithelial amyloidosis.

Amyloid tumours occur predominantly after the 20th year of life, and males are more commonly affected than females. The tumours develop subepithelially, preferably in the supraglottic region and on the vocal cords. Macroscopically they appear yellow and glisten through the mucosa. Histologically the amyloid deposits display no sharp demarcation or capsule formation. They form very fine hyaline homogeneous eosinophilic globules which tend to be confluent in the mesh of the connective tissue (Fig. 8.8a), usually in the immediate vicinity of small vessels. Sometimes these deposit are accompanied by foreign body reaction and granulation tissue (Fig. 8.8b). Since the typical tests for amyloid reaction often prove negative in "amyloid" tumours, some authors have questioned the true amyloid nature of these pseudotumours. The aetiology of local amyloid deposit is still unclear. A plasmocytoma as the cause of increased protein synthesis and deposition should be excluded by electrophoresis. The treatment is surgical removal.

"Amyloid" in vocal cord polyps is derived from depositions of fibrin and plasma proteins and is not to be considered as a true amyloid tumour.

More detailed references to the literature can be found in LEROUX-ROBERT (1962), MICHAELS and HYAMS (1979) and FERNANDES et al. (1982).

8.3.2 Gout Tophi

Uric acid deposit in the form of gout tophi can form pseudotumours. They have been observed in the region of the vocal cords and the epiglottis as well as in the laryngeal cartilages. The histological picture corresponds to that of gout tophi of other locations. References can be found in KÖHN (1969).

8.3.3 Other Metabolically Induced Pseudotumours

Pseudotumours may also arise in the larynx in the course of other metabolic disorders. In lipoid proteinosis (Urbach-Wiethe disease) nodules can appear in the larynx which are caused by pericapillary deposition of an eosinophilic hyaline substance.

Xanthomatosis or the appearance of localized fibroxanthomas, i.e. fibrohistiocytic aggregates with lipoid and cholesterol storage, may occur in the course of lipid metabolic disorders. Usually the dermis and subcutis are affected, only very rarely the larynx (review: RAUCHFUSS 1983).

8.4 Endolaryngeal Thyroid Tissue

Occasionally thyroid tissue is found in the subglottis between the cricoid cartilage and the first tracheal ring it is most likely dispersed from the thyroglossal duct into this region during embryonal development (FALK 1936, OLTERSDORF 1949, KLEIN 1967, RICHARDSON and ASSOR 1971, MICHAELS 1984). The view taken by RANDOLPH et al. (1963) and HAAS (1967), namely that constriction of the thyroid gland occurs during the fusion of the two initially paired thyroid cartilage wings, is not supported by the relatively constant site at the transition of the subglottis to the trachea. Such a development can apply only to endolaryngeal strumas in the anterior wall of the larynx near the glottis. Of the 130 cases cited by STEINBERG (1969) only seven were situated in this area, whilst almost all others were located more caudally.

As a result of pathological thyroid enlargement (struma) or following strumectomy, dispersed thyroid tissue can increase in volume and lead to symptoms of airway obstruction. This is observed almost exclusively in adults. Malignant transformation has also been described.

Histologically, ectopic thyroid tissue is usually found in the submucosa in the vicinity of seromucous glands and exhibits normal, small follicles with unremarkable colloid.

References

1 Development, Anatomy, Spatial Compartments and Regions

AJC - American Joint Committee for Cancer Staging and End Results Reporting (1972): Clinical staging system for Cancer of the Larynx. Chicago

AJC - American Joint Committee for Cancer Staging and End Results Reporting (1977): Manual of staging of Cancer. Lippincott, Philadelphia

AJCC - American Joint Committee on Cancer (1983): Manual for staging of cancer. Lippincott, Philadelphia

AREY LB (1965): Developmental anatomy. 7th edn. Saunders, Philadelphia

BARTELS P (1909): Das Lymphgefäßsystem. Fischer, Jena

BECK C, MANN W (1980): The inner laryngeal lymphatics. A lymphangioscopical and electron miroscopical study. Acta Otolaryngol (Stockh) 89: 265-270

BRAUS H, ELZE C (1956): Anatomie des Menschen. vol II: Eingeweide (einschließlich periphere Leitungsbahnen I). Springer, Berlin - Göttingen - Heidelberg

CHIEVITZ JH (1882): Untersuchungen über die Verknöcherung der menschlichen Kehlkopfknorpel. Arch Anat Physiol 1882: 303-349

CLERF LH (1944): The pre-epiglottic space - its relation to carcinoma of the epiglottis. Trans Am Laryngol Rhinol Otol Ass 1944: 127-131

CUNEO B (1902): De l'envahissement du système lymphatiques dans le cancer du larynx. Gazette des Hôpitaux 75: 1385-1391

HAST MH (1972): Early development of the human laryngeal muscles. Ann Otol Rhinol Laryngol 81: 524-530

HAST MH (1974): Applied embryology of the larynx. Can J Otolaryngol 3: 412-415

KALLIUS E (1897): Beiträge zur Entwicklungsgeschichte des Kehlkopfes. Anat Hefte 9: 303-363

KIRCHNER JA (1969): One hundred laryngeal cancers studied by serial section. Ann Otol Rhinol Laryngol 78: 689-709

KIRCHNER JA (1977): Two hundred laryngeal cancers. Patterns of growth and spread as seen in serial section. Laryngoscope 87: 474-482

KRMPOTIC-NEMANIC J, DRAF W, HELMS J (1985): Chirurgische Anatomie des Kopf-Hals-Bereiches. Springer, Berlin - Heidelberg - New York - Tokyo

LANZ T, WACHSMUTH W (1955): Praktische Anatomie. Vol I,2: Hals. Springer, Berlin - Göttingen - Heidelberg

LUND WS (1974): Classification of subglottic tumors and discussion of their growth and spread. Can J Otolaryngol 3: 469-471

MAGUIRE A, DAYAL VS (1974): Supraglottic anatomy - the pre- or the periepiglottic space. Can J Otolaryngol 3: 432-439

MEYER-BREITING E, SCHNEIDER B (1981): Plattenepithelkarzinome an der vorderen Kommissur und Penetration des Kehlkopfgerüstes. Laryng Rhinol Otol 60: 89-95

MEYER-BREITING E, POPESCU G (1986): Zur Definition der Glottischen Region. Arch Otorhinolaryngol Suppl 1986/II: 150-152

MOST A (1899): Über die Lymphgefäße und Lymphdrüsen des Kehlkopfes. Anat Anz 15: 387-393

NORRIS CM, TUCKER GF, BURNS KF, PITSER WF (1970): A correlation of clinical staging, pathological findings and five year end results in surgical treated cancer of the larynx. Ann Otol Rhinol Laryngol 79: 1033-1048

OGURA JH (1955): Surgical pathology of cancer of the larynx. Laryngoscope 65: 867-926

OLOFSSON H, NOSTRAND AWv (1973): Growth and spread of laryngeal carcinoma with reflections on the effect of preoperative irradiation. Acta Otolaryngol (Stockh) Suppl 308: 1-84

O'RAHILLY R (1973): Developmental stages in human embryos, including a survey of the Carnegie Collection. Part A: Embryos of the first three weeks (stages 1 to 9). Carnegie Institution of Washington, Washington DC

O'RAHILLY R, BOYDEN EA (1973): The timing and sequence of events in the development of the human respiratory system during the embryonic period proper. Z Anat Entwickl Gesch 141: 237-250

O'RAHILLY R, TUCKER JA (1973): The early development of the larynx in stages human embryos. Part I: Embryos of the first five weeks (to stage 15). Ann Otol Rhinol Laryngol 82: 1-27

PAFF AGE (1973): Anatomy of the head and neck. Saunders, Philadelphia

PAUWELS F (1960): Eine neue Theorie über den Einfluß mechanischer Reize auf die Differenzierung der Stützgewebe. 10. Beitrag zur funktionellen Anatomie und kausalen Morphologie des Stützapparates. Z Anat Entwickl Gesch 121: 478-515

PERNKOPF E (1952): Topographische Anatomie des Menschen. III. Band: Der Hals. Urban & Schwarzenberg, Wien

PESCH HJ, BOGENBERGER Th, RUDOLF L, THULL R (1980): Das Ossifikationsprinzip der Trachealknorpel. Röntgenologisch-morphometrische und experimentelle Untersuchungen. Arch Otorhinolaryngol 227: 457-458

PESCH HJ, GLASS Wv, STEPHAN M, THULL R (1981): Zum Ossifikationsprinzip des Schildknorpels. Arch Otorhinolaryngol 231: 829-830

POIRIER P (1887 A): Lymphatiques du larynx. Progrès méd 15: 340

POIRIER P (1887 B): Vaisseaux lymphatiques du larynx. Vaisseaux lymphatiques de la sous-glottique; Ganglion prélaryngé. Progrès méd 15: 373-375

POIRIER P, CHARPY A (1901): Traité d'Anatomie humaine. Bd II Paris

PRESSMAN JJ, SIMON MB, MONELL C (1960): Anatomical studies related to the dissemination of cancer of the larynx. Trans Am Acad Ophth Otol 64: 628-638

QUIRET H (1906): Sur les lymphatiques de la région sous-glottique du larynx. Ann Anat path Anat norm méd chir 3: 289-290

ROUVIERE H (1932): Anatomie des lymphatiques de l'homme. Masson und Cie, Paris

SCHEIER M (1901): Über die Ossifikation des Kehlkopfes. Arch mikrosk Anat 59: 220-258

SHAHEEN OH (1974): The classification of supraglottic tumors of the larynx. Can J Otolaryngol 3: 486-488

STARCK D (1975): Embryologie. 3.Aufl. Thieme, Stuttgart - New York

TILLMANN B, WUSTROW D (1982): Kehlkopf. In: BERENDES J, LINK R, ZÖLLNER F (eds), Hals-Nasen-Ohrenheilkunde in Praxis und Klinik, 2nd ed., vol 4/1. Thieme, Stuttgart - New York

TUCKER GF (1963): Some clinical inferences from the study of serial laryngeal sections. Laryngoscope 73: 728-748

TUCKER GF (1971): Human larynx coronal section atlas. Armed Forces Institute of Pathology, Washington DC

TUCKER GF (1974): The anatomy of laryngeal cancer. Can J Otolaryngol 3: 417-427

TUCKER JA, O'RAHILLY R (1972): Observations on the embryoloy of the human larynx. Ann Otol Rhinol Laryngol 81: 520-523

UICC - Union Internationale Contre le Cancer (1972): TNM-classification of malignant tumours of breast, larynx, stomach, cervix uteri, corpus uteri. Geneva

UICC - Union International Contre le Cancer (1978): Report of Committee on TNM Classification. Geneva

UICC - Union International Contre le Cancer (1986): Report of Committee on TNM Classification. Geneva

WELSH LW, WELSH JJ, BEHLKE FM (1961): Surgical alterations of the laryngeal lymphatics. Ann Otol Rhinol Laryngol 70: 52-63

WELSH LW (1964): The normal human laryngeal lymphatics. Ann Otol Rhinol Laryngol 73: 569-582

WHO - World Health Organization (1976): ICD-O (International Classification of Diseases for Oncology). 1st ed. Geneva

WHO - World Health Organization (1979): ICD-O (International Classification of Diseases for Oncology): Tumor-Lokalisationsschlüssel. Springer, Berlin - Heidelberg - New York

WUSTROW F (1963): Kehlkopf; vergleichende Anatomie und Entwick,ungsgeschichte, Mißbildungen, Anomalien und Varianten. In: BERENDES J, LINK R, ZÖLLNER F (eds), Handbuch der Hals-Nasen-Ohrenheilkunde, vol II,1. Thieme, Stuttgart

References

2 Particular Problems of Histological Preparation and Assessment: Advanced Methods

ABRAMSON M, HUANG CC, SCHILLING RW, SALOME RG (1975): Collagenase activity in epidermoid carcinoma of the oral cavity and larynx. Ann Otol Rhinol Laryngol 84: 158-163

AMTHOR M, TOMASKOWITZ H (1970): Ein Verfahren zur Herstellung histologischer Organschnitte. Z wiss Mikr 70: 130-134

ANDREASSON L, BJÖRLIN G, KORSGAARD R, MATTIASSON I, TRELL E, TRELL L (1982): Leucoplakia of the oral cavity and the arylhydrocarbon-hydrolase inducibility. Postgrad Med J 58: 138-141

BANCROFT JD, STEVENS A (1977): Theory and practice of histological techniques. Churchill Livingston, Edinburgh-London-New York

BANOCZY J (1982): Oral leukoplakia. Budapest: Akadémiai Kiadó

BICHLER E, MIKUZ G, ZINGERLE N (1985): A comment on laryngeal cytology. Arch Otorhinolaryngol 241: 209-211

BIER J, NICKLISCH U, PLATZ H (1983): The doubtful relevance of nonspecific immune reactivity in patients with squamous cell carcinoma of the head and neck. Cancer 52: 1165-1172

BJELKENKRANTZ K, OLOFSSON J, STAL O, GRÖNTOFT O (1983): Juvenile laryngeal papilloma: histologic and photometric evaluation of atypia. Laryngoscope 83: 468-474

BOS I, BURKHARDT A (1981): Epithelial and interepithelial mitoses of the oral mucosa. Light and electron microscopic study in mice after exposure to different antigens. J Invest Dermatol 76: 63-67

BRAIN EB (1966): The preparation of decalcified sections Charles C Thomas, Springfield Ill, USA

BRODERS AC (1920): Squamous-cell epithelioma of the lip. JAMA 74: 656-664

BRODERS AC (1921): Squamous-cell epithelioma of skin: A study of 256 cases. Ann Surg 73: 141-160

BRODERS AC (1922): Epithelioma of the genitourinary organs. Ann Surg 75: 574-604

BURKHARDT A (1980): Der Mundhöhlenkrebs und seine Vorstadien. Ultrastrukturelle und immunpathologische Aspekte. Fischer, Stuttgart-New York

BURKHARDT A (1984): Advanced methods in the evaluation of premalignant lesions and carcinomas of the oral mucosa. J Oral Pathol 14: 751-778

BURKHARDT A (1985): Prämaligne Veränderungen der Mundschleimhaut. Vorschläge einer internationalen Expertenkommission zur Nomenklatur. Pathologe 6: 126-132

BURKHARDT A, MAERKER R (1981): A colour atlas of oral cancers. The diagnosis of leukoplakias, precancerous conditions and carcinomas. Wolfe Medical Publications Ltd, London; Year Book Medical Publishers Inc., Chicago

CALDERON-SOLT L, SOLT DB (1985): Gamma-glutamyl transpeptidase in precancerous lesions and carcinomas of oral, pharyngeal, and laryngeal mucosa. Cancer 56: 138-143

CHODAK GW, HAUDENSCHILD C, GITTES RF, FOLKMAN J (1980): Angiogenic activity as a marker of neoplastic and preneoplastic lesions of the human bladder. Ann Surg 192: 762-771

CHRETIEN PB (1975): Unique immunobiological aspects of head and neck squamous carcinoma. Can J Otolaryngol 4: 225-235

CHRETIEN PB (1978): The effects of smoking on immunocompetence. Laryngoscope 88 (Suppl 8): 11-13

CINBERG JZ, CHANG TH, BASES R, MOLNAR J (1980): The percentage of cells in DNA synthesis in epidermoid carcinomas of the head and neck: a preliminary report. Laryngoscope 90: 920-923

CINBERG JC, CHANG TH, HEBBARD P, BASES R, VOGL SE (1983): An application of immunocytology to the analysis of the cell kinetics of upper respiratory and digestive tract squamous carcinoma. Cancer 51: 1843-1846

CLAYDEN EC (1952): A discussion on the preparation of bone sections by the paraffin wax method with special reference to the control of decalcification. J Med Lab Technol 10: 103-123

CORTESINA G, SARTORIS A, DI FORTUNATO V, CAVALLO GP, MORRA B, BUSSI M, BEATRICE F, POGGIO E, MARCATO P, RENDINE S (1984): Natural killer-mediated cytotoxicity in patients with laryngeal carcinoma. Ann Otol Rhinol Laryngol 93: 189-191

CRISSMAN JD, FU YS (1986): A clinicopathologic study of six cases with DNA analysis. Arch Otolaryngol 112: 522-528

DANIELSON JR, FRANKLIN WA (1984): Characterization of antibody-forming cells adjacent to laryngeal carcinoma. Arch Otolaryngol 110: 327-328

DAWSON DE, EVERTS ECE, VETTO RM, BURGER DR (1985): Assessment of immunocompetent cells in patients with head and neck squamous cell carcinoma. Ann Otol Rhinol Laryngol 94: 342-345

DENARO A, CARUSO R, ROSSI M, D'ARRIGO C, MALAPONTE G, MAZZARINO MC, CUTRONA D (1985): Circulating immunocomplexes and laryngeal carcinoma. Arch Otolaryngol 111: 595-597

ELÖ J (1983): Die Bedeutung des Malignitätsgrades und der Proliferationsaktivität des Larynxkarzinoms für regionäre Lymphknotenmetastasen. Laryngol Rhinol Otol 62: 244-245

EVANS AW, JOHNSON NW, BUTCHER RG (1983): A quantitative histochemical study of glucose-6-phosphate dehydrogenase activity in premalignant and malignant lesions of human oral mucosa. Histochem J 15: 483-489

EVESON JW (1981): Animal models of intra-oral chemical carcinogenesis: a review. J Oral Pathol 10: 129-146

FELIX H, TCHAO R, SCHLEICH A, HOFFMANN V (1982): Interactions of tumor cells with human amnion membrane: a model for studying tumor invasion in vitro. Scan Electron Microsc 2: 741-749

Fletcher GH, Old JW, Loquvam GS (1954): A topographic approach to the roentgenologic and pathologic examination of the laryngopharyngeal tumours. Radiology 63: 361-380

Frable WJ, Frable MA (1968): Cytologic diagnosis of carcinoma of the larynx by direct smear. Acta Cytol (Baltimore) 12: 318-324

Franklin CD, Gohari K, Smith CJ, White FH (1980): Quantitative evaluation of normal hyperplastic, and premalignant epithelium by stereological methods. In: Mackenzie JC, Dabelsteen E, Squier CA (eds), Oral premalignancy; pp 243-261. University of Iowa Press

Franz B, Neumann OG (1978): Leukoplakien des Kehlkopfes. Histologisch-zytologische Klassifizierung. Laryngol Rhinol Otol 57: 428-433

Frühwald H (1979): Zum Wert der Larynxzytologie als Screening-Untersuchung. Laryngol Rhinol Otol 58: 698-699

Gardner AF (1965): The use of acid phosphatase localization as a differential staining technique for keratin. Oral Surg 20: 218-225

Giarelli L, Silvestri F, Antonutto G, Stanta G (1977): Observation of the pathologist on precancerous lesions of the larynx. Integrated with histological data and quantitative analysis of nuclear DNA-content. Acta Otolaryngol (Suppl)(Stockh) 344: 7-18

Gierek T, Lisiewicz J, Moszczy'nski P, Pilch J, Namyslowski G (1985): Enzymatic deficiencies of the immune system cells in patients with cancer of the larynx and other malignancies. Auris Nasus Larynx (Tokyo) 12: 47-51

Glanz HK (1984): Carcinoma of the larynx; growth, p-classification and grading of squamous cell carcinoma of the vocal cords. Adv Otorhinolaryngol 32: 1-123

Golabek W, Szyszko J (1984): Lactate dehydrogenase activity in laryngeal carcinoma and surrounding mucosa. Clin Otolaryngol 9: 9-13

Grøntoft O, Hellquist A, Olofsson J, Nordström L (1978): The DNA content and nuclear size in normal, dysplastic and carcinomatous laryngeal epithelium. Acta Otolaryngol (Stockh) 86: 473-479

Grundmann E (1973): Die Bedeutung der präkanzerösen Zell- und Gewebsveränderungen in Experiment und Klinik. Arch Otorhinolaryngol 205: 55-67

Hamburger AW, Salmon SE (1977): Primary bioassay of human tumor stem cells. Science 197: 461-463

Hansemann D (1890): Über asymmetrische Zellteilung in Epithelkrebsen und deren biologische Bedeutung. Virchows Arch path Anat 119: 299-326

Hanson J, Bruchmüller W (1983): Rasterelektronenmikroskopische Schleimhautstudien an Larynx-Präkanzerosen. HNO 31: 359-365

Harabuchi Y, Yamanaka N, Kataura A (1985): Identification of lymphocyte subsets and natural killer cells in head and neck cancers. An immunohistological study using monoclonal antibodies. Arch Otorhinolaryngol 242: 89-97

Harrison DFN (1979): Intrinsic weakness of the TNM system for classification of laryngeal cancer. ORL 41: 241-251

Hellquist H, Olofsson J (1981): Photometric evaluation of laryngeal epithelium exhibiting hyperplasia, keratosis and moderate dysplasia. Acta Otolaryngol (Stockh) 92: 157-165

Herrmann JF, Schauer A, Finsterer H (1973): Zur Erkennung praeneoplastischer Veränderungen am Larynx. (Recognizing premalignant changes in the larynx). Laryngol Rhinol Otol 52: 655-660

Heyden G (1974): Histochemical investigation of malignant cells. Histochemistry 39: 327-334

Heyden G, Arwill T, Högberg M (1974): A new routine in histopathology. Br J Dermatol 90: 579-582

Hill MW (1980): Cell kinetics in premalignancy. In: Mackenzie IC, Dabelsteen E, Sqier CA (eds), Oral premalignancy; pp 191-212. University of Iowa Press

Holm LE, Jakobsson P, Killander D, Silfverswärd C, Wersäll J (1980): DNA and its synthesis in indivdual tumor cells from human upper respiratory tract squamous cell carcinomas. Laryngoscope 90: 1209-1212

Holm LE (1982): Cellular DNA amounts of squamous cell carcinomas of the head and neck region in relation to prognosis. Laryngoscope 92: 1064-1069

Holmstrup P, Dabelsteen E, Roed-Petersen B (1981): Oral leukoplakia transplanted to nude mice. Scand J Dent Res 89:275-282

Hommerich KW, Sauer H, Weede W (1971): Zur Wachstumstendenz von Larynxtumoren. Arch Otorhinolaryngol 199: 748-751

Hommerich KW (1974): Röntgenbefunde und mikroskopisches Wachstum von malignen Larynxtumoren. Laryng Rhinol Otol 53: 845-855

Hume WJ, Potten CS (1979): Advances in epithelial kinetics: an oral view. J Oral Pathol 8: 3-22

Hume WJ (1981): A theoretical consideration of some biological parameters involved in cell kinetic investigations of oral leukoplakia and abnormal stratified squamous epithelium. J Oral Pathol 10: 375-385

Jakobsson PA, Eneroth CM, Killander D et al. (1973): Histological classification and grading of malignancy in cancer of the larynx. Acta Radiol Oncol 12: 1-8

Johns ME, Mills SE (1983): Cloning efficiency. A possible prognostic indicator in squamous cell carcinoma of the head and neck. Cancer 52: 1401-1404

Johnson NW, Evans AW, Morgan PR, Butcher RG (1980): Biochemical and histochemical changes in oral premalignancy. In: Mackenzie IC, Dabelsteen E, Squier CA (eds), Oral premalignancy; pp 312-334. University of Iowa Press

Kashima HK (1976): The characteristics of laryngeal cancer correlating with cervical lymph node metastasis. In: Alberti PW, Bryce DP (eds), Centennial Conference on Langeal Cancer; pp 855-864. Appleton-Century-Crofts, New York

Kernan JD (1950): The pathology of carcinoma of the larynx studied in serial sections. Trans Am Acad Ophth Otol 55: 10-21

Kleinsasser O (1967): Wachstumsformen der Kehlkopfeingangscarcinome und Indikation zur Teilresektion. Wiss Z Karl-Marx-Univ (Lpz) 16: 723-725

Kramer IRH (1969): Precancerous conditions of the oral mucosa. Ann R Coll Surg Engl 45: 340-356

Kramer IRH, Lucas RB, El-Labban N, Lister L (1970): A computer-aided study on the tissue changes in oral keratoses and lichen planus and an analysis of case groupings by subjective and objektive criteria. Br J Cancer 24: 407-426

Kramer IRH, Lucas RB, El-Labban N, Lister L (1970): The use of discriminant analysis for examining the histological features of oral keratoses and lichen planus. Br J Cancer 24: 673-683

Kramer IRH (1980): Oral leukoplakia. J R Soc Med 73: 765-767

Leroux-Robert J (1936): Les épitheliomas intralaryngés. Formes anatomo-cliniques. Voies d'extension. Thèse pour le doctorat en médicine. Gaston Doin & Cie, Paris

LIOTTA LA, TRYGGVASON K, GARBISA S, HART I, FOLTZ CM, SHAFIE S (1980): Metastatic potential correlates with enzymatic degradation on basement membrane collagen. Nature 284: 67-68

LIOTTA LA, RAO CN, BARSKY SH (1983): Tumor invasion and the extracellular matrix. Lab Invest 49: 636-649

LÖBE L-P, QUADE R (1982): Histopathologisches Grading von Karzinomen des HNO-Gebietes. Laryngol Rhinol Otol 61: 171-173

LUNDGREN J, OLOFSSON J, HELLQUIST HB, STRAUDH HJ (1981): Exfoliative cytology in laryngology: Comparison of cytologic and histologic diagnoses in 350 microlaryngoscopic examinations - a prospective study. Cancer 47: 1336-1343

LUNDGREN J, OLOFSSON J, HELLQUIST H, GRÖNTOFT L (1983): Scanning electron microscopy of vocal cord hyperplasia, keratosis, papillomatosis, dysplasia and carcinoma. Acta Otolaryngol (Stockh) 96: 315-327

MCCOMB WS, FLETCHER GH, GALAGER HS, HEALY JE, LEHMANN OH (1967): Larynx. In: MCCOMB WS, FLETCHER GH (eds): Cancer of the head and neck. Baltimore

MCGAVRAN MH, BAUER WC, OGURA JH (1961): The incidence of cervical lymph node metastases from epidermoid carcinoma of the larynx and their relationship to certain characteristics of the primary tumor. Cancer 14: 55-66

MAGNUSSON BC, HEYDEN G, SVENSSON S-E (1974): Histochemical observations on 5'-nucleotidase activity in squamous cell carcinomas of the rat. Histochemistry 42: 1-8

MAKIMOTO K, TAMADA A, KISHIMOTO S, KANOH N, HOSHINO T (1983): Observations on immunologic parameters in laryngeal cancer patients. Arch Otorhinolaryngol 238: 241-250

MATTOX DE, VON HOFF DD (1980): In vitro stem cell assay in head and neck squamous carcinoma. Am J Surg 140: 527-530

MEYER-BREITING E, HALBSGUTH A, OPRITOIU G (1982): Die Bedeutung der Computertomographie für Diagnostik und Therapieplanung fortgeschrittener Kehlkopfkarzinome. Arch Otorhinolaryngol 235: 689-691

MEYER-BREITING E, WEITH E (1982): A whole-organ serial sectioning technique for histologic examination of laryngeal specimen. Arch Otorhinolaryngol 237: 7-15

MEYER-BREITING E, WILZ D (1988): Collagenolytic activity in head and neck cancer - study of 100 squamous cell carcinomas. In preparation

MITTERMAYER C, HÄRLE F, HAGEDORN M (1981): Versuche einer Objektivierung und Validierung der oralen Leukoplakie. In: PETERS J, MÜLLER R (eds), Präkanzerosen und Papillomatosen der Haut. Springer, Berlin-Heidelberg

MICHAELS L, GREGOR RT (1980): Examination of the larynx in the histopathology laboratory. J Clin Path 33: 705-710

MORRA B, BEATRICE F, BRUSSI M, POGGIO E, SARTORIS A, CAVALLO GP, DI FORTUNATO V, VERCELLINO M, CORTESINA G (1984): Evaluation of blocking mechanisms against immunological responses in patients with laryngeal carcinoma. Laryngoscope 94: 825-828

MÜNZEL M, MEISTER P (1976): Subepitheliale Veränderungen bei der einfachen leukoplakischen Hyperplasie der Kehlkopfschleimhaut. Laryngol Rhinol Otol 55: 96-99

OLDE KALTER P, LUBSEN H, DELEMARRE JFM, ALONS CL, VELDHUIZEN RW, MEYER CJLM, SNOW GB (1985): Quantitative morphometry of squamous cell hyperplasia of the larynx. J Clin Pathol 38: 489-495

OLDE KALTER P, DELEMARRE JFM, ALONS CL, MEYER CJLM, SNOW GB (1986): The clinical relevance of classification of squamous cell hyperplasia of the larynx by morphometry. Acta Otolaryngol (Stockh) 101: 331-340

OLOFSSON H, V NOSTRAND AW (1973): Growth and spread of laryngeal carcinoma with reflections on the effect of preoperative irradiation. Acta Otolaryngol Suppl (Stockh) 308: 1-84

PALMER DL (1978): Alcohol consumption and cellular immunocompetence. Laryngoscope 88 (Suppl 8): 13-17

PAPENHAUSEN PR, KUKWA A, CROFT CB, BOROWIECKI B, SILVER C, EMESON EE (1979): Cellular immunity in patients with epidermoid cancer of the head and neck. Laryngoscope 89: 538-549

PERENYI J (1882): Über eine neue Erhärtungsflüssigkeit. Zool Anz 5: 459-460

QUADE R, LÖBE LP (1984): Prognostische Wirksamkeit einer histologisch-zytochemischen Malignitätsgraduierung beim Plattenepithelkarzinom des Kopf-Hals-Bereiches. Acta Histochem (Suppl)(Jena) 30: 81-87

RABIN BS, JOHNSON J, CLAASSEN D (1984): Identification of subsets of lymphocytes infiltrating head and neck tumor tissue: A preliminary report. Laryngoscope 94: 688-690

RICHMAN IM, GELFAND M, HILL JM (1947): A method of decalcifying bone for histologic section. Arch Pathol Lab Med 44: 92-95

SAKU T, SATO E (1983): Prediction of malignant change in oral precancerous lesions by DNA cytofluorometry. J Oral Pathol 12: 90-102

SCHAUER A, HERRMANN J, FINSTERER H (1973): Zytologische Untersuchungen zur Erkennung praeneoplastischer und neoplastischer Larynxveränderungen. Verh Dtsch Ges Pathol 57: 370-373

SCHENK P, KONRAD K (1979): Zur Ultrastruktur der Tumor-Stromagrenze des invasiven Larynxkarzinoms. Laryngol Rhinol Otol 58: 575-582

SCHENK P (1980): Langerhanszellen bei invasivem Larynxkarzinom. Laryngol Rhinol Otol 59: 232-237

SCHENK P (1980): Die Ultrastruktur der Dyskeratose bei invasivem Larynxkarzinom. Laryngol Rhinol Otol 59: 351-355

SCHENK P (1981): Ultrastrukturelle Basallamina-Alterationen an der Tumor-Stromagrenze von invasiven Larynxkarzinomen. Laryngol Rhinol Otol 60: 573-576

SCHENK P (1983): Ultrastrukturelle Alterationen des endoplasmatischen Retikulums in malignen Keratinozyten des Larynxkarzinoms. Laryngol Rhinol Otol 62: 535-539

SCHIFF LJ, SHUGAR MA (1984): Growth of human head and neck squamous cell carcinoma stem cells in agarose. Cancer 53: 286-290

SCRAGG MA, JOHNSON NW (1980): Epithelial cell kinetics: a review of methods of study and their application to oral mucosa in health and disease. J Oral Pathol 9: 309-341

SCRAGG MA, JOHNSON NW (1982): Epithelial cell kinetics. A review of methods of study and their application to oral mucosa in health and disease. J Oral Pathol 11: 102-137

SCULLY C (1981 A): Serum alkaline desoxyribonuclease in oral cancer and premalignant lesions. Biomedicine 35: 179-180

SCULLY C (1981 B): Serum beta 2 microglobulin in oral malignancy and premalignancy. J Oral Pathol 10: 354-357

SCULLY C (1982 A): The immunology of cancer of the head and neck with particular reference to oral cancer. Oral Surg 53: 157-169

SCULLY C (1982 B): Thymidine kinase activity in oral squamous cell carcinoma. J Oral Pathol 11: 210-213

SCULLY C (1982 C): Immunological abnormalities in oral carcinoma and oral keratosis. J Maxillofac Surg 10: 113-115

SCULLY C (1983): Immunology and oral cancer. Br J Oral Surg 21: 136-146

SHKLAR G, EISENBERG E, FLYNN E (1979): Immunoenhancing agents and experimental leukoplakia and carcinoma of the hamster buccal pouch. Prog Exp Tumor Res 24: 269-282

SHKLAR G (1981): Modern studies and concepts of leukoplakia in the mouth. J Derm Surg Oncol 7: 996-1003

SILVERMAN NA, ALEXANDER JC, CHRETIEN P (1976): CEA levels in head and neck cancer. Cancer 37: 2204-2211

SUGAR J, FARAGO L (1966): Ultrastructure of laryngeal precanceroses. Acta Otolaryngol (Stockh) 62: 319-322

TAYLOR CR, KLEDZIG G (1981): Immunhistologic techniques in surgical pathology - a spectrum of "new" special stains. Hum Pathol 12: 590-596

TAYLOR SG, SAFFORD PC (1982): Antigen specifity of squamous cancers of the head and neck based on tumor site using the slide leukocyte adherence inhibition assay. J Surg Oncol 20: 41-45

THOMSEN J, OLSEN J, THOMSEN KA (1975): Exfoliative cytology in the diagnosis of laryngeal malignancy. J Laryngol Otol 89: 281-287

THOMSEN J, OLSEN J, SORENSEN H (1976): Replica cytology in cancer of the larynx:an evaluation of a replica method in the diagnosis of laryngeal malignancy. J Otolaryngol 5: 403-409

THORPE EJ, BELLOMY BB, SELLERS RF (1963): Ultrasonic decalcification of bone. J Bone Joint Surg 45 A: 1257-1259

TRELL E, BJORLING G, ANDREASSON L, KORSGAARD R, MATTIASSON I (1981): Carcinoma of the oral cavity in relation to arylhydrocarbon-hydroxylase inducibility, smoking and dental status. Int J Oral Surg 10: 93-99

TUCKER GF (1961): A histological method for the study of the spread of carcinoma within the larynx. Ann Otol Rhinol Laryngol 70: 910-921

TUCKER GF (1971): Human larynx coronal section atlas. Armed Forces Institute of Pathology, Washington D.C.

UNDERWOOD JCE (1974): Lymphoreticular infiltration in human tumours: prognostic and biological implications. Br J Cancer 30: 538-547

VISSER R, BEEK JM VD, HAVENITH MG, CLEUTJENS JPM, BOSMAN FT (1985): Immunocytochemical detection of basement membrane antigens in the histopathological evaluation of laryngeal dysplasia and neoplasia. Histopathology 10: 171-180

WAHI PN, COHEN B, LUTHRA UK, TORLONI H (1971): Histological typing of oral and oropharyngeal tumours. WHO, Geneva

WALTER RW, DANIELSON JR (1985): Defective monocyte chemotaxis in patients with epidermoid tumors of the head and neck. Arch Otolaryngol 111: 538-540

WANEBO HJ (1979): Immunobiology of head and neck cancer: basic concepts. Head Neck Surg 2: 42-55

WATANABE T, IGLEHART JD, BOLOGNESI DP, COX EB, VAUGHN A, HUDSON WR (1983): Elevated serum secretory immunoglobulin A levels in patients with head and neck carcinoma. Otolaryngol Head Neck Surg 91: 136-142

WHITACKER CW, SIEGLER EE (1956): Exfoliative cytology of the larynx - a preliminary report. Laryngoscope 66: 113-118

WOLF CT, CHRETIEN PB, ELIAS EG, MAKUCH RW, BASKIES AM, SPIEGEL HE, WEISS JF (1979): Serum glycoproteins in head and neck squamous carcinoma. Correlation with tumor extent, clinical tumor stage, and T-cell levels during chemotherapy. Am J Surg 138: 489-500

WUSTROW TPU, ZENNER H-P (1985): Natural killer cell activity in patients with carcinoma of the larynx and hypopharynx. Laryngoscope 95: 1391-1400

References

3 Benign Neoplasms

ABOULKER P, DEMALDENT JE (1966): Tumeur mixte du larynx. Ann Otolaryngol Chir Cervicofac 83: 89-90

ABOULKER P, STERKERS JM, DEMALDENT JE (1966a): Schwannome du larynx. Ann Otolaryngol Chir Cervicofac 83: 88-89

ABOULKER P, FOURESTIER M, STERKERS JM, BOURDON PC, CHAMONARD JL, FOURNIER A (1966b): Évolution filmée d'une papillomatose diffuse laryngo-trachéale évolution maligne. Ann Otolaryngol Chir Cervicofac 83: 96-98

ABRIKOSSOFF AJ (1926): Über Myome, ausgehend von der quergestreiften willkürlichen Muskulatur. Virchows Arch (A) 260: 215-233

ABRIKOSSOFF AJ (1931): Weitere Untersuchungen über Myoblastenmyome. Virchows Arch (A) 280: 723-740

ADLER D, MAIER H, PAUL K (1985): Kongenitales Chondrom des Larynx. Laryngol Rhinol Otol 64: 459-460

AGARWAL RK, BLITZER A, PERZIN KH (1979): Granular cell tumors of the larynx. Otolaryngol Head Neck Surg 87: 807-814

VON ALBERTINI A, ROULET FC (1974): Histologische Geschwulstdiagnostik. 2nd edn. Thieme, Stuttgart

ALTMEYER P, MERKEL KH (1981): Multiple systematisierte Neurome der Haut und der Schleimhaut. Hautarzt 32: 240-244

ANDREWS AH (1955): Glomus tumor (non-chromaffin paraganglioma) of the larynx. Ann Otol Rhinol Laryngol 64: 1034

ANDREWS AJ, MOSS H (1974): Experiences with the carbon dioxide laser in the larynx. Ann Otol Rhinol Laryngol 83: 462-470

ANI AN, JUNAID TA, MARTINSON FD, ADELOYE AA (1979): Chemodectomas: a review of 17 cases. Int Surg 64: 43-48

ARCIDIACONO G, MEO G (1958): Il cistoadenoma papillifero delle ghiandole salivari. Clin Otorinolaringol 10: 134

ARNOLD W (1976): Ätiologische Aspekte zur Frage der Entstehung der Larynxpapillome. Laryngol Rhinol Otol 55: 102-111

ARNOLD W, GANZER U, NASEMANN Th (1977): Zur Pathogenese und Klinik der papillomatösen Haut- und Schleimhauterkrankungen. Arch Otorhinolaryngol 214: 221-239

ARNOLD W (1979): Tubular forms of papova viruses in human laryngeal papilloma. Arch Otorhinolaryngol 225: 15-19

ARNVIG J (1959): On the treatment of papilloma of the larynx in children. J Laryngol Otol 73: 343-345

ARSLAN M, RICCI V (1966): Traitement de la papillomatose juvenile laryngée avec application directe d'ultrasons. Rev Laryngol Otol Rhinol (Bord) 89: 797-809

ASH JE, BECK MR, WILKES JD (1964): Tumors of the upper respiratory tract and ear. Atlas of Tumor Pathology, Section IV, Facsimiles 12 and 13. Armed Forces Institute of Pathology, Washington DC

BABLIK L (1959): Zur antibiotischen Therapie des Larynxpapilloms. Mschr Ohrenheilk 93: 306-308

BAGBY RA, PACKER JT, GLESIAS RG (1976): Rhabdomyoma of the larynx. Report of a case. Arch Otolaryngol 102: 101-103

BAKER DC, PENNINGTON CL (1956): Congenital hemangioma of the larynx. Laryngoscope 66: 696

BARBACCIA F, NICELLI F, TOST C (1956): Adenolinfoma della laringe. Arch Ital Otol 67: 887

BARTON RT (1972): Oncocytic adenoma of the larynx. Ann Otol Rhinol Laryngol 81: 256-257

BARTH E (1898): Zur Casuistik des Überganges gutartiger Kehlkopfgeschwülste in bösartige. Arch Otorhinolaryngol 7: 287

BASSET J-M, PARAIRE F, FRANCOIS M, FLEURY P (1982): Deux nouvelles tumeurs rares du larynx: Un lipome, un chémodectome. Ann Otolaryngol Chir Cervicofac 99: 151-158

BATSAKIS JG (1979): Tumors of the Head and Neck. Clinical and Pathological Considerations. 2nd edn. Williams & Wilkins, Baltimore

BATTIFORA HA, EISENSTEIN R, SCHILD JA (1969): Rhabdomyoma of larynx. Ultrastructural study and comparison with granular cell tumors. Cancer 23: 183-190

BAUM H (1957): Kasuistischer Beitrag zu den neurogenen Larynx-Tumoren. Monatsschr Ohrenheilkd 91: 94-98

BAXTER JD (1965): Glomus tumors (chemodektoma) of the larynx. Ann Otol Rhinol Laryngol 74: 813-815

BEHRENDT W (1965): Sogenannte Speicheldrüsenmischtumoren des Larynx. HNO 13: 118

BEK V, ABRAHAMOVA J, KOUTEK YJ, KOLIHOVA E, FAJSTAVR J (1980): Perinatal subglottic and hepatic hemangiomas as potential emergencies: effect of radiotherapy. Neoplasma 27: 337-344

BELL RD, CHAMBERLAIN D, JAHN AF (1978): Oncocytic lesions of the larynx. J Otolaryngol 7: 211-217

BENJAMIN B (1973): Juvenile laryngeal papillomatosis. J Otolaryngol Soc Aust 3: 560

BENJAMIN B (1978): Treatment of infantile subglottic hemangioma with radioactive gold grain. Ann Otol Rhinol Laryngol 87: 18-21

BERGER F (1967): Neurofibrom des Kehlkopfes unter dem Bilde eines Ventrikelprolapses. HNO 15: 316-317

BETKOWSKI A, ORLOW A, ZAJAK Z (1978): Pleomorphic adenoma of the larynx (pol). Otolaryngol Pol 32: 109-110

BEWTRA Ch, KRISHNAN R, LEE S (1982): Malignant changes in nonirradiated juvenile laryngotracheal papillomatosis. Arch Otolaryngol 108: 114-116

BIRCK HG, MANHART HE (1963): Ultrasound for juvenile laryngeal papillomatosis. A preliminary report of five cases. Arch Otolaryngol 77: 603

BIRD RJ, BRYCE DP (1980): Fibromatosis presenting as vocal cord palsy. J Otolaryngol 9: 78-83

BIRKETT HS (1934): Lipoma of the larynx intrinsic in origin. J Laryngol 49: 733-740

BJÖRK H, WEBER CH (1956): Papilloma of the larynx. Acta Otolaryngol (Stockh) 46: 499

BJÖRK H, TEIR H (1957): Beningn and malignant papilloma of the larynx in adults. Acta Otolaryngol (Stockh) 47: 95

BLANCHARD CL, SAUNDERS WH (1955): Chemodectoma of the larynx. Arch Otolaryngol 61: 472-474

BLUMENFELD F (1927): Papillomatose der Kinder. In: BLUMENFELD F, HOFFMANN R (eds), Chirurgie des Ohres und der oberen Luftwege; vol IV. Kabitzsch, Leipzig

BOEDTS D, MESTDAGH J (1979): Adult rhabdomyoma of the larynx. Arch Otorhinolaryngol 224: 221-229

BOURNE RG, TAYLOR RG (1972): Treatment of a juvenile laryngeal angioma with beta-ray therapy applicator. Radiology 103: 423-426

BOYLE WF, MCCOY EG (1970): Treatment of papilloma of the larynx in children. Laryngoscope 80: 1063-1077

BOYLE WF, RIGGS J, OSHIRO LS, LENNETH EH (1973): Electron microscopic identification of papova virus in laryngeal papilloma. Laryngoscope 83: 1102-1108

BRACH BB, KLEIN RC, MATHEWS AJ, COOK EW (1978): Papillomatosis of the respiratory tract. Upper airway obstruction and carcinoma. Arch Otolaryngol 104: 413-416

BRAUN L, KASHIMA H, EGGLESTON J, SHAH K (1982): Demonstration of papillomavirus antigen in paraffin sections of laryngeal papillomas. Laryngoscope 92: 640-643

BRIDGER GP, NASSAR VH, SKINNER HG (1970): Hemangioma in the adult larynx. Arch Otolaryngol 92: 493-498

BROYLES EN (1940): Treatment of laryngeal papilloma in children with estrogenic hormon: preliminary report. Bull Johns Hopkins Hosp 66: 319-322

BRUCH E (1931): Über große Kehlkopflipome. Laryngol Rhinol Otol 22: 94-97

BÜNGELER W (1957): Allgemeine Pathologie der Geschwülste. Monatsschr Zahnärztl Z 12: 155

BUSANNY-CASPARI WC, HAMMAR CH (1958): Zur Malignität der sog. Myoblastenmyome. Zentralbl Allg Pathol 98: 401

CADOTTE M (1974): Malignant granular cell myoblastomas. Cancer 33: 1417-1422

CAMPBELL JS (1958): Congenital subglottic hemangioma of the larynx and trachea in infants. Pedriatics 22: 727

CANCURA W (1977): Langzeitbeobachtung bei juvenilen Kehlkopfpapillomen nach chirurgischer Abtragung und Ultraschallbehandlung. Laryngol Rhinol Otol 56: 133-137

CANN-AVO C (1970): Su un caso di lipoma laringeo intrinseco. Boll Mal Orecch 88: 270-277

CHANG-LO M (1977): Laryngeal involvement in von Recklinghausen's disease: A case report and review of literature. Laryngoscope 87: 435-442

CHARACHON R, JUNIEN-LAVILLAUROY C, ACCOYER B, ROUX O, FRAPPAT P (1978): The place of cryosurgery in the treatment of subglottic angiomas of the infant. Clin Otolaryngol 2: 207-211

CHEN KTK, BALLECER RA (1986): Laryngeal myxoma. Am J Otolaryngol 7: 58-59

CHIZH GI, OGORODNIKOVA LS, ZINCHENKO VF (1980): Laryngeal liposarcoma developing from a fibrolipoma (rus). Vestn Otorinolaringol 3: 82-83

CHRISTIAENS L, DECROIX G, GAUDIER B, FONTAINE G, WALBUM R, FARRIAUX JP (1965): Les hémangiomes du larynx et de la trachée chez le nourrisson. A propos de 6 observations. Arch franc Pédiat 22: 351-355

CHUMAKOV FJ, VOINOVA VG (1973): Unusual case of teratoma of the larynx (rus). Vestn Otorinolaringol 33: 92

CLARK-NETO R (1980): Quimiodectoma da laringe. AMB 26: 61-62

CLAROS P, VISCASILLAS S, CLAROS A, CLAROS A jr (1985): Lymphangioma of the larynx as a cause of progressive dyspnea. Int J Ped Otolaryngol 9: 263-268

COHEN L (1933): Treatment of intractible laryngeal papilloma in adults, with case reports. South Med J 26: 621

COHEN SC (1984): Posterior cleft larynx associated with hamartoma. Ann Otol Rhinol Laryngol 93: 443-446

COHEN MA, BATSAKIS JG (1968): Oncocytomas of minor salivary glands. Arch Otolaryngol 88: 71-73

COHEN WR, WANG CJ (1972): Steroid treatment of hemangioma of the head and neck in children. Ann Otol Rhinol Laryngol 81: 584-590

COHEN SR, LANDING BH, ISAACS H, KOSTER KING K, HANSON V (1978a): Solitary plasmacytoma of the larynx and upper trachea associated with systemic lupus erythematosus. Ann Otol Rhinol Laryngol (Suppl) 87: 11-14

COHEN SR, LANDING BH, ISAACS H (1978b): Neurofibroma of the larynx in a child. Ann Otol Rhinol Laryngol (Suppl) 87: 29-31

COMPAGNO C, HYAMS VC, STEMARIE P (1975): Beningn granular cell tumors of the larynx. A review of 36 cases with clinicopathologic data. Ann Otol Rhinol Laryngol 84: 308-314

CORDRAY P (1951): Lymphangioma of the larynx. Arch Otolaryngol 53: 83-87

CREPEAU J, POLIQUIN J (1981): The blue rubber bleb nevus syndrome. J Otolaryngol 10: 387-390

CUMMINGS CW, MONTGOMERY WW, BALOGH K jr (1969): Neurogenic tumors of the larynx. Ann Otol Rhinol Laryngol 78: 76-95

CUNNING PS (1950): Diagnosis and treatment of laryngeal tumors. JAMA 142: 73-77

DAHMANN H (1929): Systematische Versuche zur Therapie der Papillomatose. Laryngol Rhinol Otol 17: 362-368

DAMIANI KK, TUCKER HM (1981): Chondroma of the larynx. Surgical technique. Arch Otolaryngol 107: 399-402

DAVIS EDD (1933): A lipoma of the larynx. J Laryngol Otol 48: 824-825

DECHER H (1961): Erfahrungen mit der Podophyllintherapie bei Kehlkopfpapillomen. Laryngol Rhinol Otol 40: 708-720

DEDO HH, JACKLER RK (1982): Laryngeal papilloma: results of treatment with the CO2O-laser and podophyllum. Ann Otol Rhinol Laryngol 91: 425-430

DEKELBOUM AM (1965): Papillomas of the larynx. Arch Otolaryngol 81: 390-397

DI BARTOLOMEO JR, OLSEN AR (1973): Pedunculated lipoma of the epiglottis. Arch Otolaryngol 98: 55-57

DILLARD RG (1979): Subglottic hemangioma: a new approach to management. Am J Dis Child 133: 753

DMOCHOWSKI L, GREY CE, SYKES JA, DREYER DA, LANGFORD DP, JESSE RH, MCCOMB WS (1964): A study of submicroscopic structure and of virus particles in cells of human laryngeal papillomas. Tex Rep Biol Med 22: 454-491

DOMINOK GW, KEMMER C (1966): Histologische und elektronenmikroskopische Veränderungen an juvenilen Kehlkopfpapillomen nach endolaryngealer Ultraschalltherapie. Arch Otorhinolaryngol 186: 153-160

DONALD PJ, KRAUSE CJ (1973): Papillary cystadenoma of the larynx. Laryngoscope 83: 2024-2028

DOOTERMANN J (1937/38): Über Lipome des Kehlkopfes und des Hypopharynx. Inauguraldissertation, München

DUFF TB (1971): Laryngeal papillomatosis. J Laryngol Otol 85: 947-956

DWORACEK H (1955): Über das klinische Verhalten der maligne entarteten Larynxpapillome. Monatsschr Ohrenheilkd 89: 130-132

EAGE WW (1965): Lipoma of the epiglottis and lipoma of the hypopharynx in the same patient. Ann Otol Rhinol Laryngol 74: 851-862

EBERT W, SCHOLZ H J (1979): Leiomyomas of the larynx. Zentralbl Allg Pathol 123: 580-583

EBLE JN, HULL MT, BOJRAB D (1985): Laryngeal blastoma - a light and electron microscopic study of a novel entity analogous to pulmonary blastoma. Am J Clin Pathol 84: 378-385

ECKEDAHL C, SCHNUERER LB (1969): Eosinophilic papillary cystadenoma of the larynx. Acta Otolaryngol (Stockh) 67: 467-470

ECKEL W (1957): Kehlkopfpapillome und deren carcinomatöse Entartung, entstanden jeweils während der Schwangerschaft. Ein Beitrag zur Kasuistik des Kehlkopfcarcinoms der Frau. HNO 6: 197-204

EL-GHAZALI AMS, EL-GHAZALI TMS (1982): Granular cell myoblastoma of the larynx. J Laryngol Otol 96: 1177-1180

EPPER M, MAURER R (1980): Gutartiges Larynxchondrom unter dem Bild rezidivierender Asthmaanfälle. Schweiz Med Wochenschr 110: 416-421

ESCHER A, ESCHER F, ZIMMERMANN A (1984): Zur Klinik und Pathologie chondromatöser Tumoren des Larynx. HNO 32: 269-285

EVANS P (1981): Intubation problem in a case of cystic hygroma complicated by a laryngotracheal haemangioma. Anaesthesia 36: 696-698

FABRITIUS HF (1967): Treatment of juvenile papilloma of the larynx with resin of podophyllin. Acta Otolaryngol (Suppl)(Stockh) 224: 467-468

FALSER N, SPOENDLIN H (1978): Zur Immunologie des Larynxpapilloms. Laryngol Rhinol Otol 57: 646-650

FEBLOT P, DALGROFF G (1976): Kystes et tumeurs du larynx chez le nouveau-né. Méd Infant 83: 683

FECHNER RE, MILLS StE (1982): Verruca vulgaris of the larynx. A distinct lesion of probable viral origin confused with verrucous carcinoma. Am J Surg Path 6: 357-362

FECHNER RE, GOEPFERT H, ALFORD BR (1974): Invasive laryngeal papillomatosis. Arch Otolaryngol 99: 147-151

FENDEL K (1962): Die Neurofibromatosis Recklinghausen im Hals-Nasen-Ohrengebiet. HNO 10: 1-8

FERGUSON GB (1944): Hemangioma of the adult and of the infant larynx. A review of the literature and a report of a case of respiratory obstruction in infants. Ann Otol Rhinol Laryngol 70: 1095-1112

FERGUSON CF, FLAKE CG (1961): Subglottic haemangioma as a case of respiratory obstruction in infants. Ann Otol Rhinol Laryngol 70: 1095-1112

FERLITO A (1978): Histiocytic tumors of the larynx: a clinicopathological study with review of the literature. Cancer 42: 611-622

FERLITO A, FRUGONI P (1975): Rhabdomyoma purum of the larynx. J Laryngol Otol 89: 1131-1141

FERLITO A, RECHER G (1981): Oncocytic lesions of the larynx. Arch Otorhinolaryngol 232: 107-115

FEUERSTEIN SS (1973): Subglottic haemangioma in infants. Laryngoscope 83: 466-475

FEYRTER F (1948): Über Neurome und Neurofibrome nach Untersuchungen am menschlichen Magen-Darmschlauch. Maudrich, Wien-Düsseldorf

FEYRTER F (1951): Über die Pathologie der vegetativen nervösen Peripherie und ihrer ganglionären Regulationsstätten. Maudrich, Wien-Düsseldorf

FEYRTER F (1952): Über die granulären Neurome. Virchows Arch(A) 322: 66-72

FIGI FA, ROWLAND WD, NEW GB (1944): Cystadenoma of the larynx. Arch Otolaryngol 40: 445-450

FISHBEIN AV, BORISOV AA, BARILIAK IUR (1979): Malignant laryngeal paraganglioma. Zh Ushn Nos Gorl Bolezn 4: 71-73

FLEISCHER K (1956): Drei seltene Kehlkopftumoren. Speicheldrüsenmischtumor, Teratom, Granuloblastom. Laryngol Rhinol Otol 35: 346-354

FLEURY P, BOCQUET L, BASSET J M, COMPERE J F, STERKERS O, PANSIER P, VISSUZAINE C (1979): Quatre tumeurs rares du larynx: tumeurs cellules granuleuses, Schwannome, Amylose pseudo-tumorale. Ann Otolaryngol Chir Cervicofac 96: 611-617

FLYNN JA (1933): Extrinsic lipoma of the larynx. Laryngoscope 43: 294-903

FOURNIE R, BENKIRAN D, CARESSE J, TAHIRI M (1965): A propos d'un cas de tératome goetoide anisopage endocymiens inclus de la région latero-laryngée. J Fr Otorhinolaryngol 14: 893

FRADIS M, PODOSHIN L, GRISHKAN A (1980): Granular-cell myoblastoma of the larynx. Ear Nose Throat J 59: 412-414

FRIEDBERG SA, STAGMAN R, HAAS GM (1971): Papillary lesions of the larynx in adults. A pathologic study. Ann Otol Rhinol Laryngol 80: 683-692

FRIEDMAN I (1976): Sarcomas of the larynx. In: ALBERTI PW, BRYCE DP (eds), Centennial Conference on Laryngeal Cancer; pp 122-126. Appleton-Century-Crofts, New York

GAILLARD J, GIGNOUX B, BRUNAT M (1973): Papillomatose laryngée de l'enfant. Essai de traitement par l'association Thiotepa-Bleomycine. J Fr Otorhinolaryngol 22: 423-425

GAILLARD J, HAGUENAUER JP, DUBRENIL C, ROMANET P (1978): Les tumeurs rares de la corde vocale. A propos de 2 cas: un adenome pleomorphe et un neurinome. J Fr Otorhinolaryngol 27: 714-718

GALLAGHER JC, PUZON BQ (1969): Oncocytic lesions of the larynx. Ann Otol Rhinol Laryngol 78: 307-318

GALLIVAN M, CHUN B, ROWDEN G, LACK EE (1979): Laryngeal paraganglioma. Case report with ultrastructural analysis and literature review. Am J Surg Pathol 3: 85-92

GAMMELGARD N, JUUL A (1980): Granular cell myoblastoma. A case report involving the larynx. Ugeskr Laeger 142: 247-248

GARDNER DV, CORIO RL (1983a): Multifocal adult rhabdomyoma. Oral Surg Oral Med Oral Pathol 56: 76-78

GARDNER DV, CORIO RL (1983b): Fetal rhabdomyoma of the tongue, with a discussion of the two histologic variants of this tumor. Oral Surg Oral Med Oral Pathol 56: 293-300

GARUD O, BOSTAD L, ELVERLAND HH, MAIR IWS (1984): Granular cell tumor of the larynx in a 5-year-old child. Ann Otol Rhinol Laryngol 93: 45-47

GEHANNO P, LALLEMANT Y, GROUSSARD O, BLANCHET F, VEBER F, GUEDON C, RAME JA (1980): Apudomes en ORL - propos de 6 observations (dont 1 chémodectome et 1 carcino de du larynx); critique du concept d'apudome. J Fr Otorhinolaryngol 29: 7-10

GERASCHENKO IF (1957): Laryngeal osteoma (rus). Vestn Otorinolaringol 19: 117

GESCHICKTER CF, COPELAND MM (1936): Tumors of bone. 2nd edn. New York

GIGNOUX M, MARTIN H, CAMUSET M (1963): A propos d'une tumeur dite mixte du larynx. J Fr Otorhinolaryngol 12: 679

GILBERT JG, MAZARELLA LA, FEIT LJ (1953): Primary tracheal tumors in the infant and adult. Arch Otolaryngol 58: 1-9

GISSMANN L, PFISTER H, ZUR HAUSEN H (1977): Human papilloma viruses (HPV): Characterization of four different isolates. Virology 76: 569

GOEBEL U, ARNOLD W, WAHN V, TREUNER J, JÜRGENS H,

CANTELL K (1981): Comparison of human fibroblast and leukocyte interferon in the treatment of severe laryngeal papillomatosis in children. Eur J Pediatr 137: 175-176

GOEPFERT H, GUTTERMANN J, DICHTEL W, SESSIONS R, CANGIR A, SULEK M (1982): Leucocyte interferon in patients with juvenile laryngeal papillomatosis. Ann Otol Rhinol Laryngol 91: 431-436

GOODER P, FARRINGTON T (1980): Extracranial neurilemmomata of the head and neck. J Laryngol Otol 94: 243-249

GORDON LP (1979): Case for diagnosis: subglottic hemangioma and cerebral edema. Milit Med 144: 659-664

GOTO T, NAKASHIMA Y (1973): Giant cell tumor of the larynx. Otologia (Fukuoka) 19: 507

GRACANIN S (1948): Un cas unique de leiomyome du larynx. Acta Otolaryngol (Stockh) 36: 71-74

GRANICH MS, PILCH BZ, NADOL JB, DICKERSIN GR (1983): Fetal rhabdomyoma of the larynx. Arch Otolaryngol 109: 821-826

GRANT JH (1961): Lipoma of the larynx. J Laryngol Otol 75: 765-767

GREGG JB, MYRABO AK (1959): Combined neurofibroma and carcinoma in the larynx. Arch Otolaryngol 69: 307-311

GROSS CW, CROCKER TR (1970): Current management of juvenile laryngeal papillomata. Laryngoscope 80: 532-543

GUERRIER Y (1960): Leiomyome du larynx. J Fr Otorhinolaryngol 9: 149

HAGLUND S, LUNDQUIST PG, CANTELL K, STRANDER H (1981): Interferon therapy in juvenile laryngeal papillomatosis. Arch Otolaryngol 107: 327-332

HALL-JONES J (1972): Giant cell tumor of the larynx. J Laryngol Otol 86: 371-381

HARBERT F (1951): Lipoma of the larynx. Ann Otol Rhinol Laryngol 60: 982-985

HAR-EL G, SHVIRO J, AVIDOR I, SEGAL K, SIGI J (1985): Laryngeal granular cell tumor in children. Am J Otolaryngol 6: 32-34

HARKIN JC, REED RJ (1969): Tumors of the peripheral nervous system. Armed Forces Institute of Pathology, Washington DC

HARMER L (1903): Über die Behandlung der Kehlkopfpapillome im Kindesalter mit besonderer Berücksichtigung der Laryngotomie. Arch Otorhinolaryngol 13: 58

HEALY GB, FEARON B, FRENCH R, MCGILL T (1980): Treatment of subglottic hemangioma with the carbon dioxide laser. Laryngoscope 90: 809-813

HEIBERG S (1935): Lipom des Hypopharynx. Zentralbl Hals-Nasen-Ohrenheilk 24: 437

HEIMBERG BM, TOPP WC, SCHNEIDER PS, ABRAMSON AL (1983): Laryngeal papillomavirus infection during clinical remission. N Engl J Med 308: 1261-1264

HEINZ I (1951): The adenolymphomata. Aust N Z J Surg 21: 47-51

HELIDONIS E, DOKIANAKIS G, PANTAZOPOULOS P (1978): Granular cell myoblastoma of the larynx. J Laryngol Otol 92: 525-528

HOHBACH C, MOOTZ W (1978): Chemodectoma of the larynx. A clinico-pathologic study. Virchows Arch (A) 378: 161-172

HOLBOROW CA, MOTT TJ (1973): Subglottic haemangioma in infancy. J Laryngol Otol 87: 1013-1017

HOLINGER PH, JOHNSTON KC, ANISON GC (1950): Papilloma of the larynx. A review of 109 cases with a preliminary report of Aureomycin therapy. Ann Otol Rhinol Laryngol 59: 547-564

HOLINGER PH, SCHILD JA, MAURITZ DH (1968): Laryngeal papilloma, review of etiology and therapy. Laryngoscope 78: 1462-1474

HOLINGER PH, ANDREWS AH (1974): The carbon dioxide laser in management of papilloma of the larynx. J Fr Otorhinolaryngol 23: 177-178

HOLLINGSWORTH J, KOHLMOOS H, MCNAUGHT R (1950): Treatment of juvenile papilloma with resin of podophyllum Arch Otolaryngol 52: 82-87

HOLM-JENSEN S, JACOBSEN M, THOMMESEN N, FERREIRA O (1977): Oncocytic cysts of the larynx. Acta Otolaryngol (Stockh) 83: 366-371

HOOPER R (1972): Chemodectoma of the glomus laryngicum superior. Laryngoscope 82: 686-692

HOPMANN E (1935): Fibrochondroosteom des Kehlkopfes. Laryngol Rhinol Otol 26: 268-271

HORDIJK GJ, RUITER DJ, BOSMAN FT, MAUW BJ (1981): Chemodectoma (paraganglioma) of the larynx. Clin Otolaryngol 6: 249-254

HUIZINGA E (1962): Lipoma laryngis. Pract Otorhinolaryngol (Basel) 24: 354

HYAMS VJ, RABUZZI DD (1970): Cartilaginous tumors of the larynx. Laryngoscope 80: 755-767

IKENBERG H, NEUMANN-HAEFELIN D, RICHTHAMMER B, WOLFART W, ADLER C-P, BODO G, GISSMANN L, ZUR HAUSEN H (1985): Interferon therapy for bronchial papillomatosis controlled by papillomavirus-DNA hybridization. Arch Otolaryngol 111: 96-98

ISHIDA M, HASEGAWA S, SATO T, TATEISHI R (1971): Glomus tumor (nonchromaffin-paraganglioma) of the larynx. Laryngoscope 81: 957-961

IVATURY R, SHAH D, ASCER E, SRINIVASAN K, HERAUD J, ROHMAN M (1982): Granular cell tumor of larynx and bronchus. Ann Thorac Surg 33: 69-73

JACKSON Ch, JACKSON ChL (1959): Diseases of the Nose, Throat and Ear. 2nd edn. Saunders, Philadelphia-London

JAFEK BW, STERN FA (1973): Neurofibroma of the larynx occurring with v. Recklinghausen disease. Arch Otolaryngol 98: 77-79

JAFFE BF (1973): Unusual laryngeal problems in children. Ann Otol Rhinol Laryngol 82: 637-642

JAKOBI H (1955): Diskussionsbemerkung. Arch Ohr Nas Kehlk Heilk 167: 342

JARVEY BA, LEVIN LS (1974): Subglottic hemangioma. Birth Defects 10: 320

JENKINS JC (1967): Preliminary report on the treatment of multiple juvenile laryngeal papillomata by ultrasound. J Laryngol Otol 81: 385-390

JOHNS ME, BATSAKIS JG, SHORT CD (1973): Oncocytic and oncocytoid tumors of the salivary glands. Laryngoscope 83: 1940-1952

JOHNSON JT, BARNES EL, JUSTICE W (1981): Adult onset laryngeal papillomatosis. Otolaryngol Head Neck Surg 89: 867-873

JOHNSON LF, STRONG MS (1954): Teratoma of the larynx. Arch Otolaryngol 58: 435-441

JOKINEN K, PALVA A, KÄRJÄ J (1981): Cryocauterization in the treatment of subglottic hemangioma in infants. Laryngoscope 91: 78-82

JOKINEN K, SEPPALA A, PALVA A (1974): Laryngeal pleomorphic adenoma. J Laryngol Otol 88: 1131-1134

JONES SR, MYERS EN, BARNES L (1984): Benign neoplasmas of the larynx. Otolaryngol Clin North Am 17: 151-158

JUSTRABO E, MICHIELS R, CALMETTES C, CABANNE F, BASTEIN H, HORIOT JC, GUERRIN J (1980): An uncommon apudoma: a functional chemodectoma of the larynx. Acta Otolaryngol (Stockh) 89: 135-143

Justus J, Baerthold W, Preibisch-Effenberger R (1970): Juvenile Larynxpapillomatose mit Ausbreitung über das Tracheobronchialsystem und maligne Entartung ohne Strahlentherapie. HNO 18: 349-354

Kärjä J, Palva A, Jokinen K (1979): Cryotherapy in the treatment of subglottic hemangioma in infants. Acta Otolaryngol (Suppl)(Stockh) 360: 58-60

Kapur TR (1968): Recurrent lipomata of the larynx and the pharynx with late malignant change. J Laryngol Otol 82: 761-768

Karduk A, Richter HG (1979): Lasermikrochirurgische Behandlung gutartiger Stimmlippenveränderungen und ihre funktionellen Ergebnisse. Laryngol Rhinol Otol 58: 764-769

Kastenbauer E, Federspil P (1969): Zur Klinik der Chondrome im Kehlkopfbereich. HNO 17: 245-247

Kenefick C (1978): Granular cell myoblastoma of the larynx. J Laryngol Otol 92: 521-523

Kimmelmann CP, Sugar J, Lowry LD (1979): Resident's page. Pathologic quiz case 2. Hemangioma of the vocal cord. Arch Otolaryngol 105: 500-502

Kleinsasser O (1958): Über die gut- und bösartigen Formen der Kehlkopfpapillome und deren histologisches und klinisches Bild. Arch Otorhinolaryngol 171: 44-69

Kleinsasser O (1964): Das Glomus laryngicum inferius. Ein bisher unbekanntes, nicht chromaffines Paraganglion vom Bau der sogenannten Carotisdrüse im menschlichen Kehlkopf. Arch Otorhinolaryngol 184: 214-224

Kleinsasser O (1968): Microlaryngology and endolaryngeal surgery. Saunders, Philadelphia-London

Kleinsasser O, Olivera e Cruz G (1973): Juvenile und adulte Kehlkopfpapillome. HNO 21: 97-106

Kleinsasser O, Glanz H (1979a): Spontane Kanzerisierung nicht bestrahlter juveniler Larynxpapillome. Laryngol Rhinol Otol 58: 482-489

Kleinsasser O, Glanz H (1979b): Myogenic Tumours of the Larynx. Arch Otorhinolaryngol 225: 107-119

Klose W (1938): Zwei Fälle von seltenen Kehlkopftumoren. Arch Otorhinolaryngol 145: 154-158

Köhn K (1969): Nase und Nasennebenhöhlen, Kehlkopf und Luftröhre. In: Doerr W, Seifert G, Uehlinger E (eds), Spezielle pathologische Anatomie; vol 4. Springer, Berlin - Heidelberg - New York

Konovalov SF (1977): Laryngeal lipoma. Zh Ushn Nos Gorl Bolezn 5: 105

Kotarba E, Niezabitowski A (1974): Giant cell tumor of laryngeal soft tissues. Otolaryngol Pol 28: 331-335

Kramer R, Yankauer S (1924): Lymphangioma of the larynx. Laryngoscope 83: 621-629

Kroe DJ, Pitcock JA, Cocke W (1967): Oncocytic papillary cystadenoma of the larynx. Presentation of two cases. Arch Pathol Lab Med 84: 429-432

Kubo R, Katsuda K, Nobori T (1976): Riesenzelltumor des Kehlkopfes. Otol Fukuoka 22: 776

Kveton JF, Pillsbury HC (1982): Conservative treatment of infantile subglottic hemangioma with corticosteroids. Arch Otolaryngol 108: 117-119

Lack EE, Worsham GF, Callihan MD, Crasford BC, Klappenbach S, Rowden G, Chun B (1980): Granular cell tumor: a clinico-pathologic study of 110 patients. J Surg Oncol 1980: 301-316

Lafaye M, Pottecher G, Gaillard de Collogny L, Roche G, Morin B, Wahl D (1978): Incidences respiratoires severs de la maladie de Launois et Bensaude. J Fr Otorhinolaryngol 27: 101-106

Lawson W, Zak FG (1974): The glomus bodies ("Paraganglia") of the human larynx. Laryngoscope 84: 98-111

Lazar AM, Leroy EP (1950): Hemangioma of the larynx in infants. Ear Nose Throat Monthly 29: 249

Lees CD, Levine HL, Beven EG, Tucker HM (1981): Tumors of the carotid body. Experience with 41 operative cases. Am J Surg 142: 362-365

Leikensohn JR, Benton C, Cotton R (1976): Subglottic hemangioma. J Otolaryngol 5: 487-492

Le Jenne FE, Putmann HC, Yamase HT (1980): Multiple oncocytic papillary cystadenomas of the larynx: a case report. Laryngoscope 90: 501-504

Lejeune FE (1941): The story of Warren Bell. Ann Otol Rhinol Laryngol 50: 905-910

Lemariey A, Muler H, Paquelin F, Hamon L (1964): Tumeurs sous-glottiques du nourrisson. A propos de cinq cas. Ann Otolaryngol Chir Cervicofac 81: 730-733

Lenarcic-Cepelja I, Krajina Z (1984): Interferon in der Behandlung rezidivierender Larynxpapillome. Laryngol Rhinol Otol 63: 401-402

Leroux-Robert J (1956): 3 cas de tumeurs chondromateuses du chaton cricoiden traités par cricoidectomie sous-perichondrale totale ou partielle. Ann Otolaryngol Chir Cervicofac 73: 585-590

Lesione W (1965): Der seltene Fall eines subglottischen Osteochondroms. HNO 13: 239-240

Liebermann HT, Solisch WP, Hahnefeld H (1978): Einige physikalische Eigenschaften des Virus der Larynxpapillomatose des Menschen. Arch Geschwulstforsch 48: 552-558

Lindell MM jr, Jing BS, Luna MA (1981): Glomus laryngicum superior: a case studied arteriographycally. Am J Rad Ther 136: 618-619

Lindenberger J (1982): Das onkozytäre Adenom des Kehlkopfes. Laryngol Rhinol Otol 61: 169-170

Lloyd KM, Dennis M (1963): Cowden's disease. A possible new symptom complex with multiple system involvement. Ann Intern Med 58: 136-142

Lundgren J, Olofsson J, Hellquist H (1982): Oncocytic lesions of the larynx. Acta Otolaryngol (Stockh) 94: 335-344

Lundquist PG, Frithiof L, Wersäll J (1975): Ultrastructural features of human juvenile laryngeal papillomas. Acta Otolaryngol (Stockh) 80: 137-149

Lyons GD, Schlosser JV, Lousteau R, Mouney DF, Benes EN (1978): Laser surgery and immunotherapy in the management of laryngeal papilloma. Laryngoscope 88: 1586-1588

McCabe BF, Clark KF (1983): Interferon and laryngeal papillomatosis. Ann Otol Rhinol Laryngol 92: 2-7

McHenry LC (1953): Neurolemmoma (Schwannoma) of the larynx. Ann Otol Rhinol Laryngol 62: 392-399

McIntosh WA, Kassner GW, Murray JF (1985): Fibromatosis and fibrosarcoma of the larynx and pharynx in an infant. Arch Otolaryngol 111: 478-480

McMillan RH, Fechner RE (1986): Pleomorphic adenoma of the larynx. Arch Pathol Lab Med 110: 245-247

Maconi A (1951): Lipoma of the larynx. J Laryngol Otol 65: 426-433

McSwain GR, Colpitts R, Kreutner A, O'Brien PH, Spicer S (1980): Granular cell myoblastoma. Surg Gynecol Obstet 150: 703-710

Maier I (1968): Maligne Entartung bestrahlter juveniler Larynxpapillome. Laryngol Rhinol Otol 47: 862-869

Maisel RH, Ogura JH (1974): Neurofibromatosis with laryngeal involvement. Laryngoscope 84: 132-140

Majmudar B, Thomas J, Gorelkin L, Symbas PN (1981): Respiratory obstruction caused by a multicentric granular cell tumor of the laryngotracheobronchial tree. Hum Pathol 12: 283-286

MAJOROS M, DEVINE KD, PARKHILL EM (1963): Malignant transformation of benign laryngeal papillomas in children after radiation therapy. Surg Clin North Am 43: 1049-1061
MANIGLIA AJ, XUE JDDW (1983): Plasmacytoma of the larynx. Laryngoscope 93: 741-744
MAREEV VM, SHKABROV VV (1980): Laryngo-pharyngeal lipoma and fibromyxoma (rus). Vestn Otorinolaringol 1980: 74
MARSCHIK H (1936): Neurinom des Kehlkopfes. Monatsschr Ohrenheilkd 70: 1143
MARTINSON FD (1967): Chemodectoma of the glomus laryngicum inferior. Arch Otolaryngol 86: 70-73
MATIC V, DZINIC M, RADONJIC D (1979): Schwannomas of the larynx. Med Pregl 32: 245-248
MATSCHNIG F (1954): Wiederholte Larynxpapillome: Maligne Entartung. Monatsschr Ohrenheilkd 88: 139
MATSUBA HM, THAWLEY StE, SPECTOR GJ, MAUNEY M, PIKUL FJ (1985): Laryngeal epidermoid carcinoma associated with laryngeal papillomatosis. Laryngoscope 95: 1264-1266
MATSUMOTO K, YAMAMOTO E, USHIJIMA T, FUNASAKA S (1981): A case of laryngeal leiomyoma (vascular leiomyoma)(jap). Nippon Jibiinkoka Gakkai Kaiho 84: 731-734
MATZKER J (1963): Gutartige Tumoren des Kehlkopfes. In: BERENDES J, LINK R, ZÖLLNER F (eds), Hals-Nasen-Ohren-Heilkunde; vol II/2. Thieme, Stuttgart
MAYOUX H, MARTIN, REBATTU JP (1955): A propos de deux observations de chondromes du larynx. J Fr Otorhinolaryngol 44: 127-131
MEESEN H, SCHULZ H (1957): Elektronenmikroskopischer Nachweis des Virus im Kehlkopfpapillom des Menschen. Klin Wochenschr 1957: 771-773
MEHTA P, HEROLD N (1980): Regression of juvenile laryngobronchial papillomatosis with systemic bleomycin therapy. J Pediatr 97: 479-480
MEYJERS B (1905): Drei seltene Halsgeschwülste; cited by KÖHN (1969).
MERZ W, GRAF K (1958): Haemangiofibrom der Trachea. Pract Otorhinolaryngol (Basel) 20: 77-80
MICHAELS L (1975): Neurogenic tumors, granular cell tumor and paraganglioma. Can J Otolaryngol 4: 319-327
MICHAELS L (1984): Pathology of the larynx. Springer, Berlin-Heidelberg-New York-Tokyo
MIELKE A, CHILLA R, VOLLRATH M (1980): Die Kryo- und Laserchirurgie zur Behandlung maligner und benigner Kehlkopfprozesse. HNO 28: 357-364
MINNIGERODE B (1970): Das subglottische Kehlkopfheamangiom des Neugeborenen. Laryngol Rhinol Otol 49: 585-593
MIREJAVSKY P, KONECNY L (1974): Flat proliferating hemangioma of the larynx (czech). Czech Pathol 10: 71
MITSCHKE H (1975): Chondrome des Kehlkopfes und ihre Behandlung. Wien Med Wochenschr 125: 153-155
MODLIN B (1982): Rhabdomyoma of the larynx. Laryngoscope 92: 580-582
MORAN JJ, ENTERLINE HT (1964): Benign rhabdomyoma of the pharynx. A case report, review of the literature and comparison with cardiac rhabdomyoma. Am J Clin Pathol 42: 174-181
MORGON A, GREGOIRE D, ROMANET P (1976): Traitement chimiothérapique de la papillomatose laryngée de l'enfant. J Fr Otorhinolaryngol 25: 473-476
MORI D, TORTORA R (1966): Neurinoma laringeo nel corso della neurofibromatosi multipla. Ann Laringol (Torino) 65: 802
MOSCOVIC EA, AZAR HA (1967): Multiple granular cell tumors ("myoblastomas"). Case report with electron microscopic observations and review of the literature. Cancer 20: 2032-2047
MOSTOWSKI L (1979): Case of schwannoma of the larynx. Otolaryngol Pol 33: 111-114
MOUBAYED AP, WIEBRINGHAUS H (1977): Drei Fälle eines Riesenzellfibroms des Stimmbandes. Arch Otorhinolaryngol 217: 193-198
MOULONGUET H, HAMEL S (1976): Un cas de maladie de Launois-Bensaude avec localisation laryngée. Ann Otolaryngol Chir Cervicofac 93: 513
MOUNIER-KUHN P, GAILLARD J, FONTVIELLE H, MORGON A (1964): A propos d'une statistique hospitaliere des angiomes benins a forme tumorale dans le domaine ORL. J Fr Otorhinolaryngol 13: 415
MOUNTS P, SHAH KV, KASHIMA H (1982): Viral etiology of juvenile- and adult-onset squamous papilloma of the larynx. Proc Natl Acad Sci USA 79: 5425-5429
MROSZKOWSKI E (1982): Case of laryngeal myoblastoma (pol). Otolaryngol Pol 35: 177-180
MUELFAY V, DRASOVEANU C, GUENDISCH G (1978): Comments on 6 cases of laryngeal hemangioma. Rev Chir (Otolaringol) 23: 259-265
MUENZEL M, KASTENDIEK H (1978): Neurogener Kehlkopftumor. Laryngol Rhinol Otol 57: 408-413
NACLERIO RM (1980): Pathologic quiz case 1. Arch Otolaryngol 106: 514-516
NAEIM F, WAISMAN J (1973): Calcified neurilemoma of the larynx. Ann Otol Rhinol Laryngol 82: 212-215
NAKASHIMA T, WATANABE Y (1985): Sudden airway obstruction due to a benign hemangioendothelioma of the larynx. Laryngoscope 95: 849-850
NANSON EM (1978): Neurilemoma of the larynx: a case study. Head Neck Surg 1: 69-74
NARDI S, ROSIGNOLI M (1973): Considerazioni su un voluminoso emangioma. Clin Otorinolaringol 25: 35
NARZY P et al (1980): Angiomes sous-glottiques du nourrisson. A propos de 20 observations. J Fr Otorhinolaryngol 29: 361-365
NATALI R, CORFU G, RACHINEL O, MENAGER G, MESNIL JJ (1980): Schwannome du larynx. A propos d'un cas. Ann Otolaryngol Chir Cervicofac 97: 901-903
NEEL BH, UNNI KK (1982): Cartilaginous tumors of the larynx: A series of 33 patients. Otolaryngol Head Neck Surg 90: 201-207
NEIVERT H, ROYER L (1946): Leiomyoma of the larynx. Arch Otolaryngol 44: 214-216
NEUSS O (1956): Die Bedeutung des chromophoben Paraganglioms (Chemodectoms) für die Hals-Nasen-Ohrenheilkunde. Laryngol Rhinol Otol 35: 137-141
NEVILLE BW, MCCONNEL FMS (1981): Multifocal adult rhabdomyoma. Arch Otolaryngol 107: 175-178
NIKOLAIDIS ET, TROST DC, BUCHHOLZ CL, WILKINSON EJ (1985): The relationship of histology and clinical factors in laryngeal papillomatosis. Arch Pathol Lab Med 109: 24-29
NOHTERI H (1946): A case of laryngeal cyst composed of oncocytes and the appearance of oncocytes in the mucous membrane of the nose and the larynx. Acta Pathol Microbiol Scand 23: 473-483
NOLTE E, KLEINSASSER O (1982): Granularzelltumoren des Kehlkopfes. HNO 30: 333-339
NUUTINEN J, SYRJÄNEN K (1983): Angioleiomyoma of the larynx. Report of case and review of the literature. Laryngoscope 83: 941-943
O'CALLAGHAN JP, EMKO P, PERL T (1981): Lipoma of the larynx imaged by conventional radiographic methods. J Laryngol Otol 95: 1159-1163

O'Connor AF, Freeland AP (1980): Neonatal laryngeal neurofibromatosis. Ear Nose Throat J 59: 174-177

Offenhammer K (1955): Zur Differentialdiagnose neurogener Tumoren des Larynx. Pract Otorhinolaryngol (Basel) 17: 33-45

Oliveira CA, Roth JA, Adams GL (1977): Oncocytic lesions of the larynx. Laryngoscope 87: 1718-1725

Overcash KE, Putney FJ (1973): Subglottic haemangioma of the larynx treated with steroid therapy. Laryngoscope 83: 679-682

Pahor AL (1976): Lipoma of the larynx. Ear Nose Throat J 55: 341-342

Palva T, Jokinen K, Kärjä J (1975): Neurilemmoma (Schwannoma) of the larynx. J Laryngol Otol 89: 203-207

Perrin C, Feldis JN, Gerbaux A (1975): Volumineuses localisation laryngées d'une neurofibromatose chez un jeune homme de 15 ans. Intervention par pharyngotomie laterale. Rev Otoneuroophthalmol 47: 209-212

Perrin C, Floquet J, Andre JM, Plenat JF, Petit C (1978): Reflexions a propos d'un chemodectome larygné. Rev Otoneuroophtalmol 50: 173-179

Perrino A (1958): Tumore a cellule giganti della laringe. Ann Laringol (Torino) 57: 140

Pesavento G, Ferlito A (1982): Haemangiopericytoma of the larynx. J Laryngol Otol 96: 1065-1076

Pope TH (1965): Laryngeal myoblastoma. Arch Otolaryngol 81: 80-82

Preibisch-Effenberger R (1970a): Das juvenile Larynxpapillom. HNO 18: 229-233

Preibisch-Effenberger R (1970b): Die endolaryngeale Ultraschalltherapie bei juvenilen Kehlkopfpapillomen und deren bisherige Ergebnisse. HNO 18: 234-237

Putney FJ (1955): Borderline malignant lesions of the larynx. Arch Otolaryngol 61: 381-385

Putney FJ, Morau JJ (1964): Cartilaginous tumors of the larynx. Ann Otol Rhinol Laryngol 73: 370-380

Quesada P, Medina A, Ortiz F (1978): Angioleiomioma de laringe. Ann Otorrinolaringol Ibero Am 5: 265-270

Quick CA, Faras A, Krzysek R (1978): The etiology of laryngeal papillomatosis. Laryngoscope 88: 1789-1795

Quick CA, Foucar LP, Dehner LP (1979): Frequency and significance of epithelial atypia in laryngeal papillomatosis. Laryngoscope 89: 550-560

Quick CA, Krzyzek RA, Watts SL, Faras AJ (1980): Relationship between condylomata and laryngeal papillomata; clinical and molecular virological evidence. Ann Otol Rhinol Laryngol 89: 467-471

Rabbett WF (1965): Juvenile laryngeal papillomatosis. The relation of irradiation to malignant degeneration in this disease. Ann Otol Rhinol Laryngol 74: 1149-1163

Raiz SD, Kravets SA (1980): Laryngeal Gemmahemangioma. Zh Ushn Nos Gorl Bolezn 3: 75-76

Ranger D, Thackray AC (1953): Papillary cystadenoma of the larynx. J Laryngol Otol 67: 609-614

Reinhard M (1960): Die Knorpelgeschwülste des Kehlkopfes und ihre Behandlung. HNO 8: 121-123

Ribari O, Elemer G, Balint A (1975): Laryngeal giant cell tumor. J Laryngol Otol 89: 857-861

Riccabona A v (1953): Neurinom des Pharynx. Monatsschr Ohrenheilkd 87: 60-61

Ricci V (1974): Ultrasound therapy of laryngo-tracheal papillomatosis. J Fr Otorhinolaryngol 23: 173-174

Robbins KT, Woodson GE (1984): Current concept in the management of laryngeal papillomatosis. Head Neck Surg 6: 861-866

Romualdi G, Cortesi C (1947): I mixomi della laringe. Arch Vecchi Anat Patol 9: 761-788

Rosenman D, Gertner R, Fradis M, Misslevitsch A, Boss JH (1986): Rhabdomyoma of the larynx. J Laryngol Otol 100: 607-610

Rozhinskaia IA, Chartorizhskaia NN (1980): Clear-cell adenoma of the larynx. Vestn Otorinolaringol 1: 55-56

Ruben RJ, Kucinski SA, Greenstein N (1975): Cystic lymphangioma of the vallecula. Can J Otolaryngol 4: 180-184

Rudert H (1971): Riesenzelltumor des Kehlkopfes. HNO 19: 306-309

Sakurai S, Takahashi M, Nakajima Y, Ishizaka T (1975): Juvenile papilloma of the larynx treated by local injection of Bleomycin (jap). Keio J Med 24: 11-17

Sasaki CT, Holmes RE (1976): Oncocytoma of the epiglottis. Ear Nose Throat J 55: 278

Schaefer SD, Blend BL, Denton JG (1980): Laryngeal paragangliomas: evaluation and treatment. Am J Otolaryngol 1: 451-455

Schlechter GL, Biller HF (1972): The limitations of corticosteroids and cryotherapy for subglottic hemangioma. Trans Am Acad Ophth Otol 76: 1360

Schlosnagle DC, Kratochvil FJ, Weathers DR, McConnel FMS, Campbell WG jr (1983): Intraoral multifocal adult rhabdomyoma. Arch Pathol Lab Med 107: 638-642

Schwarzbart A (1937): Beitrag zur Kasuistik gutartiger Kehlkopfgeschwülste. Monatsschr Ohrenheilkd 71: 385-390

Shapiro RS, Marlowe FI, Butcher J (1976): Malignant degeneration of nonirradiated juvenile laryngeal papillomatosis. Ann Otol Rhinol Laryngol 85: 101-104

Shevchenko AM, Egorov VP, Gladkii NI, Miroshinichenko SV (1981): Abrikosoff's granular cell tumor localized on the vocal fold (rus). Vestn Otorinolaringol 1981: 77-78

Shibata K, Komune S (1980): Laryngeal angiomyoma (vascular leiomyoma) clinicopathological findings. Laryngoscope 90: 1880-1886

Shilovtseva AS (1969): The complex treatment of patients affected with papillomatosis of the larynx and trachea. Arch Otolaryngol 89: 552-556

Shorp HS (1939): Haemangioma of the trachea in an infant. J Laryngol Otol 63: 413

Silverblatt BL (1958): The use of antibiotic-steroid combinations as nebulizing agents in the treatment of laryngeal conditions: a preliminary report. Laryngoscope 68: 1081-1086

Simon H (1968): Sofortige tödliche Blutung nach Probeexzision aus der aryepiglottischen Falte. Monatsschr Ohrenheilkd 102: 484-486

Simpson GT, McGill T, Healy GB, Strong MS (1979): Benign tumors and lesions of the larynx in children. Surgical excision by CO-2-Laser. Ann Otol Rhinol Laryngol 88: 479-485

Singh J, Black MJ, Fried J (1980): Cartilagenous tumors of the larynx: a review of literature and two case experiences. Laryngoscope 90: 1872-1879

Skabania J, Szlezak L (1978): Case of multiform adenoma of the parotid glands, peripharyngeal space and the larynx. Otolaryngol Pol 32: 647-649

Smith L, Gooding CA (1974): Pulmonary involvement in laryngeal papillomatosis. Pediatr Radiol 2: 161-166

Smoler J, Vivar G, Pinto SL (1966): Multiple neurofibromatosis with laryngeal involvement. Ann Otol Rhinol Laryngol 75: 968-974

Solomon D, Smith RRL, Kashima HK, Leventhal BG (1985): Malignant transformation in non-irradiated recurrent respiratory papillomatosis. Laryngoscope 95: 900-904

SOM LM, PEIMER R (1949): Oncocytic cystadenoma of the larynx. Ann Otol Rhinol Laryngol 58: 234-242

SOM ML, WOLFF L (1952): Lipoma of the hypopharynx producing menaging symptoms. Arch Otolaryngol 56: 524-531

SOM PM, NAGEL BD, FEUERSTEIN SS, STRAUSS L (1979): Benign pleomorphic adenoma of the larynx. A case report. Ann Otol Rhinol Laryngol 88: 112-114

SPAGNOLO DV, PARADINAS FJ (1985): Laryngeal neuroendocrine tumour with features of a paraganglioma, intracytoplasmic lumina and acinar formation. Histopathology 9: 117-131

SPEISER F (1932): Zur krebsigen Entartung der Pachydermia laryngis. Z Hals-Nasen-Ohrenheilk 30: 391-409

SPIESS A (1930): Über ein Gangliom des Kehlkopfes. Laryngol Rhinol Otol 19: 1-20

SPOENDLIN H, KISTLER G (1978): Papova-Virus in human laryngeal papillomas. Arch Otorhinolaryngol 218: 289-292

STATHEROU P (1957): Zur Kenntnis der Komplikationen der Papillomatose des Larynx. Monatsschr Ohrenheilkd 91: 300-305

STEINBERG BM, TOPP WC, SCHNEIDER PS, ABRAMSON AL (1983): Laryngeal papilloma virus infection during clinical remission. N Engl J Med 308: 1261-1264

STEINER W, JAUMANN MP, PESCH H-J (1980): Endoskopische Laserchirurgie im Larynx. Ther Umsch 37: 1103-1109

STEINER W, PESCH H-J (1976): Endoscopic-histological differential diagnosis of rare benign endolaryngeal proliferations. Laryngol Rhinol Otol 55: 111-118

STEINER W (1984): Endoskopische Chirurgie in den oberen Luft- und Speisewegen des Kindes. Laryngol Rhinol Otol 63: 198-202

SUPANCE JS, QUENELLE DJ, CRISSMAN J (1980): Endolaryngeal neurofibromas. Otolaryngol Head Neck Surg 88: 74-78

SVOBODA DA, KIRCHNER FR, PROUD GO (1963): Electron microscopic study of human laryngeal papillomatosis. Cancer Res 23: 1084

SZÖNYI F, BERENYI J (1960): Über das solitäre Kehlkopfneurinom. Zentralbl Allg Pathol 101: 338

TEFFT M (1966): The radiotherapeutic management of subglottic hemangioma in children. Radiology 86: 207-214

TERRACOL J (1965): Les tumeurs salivaires dites mixtes du larynx. Ann Otolaryngol Chir Cervicofac 82: 959-960

THOMAS AB, REES L (1969): Neurilemmoma of the larynx. J Laryngol Otol 83: 189-195

THOMAS JL, BERNARDINO ME (1981): Pheochromocytoma in multiple endocrine adenomatosis. Efficacy of computer tomography. JAMA 245: 1467-1469

THOST A (1929): Die Geschwülste des Kehlkopfes. In: DENKER A, KAHLER O (eds), Handbuch Hals-Nasen-Ohrenheilkunde; vol 5. Springer, Berlin

TOBIN HA, HARRIS HH (1972): Non-chromaffin paraganglioma of the larynx. Arch Otolaryngol 96: 154-157

TOMAS H (1971): Beitrag zum Haemangiom des Larynx beim Säugling. Monatsschr Kinderheilkd 119: 520-523

TOMECKOVA A, ODEHNAL F, CERNY K (1981): Abrikosoff's tumor (granular cell myoblastoma) with a laryngeal localization. Report of 2 cases (czech). Cesk Otolaryngol 30: 296-302

TOSO G (1971): Epithelial papillomas benign or malignant? Interesting findings in laryngeal papilloma. Laryngoscope 81: 1524-1531

TRIANTAFILIDI IG, NASYROV VA (1980): Chemodectomas with an outlet into the parapharyngeal space and larynx (rus). Vestn Otorinolaringol 1980: 83

TSUKERBERG LI, ZAKHAVORV AA (1971): Neurofibroma of the larynx (rus) Vestn Otorinolaringol 33: 107-108

TSYBYRNE GA, BOGDANSKAIA NI (1979): Osteoblastoclastoma of the larynx. A case report (rus). Vopr Onkol 25: 62-64

ULLMANN EV (1923): On the aetiology of laryngeal papilloma. Acta Otolaryngol (Stockh) 5: 317-334

URFER E (1947): Myxolipom des Kehlkopfes. Schweiz Med Wochenschr 77: 366

VETTERS JM, TONER PG (1970): Chemodectoma of larynx. J Pathol 101: 259-265

VLASIUK AN (1979): Giant cavernous hemangioma of the laryngopharynx (rus). Zh Ushn Nos Gorl Bolezn 4: 85-86

VLODYKA J (1962): The cancerogenic effect of x-ray on the larynx. Arch Otolaryngol 76: 372-376

VOSTEEN K-H (1954): Zur Genese des Adenolymphoms der Speicheldrüse. Arch Otolaryngol 166: 156-160

VOSTEEN K-H (1958): Das onkozytäre Adenom des Kehlkopfes. HNO 6: 313

WAGEMANN W (1952): Erstmalige Vorkommen einer Riesenzellgeschwulst im Kehlkopfraum. HNO 3: 93-95

WALKER JS (1947): Neurinoma of the larynx. Ann Otol Rhinol Laryngol 57: 414

WALSH TE, BEAMER PR (1950): Epidermoid carcinoma of larynx occuring in two children with papilloma of larynx. Laryngoscope 60: 1110-1124

WEBBER PA, HUSSAIN SM, RADCLIFF GJ (1986): Cartilaginous neoplasms of the head and neck (A report on four cases). J Laryngol Otol 100: 615-619

WEHMER W (1970): Beitrag zur endolaryngealen Ultraschallanwendung bei der Therapie juveniler Kehlkopfpapillomatosen. HNO 18: 168-170

WEIDAUER H (1972): Ein Beitrag zu den seltenen onkozytären Adenomen des Larynx. Laryngol Rhinol Otol 51: 163-165

WEISMAN RA, KONRAD HR, CANALIS RF (1980): Granular cell myoblastoma involving the recurrent laryngeal nerve. Arch Otolaryngol 106: 294-297

WESSELY E (1938): Cystadenoma laryngis. Monatsschr Ohrenheilkd 72: 682-686

WESSELY E (1939): Epulis laryngis. Monatsschr Ohrenheilkd 73: 751

WETMORE RF, TRONZO RD, LANE RJ, LOWRY LD (1981): Nonfunctional paraganglioma of the larynx: clinical and pathological considerations. Cancer 48: 2717-2723

WHITE A, HALLIWELL M, FAIRMAN HD (1974): Ultrasonic treatment of laryngeal papillomata. J Laryngol Otol 88: 249-260

WHITTAM DE, MORRIS TMO (1970): Neurilemmoma of the larynx. J Laryngol Otol 84: 747-750

WILHELM HJ, DIETZ R, SCHÖNDORF J (1980): Diagnostik und Therapie seltener Tumoren im Larynx-Pharynx-Bereich. Laryngol Rhinol Otol 59: 137-143

WINSTON P, EPSTEIN SS (1958): Papilloma of the larynx: A clinico-pathological study. J Laryngol Otol 72: 452-464

WINTHER LK (1976): Rhabdomyoma of the hypopharynx and larynx. Report of two cases and a review of the literature. J Laryngol Otol 90: 1041-1051

WOLTERS B, EICHHORN T, KLEINSASSER O (1984): Kritische Betrachtungen zur Therapie der juvenilen Kehlkopfpapillome. Laryngol Rhinol Otol 63: 396-400

YAMASE HT, PUTMAN HC (1979): Oncocytic papillary cystadenomatosis of the larynx. A clinicopathologic entity. Cancer 44: 2306-2311

YEE RD, HELPER RS (1973): Congenital hemangiomas of the skin with orbital and subglottic hemangiomas. Am J Ophthalmol 75: 876-879

YOSHIDA T (1983): Benign neoplasms of the larynx. A ten-year review. Auris Nasus Larynx Suppl 10: 61-71
YURICH E, BEEKHUIS GJ (1960): Multiple Neurofibromatosis involving the larynx. Laryngoscope 70: 46-54
ZAGARSKIKH A (1971): Ganglioneurofibroma of the larynx in a child aged one year and one month (rus). Vestn Otorinolaringol 33: 102-103
ZAK FG, LAWSON W (1982): The paraganglionic chemoreceptor system. Physiology, pathology and clinical medicine. Springer, Berlin-Heidelberg-New York
ZAKRZEWSKI A (1965): Subglottic lipoma of the larynx. Case report and literature review. J Laryngol Otol 79: 1039-1048
ZAKRZEWSKI A, PRZYBORA L, SZMEJA Z, SOBIESZCZYK A (1977): Case of malignant transformation of laryngeal neurilemmoma (pol). Otolaryngol Pol 31: 551-555
ZAKRZEWSKI A, SZEMJA Z, GABRYEL P (1963): Subglottic hemangioma of larynx in an infant cured operatively. Acta Otolaryngol (Stockh) 56: 599-602
ZAKZOUK MS (1985): Pleomorphic adenoma of the larynx. J Laryngol Otol 99: 611-616
ZALIN H (1948): Treatment of laryngeal papillomata in childhood. J Laryngol Otol 62: 621-626
ZAPF B, LEHMANN WB, SNYDER G (1981): Hamartoma of the larynx: an unusual cause for stridor in an infant. Otolaryngol Head Neck Surg 89: 797-799
ZEHNDER PR, LYONS GD (1975): Carcinoma and juvenile papillomatosis. Ann Otol Rhinol Laryngol 84: 614-618
ZEITLHOFER J (1955): Ungewöhnlicher Tumor im Larynx (Chromophobes Paragangliom). Monatsschr Ohrenheilkd 69: 133-136
ZÖLLNER F (1963): Die Operabilität kavernöser Hämangiome der Zunge und des Kehlkopfeingangs. Laryngol Rhinol Otol 42: 1-7

References

4 General Conditions and Risk Factors of Carcino genesis, Precancerous Lesions

ALTMAN F, GINSBERG I, STOUT AP (1952): Intraepithelial carcinoma (cancer in situ) of the larynx. Arch Otolaryngol 56: 121-133

ANDREASSON L, BJÖRLIN G, KORSGAARD R, MATTIASSON I, TRELL E, TRELL L (1982): Leucoplakia of the oral cavity and the arylhydrocarbon-hydrolase inducibility. Postgrad Med J 58: 138-141

AUERBACH O, HAMMOND EC, GARFINKEL L (1970): Histologic changes in the larynx in relation to smoking habits. Cancer 25: 92-104

AXELL T, HOLMSTRUPP P, KRAMER IRH, PINDBORG JJ, SHEAR M (1984): International seminar on oral leukoplakia and associated lesions related to tobacco habits. Commun Dent Oral Epidemiol 12: 145-154

BANOCZY J (1977): Follow-up studies in oral leukoplakia. J Maxillofac Surg 5: 69-75

BARNES L, GNEPP DR (1985): Diseases of the larynx, hypopharynx, and esophagus. In: Barnes L (ed), Surgical Pathology of the Head and Neck; vol 1, pp 141-226. Marcel Dekker Inc., New York - Basel

BAUER WC (1976): Concomitant carcinoma in situ and invasive carcinoma of the larynx. In: ALBERTI PW, BRYCE DP (eds), Centennial Conference on Laryngeal Cancer, pp 127-136. Appleton-Century-Crofts, New York

BJELKENKRANTZ K, OLOFSSON J, STAL O, GRÖNTOFT O (1983): Juvenile laryngeal papilloma: histologic and photometric evaluation of atypia. Laryngoscope 83: 468-474

BLACK RJ, GLUCKMAN JL, SHUMRICK DA (1983): Multiple primary tumours of the upper aerodigestive tract. Clin Otolaryngol 8: 277-281

BOHNDORF W, HÖCKER G (1976): Würzburger Ergebnisse beim Larynxkarzinom. Strahlentherapie 151: 132-143

BOSSART A (1977): Precancerous lesions of the larynx. Round table. Acta Otolaryngol Suppl (Stockh) 344: 1-32

BRICHACEK B, HIRSCH I, SIBL O, VILIKUSOVA E, CONKA V (1983): Association of some supraglottic laryngeal carcinomas with EB-virus. Int J Cancer 32: 193-197

BRODERS AC (1932): Practical points on the microscopic grading of carcinoma. N Y State J Med 32: 667-671

BROWN M (1978): Second primaries in cases of cancer of the larynx. J Laryngol Otol 92: 991-996

BRUGERE J, GUENEL P, LECLERC A, RODRIGUEZ J (1986): Differential effects of tobacco and alcohol in cancer of the larynx, pharynx and mouth. Cancer 57: 391-395

BUNDESAMT FÜR STATISTIK (1984): Geografische Verteilung der Krebssterblichkeit in der Schweiz 1979/1981. Beitr schweiz Statistik, Heft 119

BURCH JD, HOWE GR, MILLER AB, SEMENCIW R (1981): Tobacco, alcohol, asbestos and nickel in the etiology of cancer of the larynx: a case-control study. JNCI 67: 1219-1224

BURGHARDT E (1972): Histologische Frühdiagnose des Zervixkrebses. Thieme, Stuttgart

BURKHARDT A (1980): Der Mundhöhlenkrebs und seine Vorstadien. Ultrastrukturelle und immunpathologische Aspekte. Fischer, Stuttgart-New York

BURKHARDT A (1985): Prämaligne Veränderungen der Mundschleimhaut. Vorschläge einer internationalen Expertenkommission zur Nomenklatur. Pathologe 6: 126-132

BURKHARDT A, MAERKER R (1981): Vor- und Frühstadien des Mundhöhlenkarzinoms. Ein Farbatlas zur Diagnostik und Klassifizierung oraler Leukoplakien, Präkanzerosen und Karzinome. Carl Hauser Verlag, München

CAHAN WG (1955): Lung cancer associated with primary in other sites. Am J Surg 89: 494-514

CRISSMAN JD (1979): Laryngeal keratosis and subsequent carcinoma. Head Neck Surg 1: 386-391

CRISSMAN JD (1982): Laryngeal keratosis preceding laryngeal carcinoma. A report of fours cases. Arch Otolaryngol 108: 445-448

CRISSMAN JD, FU YS (1986): Intraepithelial neoplasia of the larnyx. A clinicopathologic study of six cases with DNA analysis. Arch Otolaryngol 112: 522-528

DEITMER T (1983): Pathogenesis of laryngeal cancer in women. Laryngol Rhinol Otol 62: 68-73

DEVESA S, SILVERMAN D (1978): Trends in cancer incidence and mortality in the United States: 1935-1974. J Natl Cancer Inst 60: 393-400

DUCHON J, CZIGNER J, PUPP L (1972): Pachydermia laryngis and smoking. Laryngol Rhinol Otol 51: 253-257

FECHNER RE (1974): Laryngeal keratosis and atypia. Can J Otolaryngol 3: 516-521

FERLITO A (1976): Histological Classification of Larynx and Hypopharynx Carcinoma and their Clinical Implications. Pathologic Aspects of 2052 Malignant Neoplasms Diagnosed at the ORL Department of Padua University from 1966 to 1976. Acta Otolaryngol (Stockh) Suppl 342: 1-88

FERLITO A (1980): Double primary synchronous and metachronous cancer of the larynx and hypopharynx with dissimilar histology. Arch Otorhinolaryngol 229: 107-119

FERLITO A, POLIDARO F, ROSSI M (1981): Pathological basis and clinical aspects of treatment policy in carcinoma-in-situ of the larynx. J Laryngol Otol 95: 141-154

FISHER HR (1976): The delineation of carcinoma in situ of the larynx. In: ALBERTI PW, BRYCE DP (eds), Centennial Conference on Laryngeal Cancer; pp 116-119. Appleton-Century-Crofts, New York

FISHER HR, MILLER AH (1958): Cancer in situ of the larynx: a ten year study of its histopathological classification prognosis and treatment. Ann Otol Rhinol Laryngol 67: 695-702

FLANDERS WD, ROTHMAN KJ (1982): Occupational risk for laryngeal cancer. Am J Public Health 72: 369-372

FLANDERS WD, CANN CI, ROTHMAN KJ, FRIEDMP (1984): Work-related risk factors of laryngeal cancer. Am J Epidermiol 119: 23-32

Franz B, Neumann OG (1978): Leukoplakien des Kehlkopfes. Histologisch-zytologische Klassifizierung. Laryngol Rhinol Otol 57: 428-433

Friedmann I (1976): Precancerous lesions of the larynx. In: Alberti PW, Bryce DP (eds), Centennial Conference on Laryngeal Cancer; pp 122-126. Appleton-Century-Crofts, New York

Furfaro M, Baricalla R (1971): Precancerous changes of the larynx. Pathologica 63: 151-159

Gabriel CE, Jones DG (1960): The importance of chronic laryngitis. J Laryngol Otol 74: 349-357

Gabriel CE, Jones DG (1976): Carcinoma in situ of the larynx - an unsatisfactory diagnosis. Clin Otolaryngol 1: 271-276

Giarelli L, Silvestri F, Antonutto G, Stanta G (1977): Observation of the pathologist on precancerous lesions of the larynx. Integrated with histological data and quantitative analysis of nuclear DNA-content. Acta Otolaryngol Suppl (Stockh) 344: 7-18

Gillis TM, Incze J, Strong MS, Vaughan CW, Simpson GT (1983): Natural history and management of keratosis, atypia, carcinoma-in-situ and microinvasive cancer of the larynx. Am J Surg 146: 512-516

Glanz HK, Kleinsasser O (1976): Chronische Laryngitis und Carcinom. Arch Otorhinolaryngol 212: 57-75

Glanz HK, Kleinsasser O (1978): Verrucous acanthosis (verrucous carcinoma) of the larynx. Laryngol Rhinol Otol 57: 835-843

Goldsher M, Bartal A, Eliachar J, Robinson E (1977): Laryngeal carcinoma associated with multiple additional primary tumors. Arch Otolaryngol 103: 550-552

Goodman ML (1984): Keratosis (leukoplakia) of the larynx. Otolaryngol Clin North Am 17: 179-183

Graham S, Metlin C, Marshall J, Priore R, Rzepka Th, Shedd D (1981): Dietary factors in the epidemiology of cancer of the larynx. Am J Epidemiol 123: 675-680

Greenspan D, Silverman S, Greenspan JS (1984): Oral leukoplakia in ARC (Aids related complex). Abstracts of the second meeting of the international meeting of the international association of oral pathologists. J Oral Pathol 14: 74

Grundmann E (1973): Die Bedeutung der präkanzerösen Zell- und Gewebsveränderungen in Experiment und Klinik. Arch Otorhinolaryngol 205: 55-67

Haidoutova R, Melamed M, Dimitrova S, Kyossovska R (1985): Investigations of serum testosterone levels in patients with laryngeal cancers. Arch Otorhinolaryngol 241: 213-217

Hellquist H, Olofsson J, Gröntoft O (1981): Carcinoma in situ and severe dysplasia of the vocal cords; a clinicopathological and photometric investigation. Acta Otolaryngol (Stockh) 92: 543-555

Hellquist H, Lundgren J, Olofsson J (1982): Hyperplasia, keratosis, dysplasia and carcinoma in situ of the vocal cords - a follow-up study. Clin Otolaryngol 7: 11-27

Henry RC (1979): The transformation of laryngeal leukoplakia to cancer. J Laryngol Otol 93: 447-459

Herity B, Moriarty M, Daly L, Dunn J, Bourke GJ (1982): The role of tobacco and alcohol in the aetiology of lung and larynx cancer. Br J Cancer 46: 961-964

Hyams VJ (1976): Discussion to Bauer WC (1976): Concomitant carcinoma in situ and invasive carcinoma of the larynx. In: Alberti PW, Bryce DP (eds), Centennial Conference on Laryngeal Cancer, pp 134-135. Appleton-Century-Crofts, New York

Hussl B, Loewit K, Richter E, Schwarz S (1978): First clinical experiences with hormone-therapy of pachydermia laryngis. Arch Otorhinolaryngol 221: 221-225

Johnson JT, Barnes EL, Justice W (1981): Adult onset laryngeal papillomatosis. Otolaryngol Head Neck Surg 89: 867-873

Kahn T, Schwarz E, zur Hausen H (1986): Molecular cloning and characterization of the DNA of a new human papillomavirus (HPV 30) from a laryngeal carcinoma. Int J Cancer 37: 61-65

Kambic V (1977): Macro-microscopical findings and prognosis of hyperplastic aberrations of the laryngeal mucous membrane. Acta Otolaryngol (Suppl)(Stockh) 344: 19-21

Kambic V (1978): Difficulties in manegement of vocal cord precancerous lesions. J Laryngol Otol 92: 305-315

Kambic V, Lenart J (1971): Our classification of hyperplasia of laryngeal epithelium. J Fr Otorhinolaryngol 20: 1145-1150

Kambic V, Radsel Z, Prezelj J Zargi M (1984): The role of testosterone in laryngeal carcinogenesis. Am J Otolaryngol 5: 344-349

Kleinsasser O (1958): Über die gut- und bösartigen Formen der Kehlkopfpapillome und deren histologisches und klinisches Bild. Arch Otorhinolaryngol 171: 44-69

Kleinsasser O (1959): Über verschiedene Formen der Plattenepithelhyperplasien im Kehlkopf und ihre Beziehungen zum Carcinom. Arch Otorhinolaryngol 174: 290-313

Kleinsasser O (1963a): Eine Analyse der Vorgeschichte von Kehlkopfkrebskranken. Laryngol Rhinol Otol 42: 14-31

Kleinsasser O (1963b): Die Klassifikation und Differentialdiagnose der Epithelhyperplasien der Kehlkopfschleimhaut auf Grund histomorphologischer Merkmale. Laryngol Rhinol Otol 42: 339-362

Kleinsasser O (1963c): Über den Krankheitsverlauf bei Epithelhyperplasien der Kehlkopfschleimhaut und die Entstehung von Karzinomen. IV. Mitteilung. Laryngol Rhinol Otol 42: 541-558

Kleinsasser O (1983): Bösartige Geschwülste des Kehlkopfes und des Hypopharynx. In: Berendes J, Link R, Zöllner F (eds), Hals-Nasen-Ohrenheilkunde in Praxis und Klinik; vol 4.2, pp. 12.1-12.337 Kehlkopf II. Thieme, Stuttgart - New York

Kleinsasser O, Heck KH (1959): Über das sogenannte Carcinoma in situ des Kehlkopfes. Arch Otorhinolaryngol 174: 210-242

Koss LG (1978): Dysplasia. A real concept or a misnomer? Obstet Gynecol 51: 374-379

Kramer IRH (1973): Carcinoma in situ of the oral mucosa. Int Dent J 23: 94-99

Krespi YP, Wurster CF, Ossoff RM, Sisson GA (1983): Four separate and simultaneous pharyngolaryngeal squamous cell carcinomas. Otolaryngol Head Neck Surg 91: 704-708

Krompecher E (1924): Basalzellen,Metaplasie und Regeneration. Beitr path Anat 72: 163-183

Lamprecht J, Lamprecht A, Morgenstern C (1983): Mehrfachtumoren im oberen Aerodigestivtrakt - eine retrospektive Studie. Laryngol Rhinol Otol 62: 499-501

Laniado K, Thann W, Metzner A (1981): Untersuchungen zur Entstehung eines Karzinoms aus einer Epitheldysplasie der Kehlkopfschleimhaut. Laryngol Rhinol Otol 60: 571-572

Liapis EG, Papacharalampous NX (1969): Die Hyperplasie des Kehlkopfschleimhautepithels und ihre präkanzeröse Bedeutung. Laryngol Rhinol Otol 48: 902-909

Link R, Pascher W (1969): Klinische Gesichtspunkte zum Stimmbandkarzinom. In: Becher J, Gauwerky F (eds), Tumoren der Mundhöhle, des Rachens und des Kehlkopfes. Urban & Schwarzenberg, München-Berlin-Wien

LIPKIN A, MILLER RH, WOODSON GE (1985): Squamous cell carcinoma of the oral cavity, pharynx, and larynx in young adults. Laryngoscope 95: 790-793

LOEWIT K, SCHWARZ S, HUSSL B, RICHTER E (1979): Urinary androgen and estrogen excretion in men with pachydermia laryngis and cancer of the larynx. Endokrinologie 73: 151-156

MARAN AGD, MACKENZIE IJ, STANLEY RE (1984): Carcinoma in situ of the larynx. Head Neck Surg 7: 28-31

MARTIN G, GLANZ H, KLEINSASSER O (1979): Multiple maligne Tumoren bei Patienten mit Larynxkarzinomen. Laryng Rhinol Otol 58: 756-763

McCoy GD, HECHT STS, WYNDER EL (1980): The roles of tobacco, alcohol, and diet in the etiology of upper alimentary and respiratory tract cancers. Prev Med 9: 622-629

MCMICHAEL AJ (1978): Increases in laryngeal cancer in Britain and Australia in relation to alcohol and tobacco consumption trends. Lancet 1: 1244-1247

MCNELIS FL (1974): Carcinoma in situ of the larynx. RI Med J 57: 22-23

MICHAELS L (1982): Precancerous changes in the larynx. Clin Otolaryngol 7: 1-2

MICHAELS L (1984): Pathology of the larynx. Springer, Berlin-Heidelberg-New York-Tokyo

MILLER AH (1976): Premalignant laryngeal lesions, carcinoma in situ, superficial carcinoma-definiton and management. In: ALBERTI PW, BRYCE DP (eds), Centennial Conference on Laryngeal Cancer, pp 167-169. Appleton-Century-Crofts, New York

MINCER HH, COLEMAN AS, HOPKINS P (1972): Observations on the clinical characteristics of oral lesions showing histologic epithelial dysplasia. Oral Surg Oral Med Oral Pathol 33: 389-399

MIYAHARA H, YOSHINO K, UMATANI K, SATO T (1985): Multiple primary tumours in laryngeal cancer. J Laryngol Otol 99: 999-1004

MÜLLER KM, KROHN BR (1980): Smoking habits and their relationship to precancerous lesions of the larynx. J Cancer Res Clin Oncol 96: 211-217

MÜNZEL M, MEISTER P (1976): Subepitheliale Veränderungen bei der einfachen leukoplakischen Hyperplasie der Kehlkopfschleimhaut. Laryngol Rhinol Otol 55: 96-99

NEUMANN OG, FRANZ B (1977): Leukoplakien des Kehlkopfes. (I. klinische und histologische Klassifizierung). Laryngol Rhinol Otol 56: 828-831

NEUMANN OG, KOPP L (1980): Classification of laryngeal papillomas, larynxpapillomas and papillomatosis. Laryngol Rhinol Otol 59: 57-65

NIELSEN KO, BAK-PEDERSEN K (1984a): Mucous-producing elements in the laryngeal mucosa in smokers with cancer of the larynx. Cancer 54: 61-64

NIELSEN KO, BAK-PEDERSEN K (1984b): Goblet cells in the laryngeal mucosa in cancer of the larynx. Laryngoscope 94: 1230-1234

OLDE KALTER P, LUBSEN H, DELEMARRE JFM, ALONS CL, VELDHUIZEN RW, MEYER CJLM, SNOW GB (1985): Quantitative morphometry of squamous cell hyperplasia of the larynx. J Clin Pathol 38: 489-495

OLDE KALTER P, DELEMARRE JFM, ALONS CL, MEYER CJLM, SNOW GB (1986): The clinical relevance of classification of squamous cell hyperplasia of the larynx by morphometry. Acta Otolaryngol (Stockh) 101: 331-340

OLOFSSON H, VAN NOSTRAND AW (1973): Growth and spread of laryngeal carcinoma with reflections on the effect of preoperative irradiation. Acta Otolaryngol (Stockh) Suppl 308: 1-84

OLSEN J, SABROE S, LAJER M (1984): Welding and cancer of the larynx: a case-control study. Eur J Cancer Clin Oncol 20: 639-643

OLSEN J, SABROE S (1984): Occupational causes of laryngeal cancer. J Epidemiol Community Health 38: 117-121

PESCH HJ, STEINER W (1979): Die Bedeutung der Dysplasien an der Kehlkopfschleimhaut. Verh Dtsch Ges Pathol 63: 105-111

PESCH HJ, STEINER W, MAAK G (1976): Simultanes Wachstum von Carcinoma und Präcancerose im Kehlkopf - eine stratigraphische histomorphologische Analyse. Arch Otorhinolaryngol 213: 419-420

PESCH HJ, STEINER W, MAAK G (1978): Karzinom und Präkanzerose im Kehlkopf. Stratigraphisch-histomorphologische Untersuchungen zum simultanen Wachstum. Verh Dtsch Ges Pathol 62: 335

PETERSEN (1901): Beiträge zur Lehre vom Karzinom. Bruns' Beitr 32: 543-654

PINDBORG JJ (1980): Oral cancer and precancer. Bristol, John Wright

PINDBORG JJ, DAFTARY DK, MEHTA FS (1977): A follow-up study of sixty-one oral dysplastic precancerous lesions in Indian villagers. Oral Surg Oral Med Oral Pathol 43: 383-390

QUANTE M, STRAUSS P, KORTE W, EDINGER D (1976): Observations on the course of leukoplakia in the larynx. Laryngol Rhinol Otol 55: 99-102

QUICK CA, FOUCAR E, DEHNER, LP (1979): Frequency and significance of epithelial atypsia in laryngeal papillomatosis. Laryngoscope 89: 550-560

RABBETT WF (1962): Multiple foci of carcinoma of the larynx. Laryngoscope 72: 1760-1776

RAMADAN MF, MORTON RP, STELLE PM, PHAROAH POD (1982): Epidemiology of laryngeal cancer. Clin Otolaryngol 7: 417-428

ROBBETT WF (1972): Premalignant changes in the vocal cord. Laryngoscope 82: 1007-1012

ROTHMAN KJ, CANN ChJ, FLANDERS D, FRIED MP (1980): Epidemiology of laryngeal cancer. Epidemiol Rev 2: 195-209

RYWLIN AM (1984): Terminology of premalignant lesions in light of the multistep theory of carcinogenesis. Hum Pathol 15: 806-807

SAKULA A (1974): Multiple primary carcinomas of respiratory tract: primary carcinoma of larynx followed by primary carcinomas involving two lungs consecutively. Br J Dis Chest 68: 128-136

SCHOTTENFELD D, GAUTT RC, WYNDER EL (1974): The role of alcohol and tobacco in multiple primary cancers of the upper digestive system, larynx and lung: a prospective study. Prev Med 3: 277-293

SCHWAB W, ZUM WINKEL J (1975): Möglichkeiten der Strahlentherapie in der Hals-Nasen-Ohrenheilkunde. Thieme, Stuttgart

SCOTT GBD (1976): A quantitative study of microscopical changes in the epithelium and subepithelial tissue of the laryngeal folds, sinus and saccule. Clin Otolaryngol 1: 257-264

SEIFERT LB, GLANZ HK (1971): Carcinoma in situ laryngis. Klinik und Pathologie. Laryngol Rhinol Otol 50: 827-851

SHANMUGARATNAM K, SOBIN LH (1978): Histological typing of upper respiratory tract tumors. International histological classification of tumors, No. 19. WHO, Geneva

SHAW HJ (1977): Precancerous lesions of the larynx. Acta Otolaryngol (Suppl)(Stockh) 344,22-23

SHEAR M, PINDBORG JJ (1980): Verrucous hyperplasia of the oral mucosa. Cancer 46: 1855-1862

SILVERMAN S, GORSKY M, LOZADA F (1984): Oral leukoplakia and malignant transformation. A follow-up study of 257 patients. Cancer 53: 563-

SLAUGHTER DP, SOUTHWICK HW, SMEJKAL W (1953): "Field cancerization" in oral stratified squamous epithelium. Cancer 5: 963-968

SOSKOLONE CL, ZEIGHAMI EA, HANIS NM, KUPPER LL, HERRMANN N, AMSEL J, MAUSNER JS, STELLMANN JM (1984): Laryngeal cancer and occupational exposure to sulfuric acid. Am J Epidemiol 120: 358-369

STATISTISCHES BUNDESAMT (1984): Statistisches Jahrbuch 1984 für die Bundesrepublik Deutschland. Kohlhammer 1984

STEINER W (1984): Endoskopische Chirurgie in den oberen Luft- und Speisewegen des Kindes. Laryngol Rhinol Otol 63: 198-202

STELL PM (1972): Smoking and laryngeal cancer. Lancet 1: 617-618

STELL PM, GREGORY I, WATT J (1980): Morphology of the human larynx. II: The subglottis. Clin Otolaryngol 5: 389-395

STOUT AP (1953): Intramucosal epithelioma of the larynx. AJR 69: 1-13

SUGAR J (1970): The histology of precancerous changes of the larynx. Arch Otorhinolaryngol 197: 142-153

SYRJÄNEN KJ, SYRJÄNEN SM (1981): Histological evidence for the presence of condylomatous epithelial lesions in association with laryngeal squamous cell carcinoma. ORL 43: 181-194

SYRJÄNEN K, SYRJÄNEN S, PYRHÖNEN S (1982): Human papilloma virus (HPV) antigens in lesions of laryngeal squamous cell carcinomas. ORL 44: 323-334

SZMEJA Z, KONCZEWSKA H (1986): Der Magnesiumgehalt bei Larynxpräkanzerosen und Larynxkarzinomen. HNO 34: 85-87

THOMA GW (1964): The incidence and significance of multiple primary malignant tumors. Am J Med Sci 247: 427-430

TRELL E, BJORLING G, ANDREASSON L, KORSGAARD R, MATTIASSON I (1981): Carcinoma of the oral cavity in relation to arylhydrocarbon-hydroxylase inducibility, smoking and dental status. Int J Oral Surg 10: 93-99

TRENTINI GP, GAETANI CF, CRISTIANI G (1973): Precancerous lesions of the larynx. Arch De Vecchi Anat Patol 59: 55-90

WAGENFELD DJ, HARWOOD AR, BRYCE DP, VAN NOSTRAND AWP, DEBOER G (1980): Second primary respiratory tract malignancies in glottic carcinoma. Cancer 46: 1883-1886

WALLACE AF (1957): Multiple malignant primary neoplasms. Br J Surg 45: 165-169

WENIG BL, ABRAMSON AL (1983): Prostatic and laryngeal malignancies: common or uncommon multiple occurence? Laryngoscope 93: 357-361

WHO COLLABORATING CENTER FOR ORAL PRECANCEROUS LESIONS (1978): Definition of leukoplakia and related lesions: an aid to studies on oral precancer. Oral Surg Oral Med Oral Pathol 46: 518-539

WYNDER EL, COVEY LS, MABUCHI K, MOSHINSKI M (1976): Enviromental factors in cancer of the larynx. Cancer 38: 1591-1601

ZUPPINGER A (1938): Betrachtungen zu sekundären Oesophagustumoren. Z Krebsforsch 47: 413-420

ZUR HAUSEN H (1978): Human papillomaviruses and their possible role in squamous cell carcinomas. Curr Top Microbiol Immunol 78: 1-30

References

5 Squamous Cell Carcinomas

AJC - American Joint Committee for Cancer Staging and End Results Reporting (1972): Clinical Staging System for Cancer of the Larynx. Chicago

AJC - American Joint Committee for Cancer Staging and End Results Reporting (1977): Manual of Staging of Cancer. Lippincott, Philadelphia

AJCC - American Joint Committee on Cancer (1983): Manual for staging of cancer. Lippincott, Philadelphia

ALBERTI PW, BRYCE DP (1976): Centennial Conference on Laryngeal Cancer. Appleton-Century-Crofts, New York

VON ALBERTINI A, ROULET FC (1974): Histologische Geschwulstdiagnostik. 2nd edn. Thieme, Stuttgart

BECK C, MANN W (1980): The inner laryngeal lymphatics. A lymphangioscopical and electron miroscopical study. Acta Otolaryngol (Stockh) 89: 265-270

BOCCA E (1968): Supraglottis surgery of the larynx. Ann Otol Rhinol Laryngol 77: 1005-1026

BOCCA E (1975): Limitations of supraglottic laryngectomy and conservative neck dissection. Can J Otolaryngol 4: 403-419

BOCCA E (1975): Supraglottic cancer. Laryngoscope 85: 1318-1326

BOHNDORF W, HÖCKER G (1976): Würzburger Ergebnisse beim Larynxkarzinom. Strahlentherapie 151: 132-143

BRIDGER GP (1974): Mucous gland involvement in cancer at the anterior commissure. Can J Otolaryngol 3: 507-511

BRIDGER GP, NASSAR VH (1972): Cancer spread in the larynx. Arch Otolaryngol 95: 497-505

BRODERS AC (1920): Squamous-cell epithelioma of the lip. JAMA 74: 656-664

BRODERS AC (1921): Squamous-cell epithelioma of skin: A study of 256 cases. Ann Surg 73: 141-160

BRODERS AC (1922): Epithelioma of the genitourinary organs. Ann Surg 75: 574-604

BRODERS AC (1925): Cancer's selfcontrol. Med J Rec 121: 133-135

BRODERS AC (1932a): Practical points on the microscopic grading of carcinoma. N Y State J Med 32: 667-671

BRODERS AC (1932b): Carcinomas in situ contrasts with benign penetrating epithelium. JAMA 99: 1670-1674

BRODERS AC (1940): Grading of cancer. In: PACK GT, LIVINGSTON EM (eds), Treatment of cancer and allied diseases; 1st edn. Hoeber, New York

BROYLES EN (1943): The anterior commissure tendon. Ann Otol Rhinol Laryngol 52: 342-345

BRYCE DP (1972): Convential pharyngolaryngectomy in the surgical management of hypopharyngeal cancer. Can J Otolaryngol 1: 231-244

BURKHARDT A (1980): Der Mundhöhlenkrebs und seine Vorstadien. Ultrastrukturelle und immunpathologische Aspekte. Fischer, Stuttgart-New York

CANN CI, FRIED P (1984): Determinants and prognosis of laryngeal cancer. Otolaryngol Clin North Am 17: 139-150

CHUNG CK, STRYKER JA, ABT AB, CUNNINGHAM DE, STRAUSS M, CONNOR GH (1980): Histologic grading in the clinical evaluation of laryngeal carcinoma. Arch Otolaryngol 106: 623-624

COATES HL, DESANTO LW, DEVINE KD, ELVEBACK LR (1976): Carcinoma of the supraglottic larynx. A review of 221 cases. Arch Otolaryngol 102: 686-689

CINBERG JZ, CHANG TH, BASES R, MOLNAR J (1980): The percentage of cells in DNA synthesis in epidermoid carcinomas of the head and neck: a preliminary report. Laryngoscope 90: 920-923

DENOIX PF (1944): Bull Inst Nat Hyg (Paris) 1: 1-69; 5: 52-82

EDMUNDSON WF (1948): Microscopic grading of cancer and its practical implication. Arch Derm Syphil 57: 141-160

FLEISCHER I (1977): Morphologische Untersuchungen an subglottischen Kehlkopfkarzinomen. Inauguraldissertation, Marburg

GANZER U, MEYER-BREITING E, EBBERS J, VOSTEEN K-H (1982): Der Einfluß von Tumorgröße, Lymphknotenbefall und Behandlungsart auf die Prognose des Hypopharynxkarzinoms. Laryngol Rhinol Otol 61: 622-628

GANZER U, SENDROWSKI P, VOSTEEN K-H, MEYER-BREITING P (1981): Die kombinierte radiochirurgische Behandlung des fortgeschrittenen Kehlkopfkarzinoms (T3-4, NO-3). Ein retrospektiver Vergleich zwischen Sandwich-Technik und postoperativer Bestrahlung. Laryngol Rhinol Otol 60: 63-70

GLANZ HK (1981): Die prognostische Bedeutung des histologischen gradings von Stimmlippenkarzinomen. Arch Otorhinolaryngol 231: 745-746

GLANZ HK (1984): Carcinoma of the larynx; growth, p-classification and grading of squamous cell carcinoma of the vocal cords. Adv Otorhinolaryngol 32: 1-123

GLANZ HK, EICHHORN Th (1985): Die Bedeutung des histologischen "gradings" von Stimmlippenkarzinomen. HNO 33:103-111

GRAEM N, HELWEG-LARSEN K, KEIDING N (1980): Precision of histological grading of malignancy. Acta Pathol Microbiol Immunol Scand (A) 88: 307-317

GUDZIOL H, BELEITES E (1983): Über die Häufigkeit regionärer Metastasen beim supraglottischen Karzinom. Laryngol Rhinol Otol 62: 35-37

GÜNNEL F, BAERTHOLD W (1967): Zur Frage der Teilresektion bei Kehlkopfkrebsen. Arch Otorhinolaryngol 189: 195-209

HAMPERL H (1967): Early invasive growth as seen in uterine cancer and the role of the basal membrane. In: DENOIX P (edr), Mechanisms of invasion in cancer. UICC Monography, vol 6. Springer, Berlin-Heidelberg-New York

HANSEMANN D (1890): Über asymmetrische Zellteilung in Epithelkrebsen und deren biologische Bedeutung. Virchows Arch(A) 119: 299-326

HARRISON DFN (1972): Thyroid gland in the management of laryngopharyngeal cancer. Arch Otolaryngol 7: 301-302

HARRISON DFN (1979): Intrinsic weakness of the TNM system for classification of laryngeal cancer. ORL 41:241-251

HAST MH (1974): Applied embryology of the larynx. Can J Otolaryngol 3: 412-415

HELWEG-LARSEN K, GRAEM N, MEISTRUP-LARSEN K-I, MEISTRUP-LARSENK U (1978): Clinical relevance of histological grading of cancer of the larynx. Acta Pathol Microbiol Immunol Scand (A) 86: 499-504

HERMANEK P, SOBIN LH (1987): TNM classification of malignant tumours. 4th fully revised edition. Springer, Berlin - Heidelberg - New York - Paris - Tokyo

HOFFMANN I (1968): Morphologische Untersuchungen an 60 Kehlkopfeingangskarzinomen. Inauguraldissertation, Köln

HOLM LE, JAKOBSSON P, KILLANDER D, SILFVERSWÄRD C, WERSÄLL J (1980): DNA and its synthesis in indivdual tumor cells from human upper respiratory tract squamous cell carcinomas. Laryngoscope 90: 1209-1212

HOMMERICH KW, SAUER H, WEEDE W (1971): Zur Wachstumstendenz von Larynxtumoren. Arch Otorhinolaryngol 199: 748-751

JAKOBSSON PA, ENEROTH CM, KILLANDER D et al (1973): Histological classification and grading of malignancy in cancer of the larynx. Acta Radiol Oncol 12: 1-8

JOERGENSEN K, SELL A (1971): Carcinoma of the larynx II. Treatment by 60-Co supervoltage irradiation. Acta Radiol (Oncol) 10: 161-173

KASHIMA HK (1976): The characteristics of laryngeal cancer correlating with cervical lymph node metastasis. In: ALBERTI PW, BRYCE DP (eds), Centennial Conference on Laryngeal Cancer, pp 855-864. Appleton-Century-Crofts, New York

KIRCHNER JA (1969): One hundred laryngeal cancers studied by serial section. Ann Otol Rhinol Laryngol 78: 689-709

KIRCHNER JA (1970): Cancer at the anterior commissure of the larynx. Arch Otolaryngol 91: 524-525

KIRCHNER JA (1975a): Pyriforms sinus cancer: A clinical and laboratory study. Ann Otol Rhinol Laryngol 84: 793-804

KIRCHNER JA (1975b): Staging as seen in serial sections. Laryngoscope 85: 1816-1821

KIRCHNER JA (1977): Two hundred laryngeal cancers. Patterns of growth and spread as seen in serial section. Laryngoscope 87: 474-482

KIRCHNER JA, FISCHER JJ (1975): Anterior commissure cancer - A clinical and laboratory study of 39 cases. Can J Otolaryngol 4: 637-643

KIRCHNER JA, OWEN JR (1977): Five hundred cancers of the larynx and pyriform sinus. Results of treatment by radiation and surgery. Laryngoscope 87: 1288-1303

KIRCHNER JA, SOM ML (1971): Clinical and histological observations on supraglottic cancer. Ann Otol Rhinol Laryngol 80: 638-645

KIRCHNER JA, CORNOG JL, HOMES RE (1974): Transglottic cancer. Arch Otolaryngol 99: 247-251

KLEINSASSER O (1967): Wachstumsformen der Kehlkopfeingangscarcinome und Indikation zur Teilresektion. Wiss Z Karl-Marx-Univ (Lpz) 16: 723-725

KUS J, MIODONSKI A, OLSZEWSKI E, TYRANKIESWICZ R (1981): Morphology of arteries, veins, and capillaries in cancer of the larynx. J Cancer Res Clin Oncol 100: 271-283

LAM KH (1983): Three preepiglottic and paraglottic spaces in relation to spread of carcinoma of the larynx. Am J Otolaryngol 4:81-91

LAM KH (1983): Extralaryngeal spread of cancer of the larynx: a study with whole-organ sections. Head Neck Surg 5: 410-424

LÖBE L-P, QUADE R (1982): Histopathologisches Grading von Karzinomen des HNO-Gebietes. Laryngol Rhinol Otol 61: 171-173

LOTT S, EL-MAHDI AM, HAZRA T (1972): Supervoltage radiotherapy for carcinoma of the larynx. The Johns Hopkins Hospital results 1961-1967. Johns Hopkins Med J 130: 244-253

LUND C, SOGAARD H, JORGENSEN K, HJELM-HANSEN M (1975): Epidermoid carcinoma of the larynx. Radiol Ther Physics Biol 15: 293

MARTENSSON B, FLUUR E, JAKOBSSON F (1967): Aspects on treatment of cancer of the larynx. Ann Otol Rhinol Laryngol 76: 313-329

MCCOMB WS, FLETCHER GH, GALAGER HS, HEALY JE, LEHMANN OH (1967): Larynx. In: MCCOMB WS, FLETCHER GH (eds), Cancer of the head and neck. Baltimore

MCGAVRAN MH, BAUER WC, OGURA JH (1961): The incidence of cervical lymph node metastases from epidermoid carcinoma of the larynx and their relationship to certain characteristics of the primary tumor. Cancer 14: 55-66

MENDONCA DR, BRYCE DP (1973): Transglottic cancer of the larynx. Can J Otolaryngol 2: 271-276

MEYER-BREITING E (1981a): Zur Histopathologie bestrahlter und nicht bestrahlter Kehlkopfkarzinome. Habilitationsschrift, Frankfurt

MEYER-BREITING E (1981b): Histologisches Verhalten und Prognose fortgeschrittener Plattenepithelkarzinome. Arch Otorhinolaryngol 231: 746-750

MEYER-BREITING E, VON ILBERG Ch (1979): Spread and mode of metastasis of supraglottic laryngeal carcinoma. ORL 41: 288-300

MEYER-BREITING E, POPESCU G (1986): Zur Definition der Glottischen Region. Arch Otorhinolaryngol Suppl 1986/II: 150-152

MEYER-BREITING E, SCHNEIDER B (1981): Plattenepithelkarzinome an der vorderen Kommissur und Penetration des Kehlkopfgerüstes. Laryngol Rhinol Otol 60: 89-95

MEYER-BREITING E, SCHORM-EWERS P (1987): Zur T-Klassifikation des Larynxkarzinoms - eine klinisch pathohistologische Studie. In: MAJER EH, ZRUNEK M (eds), Die Oto-Rhino-Laryngologie in Kooperation mit Nachbardisziplinen; pp 222-225. Facultas, Wien

MITTAL B, MARKS JE, OGURA JH (1984): Transglottic carcinoma. Cancer 53: 151-161

MÜLLER E (1966): Über den Befall des Gerüstes beim inneren Kehlkopfkarzinom. Laryngol Rhinol Otol 45: 512-523

NORRIS CM, TUCKER GF, BURNS KF, PITSER WF (1970): A correlation of clinical staging, pathological findings and five year end results in surgically treated cancer of the larynx. Ann Otol Rhinol Laryngol 79: 1033-1048

OGURA JH (1955): Surgical pathology of cancer of the larynx. Laryngoscope 65: 867-926

OGURA JH (1958): Supraglottic subtotal laryngectomy and radical neck dissection for carcinoma of the epiglottis. Laryngoscope 68: 983-1003

OLOFSSON H, VAN NOSTRAND AWP (1973): Growth and spread of laryngeal carcinoma with reflections on the effect of preoperative irradiation. Acta Otolaryngol (Stockh) Suppl 308: 1-84

OLOFSSON J, WILLIAMS GT, RIDER WD, BRYCE DP (1972): Anterior commissure carcinoma. Arch Otolaryngol 95: 230-239

PARK WW (1980): The histology of borderline cancer with notes on prognosis. Springer, Berlin-Heidelberg-New York

PIETRANTONI L, AGAZZI C, FIOR (1961): Le problème ganglionnaire dans le traitement des cancers du larynx et résultats après 5 ans. Adv Otorhinolaryngol 9: 275-323

PRESSMAN JJ, SIMON MB, MONELL C (1960): Anatomical studies related to the dissemination of cancer of the larynx. Trans Am Acad Ophthalmol Otolaryngol 64: 628-638

ROSEMANN G (1963): Über das Vorkommen multizentrischer Carcinomata in situ und Karzinome der Epiglottis. Laryngol Rhinol Otol 42:641-654

ROUVIERE H (1932): Anatomie des lymphatiques de l'homme. Masson und Cie., Paris

ROUVIERE H (1938): Anatomy of the human lymphatic system. Edwards Brothers, Inc., Ann Arbor

SCHWAB W, ZUM WINKEL J (1975): Möglichkeiten der Strahlentherapie in der Hals-Nasen-Ohrenheilkunde. Thieme, Stuttgart

SMITH RR, CAULK RM, RUSSEL WO, JACKSON CL (1961): End results in 1600 laryngeal cancers using the American Joint Committee's proposed method of stage classification and end results reporting. Surg Gynecol Obstet 113: 435-444

SMITH RR, CAULK R, FRAZELL E, HOLINGER PH, McCOMB WS, RUSSELL WO et al (1973): Revision of the clinical staging system for cancer of the larynx. Cancer 31: 72-80

SZLESAK L (1966): Histological serial block examination of 57 cases of laryngeal cancer. Oncologia 20: 178-194

TASKINEN PJ (1969): Radiotherapy and TNM-classification of cancer of the larynx. Acta Radiol (Suppl)(Stockh) 287

TUCKER GF (1963): Some clinical inferences from the study of serial laryngeal sections. Laryngoscope 73: 728-748

TUCKER GF (1971): Human larynx coronal section atlas. Armed Forces Institute of Pathology, Washington DC

TUCKER GF (1973): The anterior commissure revisited. Ann Otol Rhinol Laryngol 625-636

TUCKER GF (1974): The anatomy of laryngeal cancer. Can J Otolaryngol 3: 417-427

UICC (International Union Against Cancer) (1958): Clinical stage classification and presentation of results. Malignant tumours of the breast and larynx. Paris

UICC Union Internationale Contre le Cancer (1968): TNM classification of malignant tumours. (Larynx and Hypopharynx). Classified 1962. Genf

UICC Union Internationale Contre le Cancer (1972): TNM-classification of malignant tumours of breast, larynx, stomach, cervix uteri, corpus uteri. Genf

UICC Union Internationale Contre le Cancer (1978): Report of Committee on TNM Classification. Geneva

UICC Union Internationale Contre le Cancer (1979): TNM-Klassifikation der malignen Tumoren. 3. Aufl. Springer, Berlin-Heidelberg-New York

WAHI PN, COHEN B, LUTHRA UK, TORLONI H (1971): Histological typing of oral and oropharyngeal tumours. WHO, Geneva

WEEDE W (1974): Histolgische Untersuchungen über die Wachstumstendenzen supraglottischer Kehlkopftumoren. Inauguraldissertation, Berlin

WELSH LW (1964): The normal human laryngeal lymphatics. Ann Otol Rhinol Laryngol 73: 569-582

WELSH LW, WELSH JJ, BEHLKE FM (1961): Surgical alterations of the laryngeal lymphatics. Ann Otol Rhinol Laryngol 70: 52-63

WHO - World Health Organization (1976): ICD-O (International Classification of Diseases for Oncology). 1st edn. WHO, Geneva

WHO - World Health Organization (1979): ICD-O (International Classification of Diseases for Oncology): Tumor-Lokalisationsschlüssel. Springer, Berlin - Heidelberg - New York

YEAGER VL, ARCHER CR (1982): Anatomical routes for cancer invasion of laryngeal cartilages. Laryngoscope 92: 449-452

References

6 Management of Laryngeal Cancer and Histopathological Inferences

ACKERMAN LV (1948): Verrucous carcinoma of the oral cavity. Surgery 23: 670-678

ALAJMO E, FINI-STORCHI O, POLLI G (1976): Five-year results of 1.000 patients operated on for a cancer of the larynx. Acta Otolaryngol (Stockh) 82: 437-439

ALBERTINI A VON, ROULET FC (1974): Histologische Geschwulstdiagnostik. 2nd edn. Thieme, Stuttgart

ALONSO JM (1947): Conservative surgery of cancer of the larynx. Trans Am Acad Ophthalmol Otolaryngol 51: 663-642

ALONSO JM (1961): Cancer du larynx: Introduction et classification. Adv Otorhinolaryngol 9: 1-43

ALTMANN KI, GERBER GB, OKADA S (1970): Radiation-Biochemistry. Academic Press, New York - London

ARCHER CR, YEAGER VL, HERBOLD DR (1983): Computed tomography vs. histology of laryngeal cancer: their value in predicting laryngeal cartilage invasion. Laryngoscope 93: 140-147

BERGONIÉ J, TRIBONDEAU L (1906): Interprétation de quelques résultats de la radiothérapie - essai de fixation d'une technique rationelle. C R Acad Science (Paris) 143: 983-985

BILLER HF, OGURA JH, DAVIS WH, POWERS WE (1969): Planned pre-operative irradiation for carcinoma of the larynx and laryngopharynx treated by total and partial laryngectomy. Laryngoscope 79: 1387-1395

BILLER HF, OGURA JH, BAUER WC (1971): Verrucous cancer of the larynx. Laryngoscope 81: 1323-1329

BOCCA E (1968): Supraglottis surgery of the larynx. Ann Otol Rhinol Laryngol 77: 1005-1026

BOCCA E (1975): Limitations of supraglottic laryngectomy and conservative neck dissection. Can J Otolaryngol 4: 403-419

BOCCA E, PIGNATARO O (1984): Functional neck dissection. In: ROB C, SMITH R, WILSON JSP (eds), Operative Surgery - Head and neck, part II, pp 270-286. Butterworths, London - Toronto

BRIDGER GP (1974): Mucous gland involvement in cancer at the anterior commissure. Can J Otolaryngol 3: 507-511

BRYCE DP, RIDER WD (1971): Pre-operative irradiation in the treatment of advanced laryngeal carcinoma. Laryngoscope 81: 1481-1490

BYERS RM (1979): Symposium: Adjuvant cancer therapy of head and neck tumors. The use of postoperative irradiation. Its Goals and 1978 Attainments. Laryngoscope 89: 567-572

BURKHARDT A, HÖLTJE W-J (1975): The effects of intraarterial bleomycin therapy on squamous cell carcinoma of the oral cavity. Biopsy and autopsy examinations. J Max-Fac Surg 3: 217-230

BURKHARDT A, BOMMER G, GEBBERS J-O, HÖLTJE W-J (1976): Riesenzellbildung bei Bleomycintherapie oraler Plattenepithelcarcinome. Enzymhistochemische, elektronenmikroskopische und ultrahistochemische Untersuchungen. Virchows Arch (A) 369: 197-214

BURKHARDT A, GEBBERS J-O (1977): Giant cell stromal reaction in squamous cell carcinomata. Electronmicroscopic and ultrahistochemical observations on the genesis and functional activity of multinucleated giant cells in bleomycin-induced tumor regression. Virchows Arch (A) 375: 263-280

BURKHARDT A (1980): Der Mundhöhlenkrebs und seine Vorstadien. Ultrastrukturelle und immunpathologische Aspekte. Fischer, Stuttgart - New York

CARPENTER RJ, DE SANTO LW, DEVINE KD, TAYLOR WP (1976): Cancer of the hypopharynx. Analysis of treatment and results in 162 patients. Arch Otolaryngol 102: 716-721

CATLIN D, STRONG EW (1967): Preoperative irradiation for neck dissection. Surg Clin North Am 47: 1131-1139

COATES HL, DESANTO LW, DEVINE KD, ELVEBACK LR (1976): Carcinoma of the supraglottic larynx. A review of 221 cases. Arch Otolaryngol 102: 686-689

CONLAY J (1970): Concepts in head and neck surgery. Thieme, Stuttgart

CONSTABLE WC, WHITE RL, EL-MAHDI AM, FITZ-HUGH GS (1975): Intermediate dose preoperative radiotherapy for cancer of the larynx. End results. Can J Otolaryngol 4: 246-250

COTTIER H (1980): Pathogenese, Bd. I und II Springer, Berlin - Heidelberg - New York

CROSSLAND PM (1962): Effects of x-ray therapy on basal cell carcinoma. I. A histologic study of serial biopsy specimens. Arch Derm 86: 745-752

DEMIAN S, BUSHKIN R, ECHEVERIA R (1973): Perineural invasion and anapalstic transformation of verrucous carcinoma. Cancer 32: 395-401

DENECKE HJ (1980): Die oto-rhino-laryngologischen Operationen im Mund- und Halsbereich. In: ZENKER R, HEBERER G, PICHLMAYR R (eds), Allgemeine und spezielle Operationslehre; vol V,3. Springer, Berlin - Heidelberg - New York

DENEKAMP J (1970): Cellular proliferation kinetics of animal tumours. Cancer Res 30: 393-400

ELLIOT GB, DOUGALL JA, ELLIOT JD (1973): Problems of verrucous squamous carcinoma. Ann Surg 177: 21-29

FLEISCHER I (1977): Morphologische Untersuchungen an subglottischen Kehlkopfkarzinomen. Inauguraldissertation, Marburg

FONTS EA, GREENLAW RH, RUSH BF, ROVIN S (1969): Verrucous squamous cell carcinoma of the oral cavity. Cancer 23: 152-160

FOWLER JF, DENEKAMP J, HEGAZY MAH (1971): Fraktionierung in der Strahlentherapie: Folgerungen aus tierexperimentellen Studien über die Zellkinetik in Tumoren und der Haut. In: HUG O (edr), Präoperative Tumorbestrahlung. Urban & Schwarzenberg, München, p 22-35

GANZER U, SENDROWSKI P, VOSTEEN K-H, MEYER-BREITING P (1981): Die kombinierte radiochirurgische Behandlung des fortgeschrittenen Kehlkopfkarzinoms (T3-4, NO-3). Ein retrospektiver Vergleich zwischen Sandwich-Technik und postoperativer Bestrahlung. Laryngol Rhinol Otol 60: 63-70

GANZER U, MEYER-BREITING E, EBBERS J, VOSTEEN K-H (1982): Der Einfluß von Tumorgröße, Lymphknotenbefall und Behandlungsart auf die Prognose des Hypopharynxkarzinoms. Laryng Rhinol Otol 61: 622-628

GARAS J, KARAIOSSIFIDIS K, AGNANTI N, BESBEAS S, GEORGAKA A, MARAGOUDAKIS S, LIARIKOS S, GROPAS G, PAPAHARALAMBOUS N (1975): Histological changes of squamous cell carcinoma induced by continuous intra-arterial infusion of high doses of methotrexate. Panminerva Medica 17: 331-336

GLANZ HK (1981): Die prognostische Bedeutung des histologischen gradings von Stimmlippenkarzinomen. Arch Otorhinolaryngol 231: 745-746

GLANZ HK (1984): Carcinoma of the larynx; growth, p-classification and grading of squamous cell carcinoma of the vocal cords. Adv Otorhinolaryngol 32: 1-123

GLUCK T, SOERENSEN J (1922): Die Exstirpation und Resektion des Kehlkopfes. In: KATZ L, BLUMENFELD F (eds), Handbuch der speziellen Chirurgie des Ohres und der oberen Luftwege; Kabitzsch, Leipzig

GLÜCKSMANN A, CHERRY CP (1959): The histological criteria of radiation response. Acta Cytol (Baltimore) 3: 381, 385-387

GOLDMAN JL, SILVERSTONE S, ROSIN HD, CHEREN RR, ZAK FG (1964): Combined radiation and surgery for cancer of the larynx and laryngopharynx. Laryngoscope 74: 1111-1134

GOLDMAN JL, CHEREN RV, ZAK FG, GUNSBERG MJ (1966): Histopathology of larynges and radical neck specimens. Ann Otol Rhinol Laryngol 75: 313-335

GOLDMAN JL, BLOOM BS, FRIEDMAN WH, GUNSBERG MJ, SILVERSTONE SM (1969): Serial studies of radical neck dissections. Arch Otolaryngol 89: 620-628

GOLDMAN JL, ZAK FG, ROFFMAN JD, BIRKEN EA (1972): High dosage preoperative radiation and surgery for carcinoma of the larynx and laryngopharynx. Ann Otol Rhinol Laryngol 81: 488-495

GOLDMAN JL, ROFFMAN JD (1975): Combined preoperative irradiation and surgery for advanced cancer of the larynx and laryngopharynx. Can J Otolaryngol 4: 251-260

GOLDMAN JL, SILVERSTONE SM (1980): The role of radiation therapy in carcinoma of the larynx. Ann Otol Rhinol Laryngol 69: 890-906

GRAY LH, CONGER AD, EBERT M, HORNSEY S, SCOTT OCA (1953): The concentration of oxygen dissolved in tissue at the time of irradiation as a factor in radiotherapy. Br J Radiol 26: 638-648

GROSSENBACH R (1985): Laserchirurgie in der Oto-Rhino-Laryngologie. Thieme, Stuttgart - New York

HALL JW, FRIEDMAN M (1948): Histological changes in squamous cell carcinoma of the mouth and oropharynx produced by fractionated external roentgen irradiation. Radiology 50: 318-350

HANSEMANN D (1890): Über asymmetrische Zellteilung in Epithelkrebsen und deren biologische Bedeutung. Virchows Arch(A) 119: 299-326

HAYES DM, MILKINS FB MEREDITH JH (1964): Regional arterial infusion for localized malignancies. Arch Surg 88: 1070-1076

HEGEMANN G (1967): Wundheilung und Wundbehandlung. In: HELLNER H, NISSEN R, VOSSSCHULTE K (eds), Lehrbuch der Chirurgie; 5th edn. Thieme, Stuttgart

HERMANEK P, SOBIN LH (1987): TNM classification of malignant tumours. 4th fully revised edition. Springer, Berlin - Heidelberg - New York - Paris - Tokyo

HERMENS AF, BARENDSEN GW (1969): Changes of cell proliferation kinetics in a rat rhabdomyosarcoma before and after X-irradiation. Eur J Cancer Clin Oncol 5: 173-189

HOLTHUSEN H (1921): Beiträge zur Biologie der Strahlenwirkung. Untersuchungen an Askarideneiern. Pflügers Arch ges Physiol 187: 1-24

HOMMERICH KW (1974): Röntgenbefunde und mikroskopisches Wachstum von malignen Larynxtumoren. Laryngol Rhinol Otol 53: 845-855

HOWARD A, PELC SR (1963): Synthesis of DNA in normal and irradiated cells and its relation to chromosome breakage. Heredity 6: 261-273

HOYE RC, SMITH RR (1961): The effectiveness of small amounts of preoperative irradiation in preventing the growth of tumor cells disseminated at surgery. An experimental study. Cancer 11: 284-291

HUDSON WR, CAVANAUGH PJ (1965): Combined surgical and radiation management of carcinoma of the laryngopharynx. Laryngoscope 75: 1123-1138

INCH WR, MCCREDIE JA (1963): Effects of a small dose of X-radiation on local recurrence of tumors in rats and mice. Cancer 16: 595-598

INCH WR, MCCREDIE JA, SUTHERLAND RM (1970): Effect of X-radiation to tumor bed on local recurrence. Front Radiat Ther Oncol 5: 30-39

KIRCHNER JA (1970): Cancer at the anterior commissure of the larynx. Arch Otolaryngol 91: 524-525

KIRCHNER JA, FISCHER JJ (1975): Anterior commissure cancer - A clinical and laboratory study of 39 cases. Can J Otolaryngol 4: 637-643

KIRCHNER JA, OWEN JR (1977): Five hundred cancers of the larynx and pyriform sinus. Results of treatment by radiation and surgery. Laryngoscope 87: 1288-1303

KLEINSASSER O (1961): Kritische Betrachtung der Behandlungsergebnisse bei 410 Kehlkopfkarzinomen unter besonderer Berücksichtigung der Indikation zur Radical Neck Dissection. Laryngol Rhinol Otol 40: 652-674

KLEINSASSER O (1968): Microlaryngology and endolaryngeal surgery. Saunders, Philadelphia - London

KLEINSASSER O, MADJD S (1969): Rückblick auf die Ergebnisse von 224 Totalexstirpationen des Kehlkopfes. Laryngol Rhinol Otol 48: 161-178

KLEINSASSER, O (1980): Personal communication

KOLLMORGEN GM, BEDFORD JS (1973): Cellular radiation biology. In: DALRYMPLE GV, GAULDEN ME, KOLLMORGEN GM, VOGEL HH (eds), Medical radiation biology; pp 100-128. Saunders, Philadelphia - London

KRAUS FT, PEREZ-MESA C (1966): Verrucous carcinoma. Clinical and pathologic study of 105 cases involving oral cavity, larynx and genitalia. Cancer 19: 28-38

KROKOWSKI EH (1971): Drei grundsätzliche Vorbestrahlungsmodi. In: HUG O (edr), Präoperative Tumorbestrahlung; p 52-57. Urban & Schwarzenberg, München

LEICHER H (1961): Indikation- und 5-Jahresheilungen bei radiochirurgischer Behandlung des Kehlkopf- und Hypopharynxkarzinoms. Adv Otorhinolaryngol 9: 220-274

LELBACH WK (1955): Histologische Veränderungen an bestrahlten Carcinomen. In: LANGENDORFF H, LELBACH WK, JANKER R, ROSSMANN K (eds), Grundlagen und Praxis der Bewegungsbestrahlung. Girardet, Wuppertal-Elberfeld

LEROUX-ROBERT J (1936): Les épithéliomas intralaryngés.

Formes anatomo-cliniques. Voies d'extension. Thêse pour le doctorat en médicine. Thêse pour le doctorat en médicine. G Doin & Cie, Paris

LEROUX-ROBERT J (1957): La chirurgie par laryngofissure ou laryngectomie partielle dans les cancers du larynx (Résultats de 150 cas personnels avec reçul de plus de 5 ans). Ann Otolaryngol Cervicofac 74: 40-74

LEROUX-ROBERT J (1961): Indications et résultats après 5 ans de la chirurgie conservatrice fonctionelle des cancers du larynx et de l'hypopharynx. Adv Otorhinolaryngol 9: 44-130

LÖNING T, BURKHARDT A (1979): Plasma cells and immunoglobulinsynthesis in oral precancer and cancer. Correlation with dysplasia, cancer differentiation, radio- and chemotherapy. Virchows Arch (A) 384: 109-120

LÖRZ M, MEYER-BREITING E (1988): Evaluation of Proliferative Activity in Human Head and Neck Tumors Using the Monoclonal Antibody Ki-67. ORL (in press)

LORÉ JM jr (1962): An atlas of head and surgery. Saunders, Philadēlphia - London

LORENZ W (1957): Experimentalbeitrag zur präoperativen Bestrahlung. Strahlentherapie 103: 456-466

MCGAVRAN MH, BAUER WC, OGURA JH (1961): The incidence of cervical lymph node metastases from epidermoid carcinoma of the larynx and their relationship to certain characteristics of the primary tumor. Cancer 14: 55-66

MANCUSO AA, HANAFEE WN (1979): A comparative evaluation of computed tomography and laryngography. Radiology 133: 131-138

MANCUSO AA, HANAFEE WN, JUILLARD GJF, WINTER J, CALCATERRA TC (1977): The role of computed tomography in the management of cancer of the larynx. Radiology 124: 243-244

MEYER-BREITING E (1977): Vergleich histologischer Untersuchungsergebnisse bei vorbestrahlten supraglottischen und glottischen Kehlkopfkarzinomen. Arch Otorhinolaryngol 210: 566-567

MEYER-BREITING E (1978): Katamnestische Untersuchungen zur kombinierten Therapie des Larynxkarzinoms. Arch Otorhinolaryngol 219: 389-390

MEYER-BREITING E, ILBERG CH VON (1979): Spread and mode of metastasis of supraglottic laryngeal carcinoma. Orl J Otorhinolaryngol Relat Spec 41: 288-300

MEYER-BREITING E, ILBERG CH VON (1981): Behandlungsergebnisse der Chirurgie früher Stimmbandkarzinome. HNO 29: 41-46

MEYER-BREITING E (1981): Zur Histopathologie bestrahlter und nicht bestrahlter Kehlkopfkarzinome. Habilitationsschrift, Frankfurt

MEYER-BREITING P (1981): Katamnestische Untersuchungsergebnisse zur radiochirurgischen Kombinationstherapie fortgeschrittener innerer und äußerer Kehlkopfkarzinome. Inauguraldissertation, Frankfurt am Main

MEYER-BREITING E, HALBSGUTH A, OPRITOIU G (1982): Die Bedeutung der Computertomographie für Diagnostik und Therapieplanung fortgeschrittener Kehlkopfkarzinome. Arch Otorhinolaryngol 235: 689-691

MEYER-BREITING E (1984): The value of computerized tomography in conservative surgery of glottic cancer. In: WIGAND ME, STEINER W, STELL PM (eds), Functional partial laryngectomy. Conservation surgery for carcinoma of the larynx; pp 63-65. Springer, Berlin - Heidelberg - New York - Tokyo

MICHAELS L (1975): Differentiation of squamous carcinoma of the larynx as a determinant of prognosis. Can J Otolaryngol 4: 873-880

MONTGOMERY WW (1979): Surgery of the upper respiratory system; vol 1, 2nd edn. Lea & Febiger, Philadelphia

MOST A (1899): Über die Lymphgefäße und Lymphdrüsen des Kehlkopfes. Anat Anz 15: 387-393

NAUMANN HH (1972): Chirurgie der malignen Tumoren des Larynxinneren. In: NAUMANN HH (edr), Kopf- und Halschirurgie, vol 1. Thieme, Stuttgart

NUSSBAUM M, SOM M, CHO H (1981): Conservation surgery of the larynx. In: ROB C, SMITH R, WILSON JSP (eds), Operative Surgery - Head and neck, part II; p 686-699. Butterworths, London - Boston

OGURA JH (1955): Surgical pathology of cancer of the larynx. Laryngoscope 65: 867-926

OGURA JH (1970): Personal communication cited by ILBERG Ch VON.

OLOFSSON J, WILLIAMS GT, RIDER WD, BRYCE DP (1972): Anterior commissure carcinoma. Arch Otolaryngol 95: 230-239

OLOFSSON H, VAN NOSTRAND AW (1973): Growth and spread of laryngeal carcinoma with reflections on the effect of preoperative irradiation. Acta Otolaryngol (Stockh) Suppl 308: 1-84

OLOFSSON J (1984): Computed tomography in the diagnosis of laryngeal carcinoma. In: WIGAND ME, STEINER W, STELL PM (eds), Functional partial laryngectomy. Conservation surgery for carcinoma of the larynx; pp 66-68. Springer, Berlin - Heidelberg - New York - Tokyo

OMBRÉDANNE M (1930): Traitment du cancer endolaryngé - l'hémilaryngectomie - technique A.Hautant. Masson, Paris

POWERS WE, PALMER LA (1968): Biologic basis of preoperative radiation treatment. AJR 102: 176-192

PRESSMAN JJ, SIMON MB, MONELL C (1960): Anatomical studies related to the dissemination of cancer of the larynx. Trans Am Acad Ophthalmol Otolaryngol 64: 628-638

RIDER WD (1976): Toronto experience of verrucous carcinoma of the larynx. In: ALBERTI PW, BRYCE DP (eds) Centennial Conference on Laryngeal Cancer. Appleton-Century-Crofts, New York, p 460-461

RUDERT H (1985): Kehlkopfkarzinom: Möglichkeiten und Grenzen der Therapie imt dem CO2-Laser. Dtsch Ärztebl 82: 2104-2107

RYAN RE, DE SANTO LW, DEVINE KD, WEILAND LH (1977): Verrucous carcinoma of the larynx. Laryngoscope 87: 1989-1994

SCHERER E (1980): Operation, Bestrahlung, Chemotherapie und Organisationsfragen. In: SCHERER E (edr) Strahlentherapie, Radiologische Onkologie, 2nd edn. Springer, Berlin - Heidelberg - New York

SCHNEIDER JJ, FLETCHER GH, BARKLEY HT (1975): Control by irradiation of non fixed clinically positive lymphnodes from squamous cell carcinoma of the oral cavity, oropharynx, supraglottic larynx and hypopharynx. AJR 123: 42-48

SCHULLER DE, MCGUIRT WF, KRAUSE CJ, MCCABE BF, PFLUG BK (1979): Adjuvant cancer therapy of head and neck tumours: Increased survival with surgery alone vs. combined therapy. Laryngoscope 89: 582-594

SCHULTZE B (1968): Die Orthologie und Pathologie des Nuklein- und Eiweißstoffwechsels der Zelle im Autoradiogramm. In: Handbuch der Allgemeinen Pathologie, vol II,5, Die Zelle. Springer, Berlin - Heidelberg - New York

SCHUMANN K, LANIADO K, MITTERMAYER CH, WANNENMACHER W, DAUMANN G (1980): Die präoperative Bestrahlung bei Plattenepithelkarzinomen der Tonsille, des Zungengrundes und des Hypopharynx. Laryngol Rhinol Otol 59: 335-340

SCHWADE JG, WARA WM, DEDO HH, PHILIPPS TL (1976): Radiotherapy of verrucous carcinoma. Radiology 120: 677-679
SERAFINI I (1984): Results of Supraglottic Horizontal Partial Laryngectomy. In: WIGAND ME, STEINER W, STELL PM (eds), Functional partial laryngectomy. Conservation surgery for carcinoma of the larynx; pp 223-225. Springer, Berlin - Heidelberg - New York - Tokyo
SHIRAKAWA S, LUCE JK, TANNOCK JF, FREI JE (1970): Cell proliferation in human melanome. J Clin Invest 49: 1188-1199
SHAW HJ (1981): Pharyngolaryngectomy. In: Wilson JSP (edr), Operative Surgery - Head and Neck, vol II p 754-764. Butterworth, London - Boston
SHKLAR G, CATALDO E, FITZGERALD AL (1966): The effect of methotrexate on chemical carcinogenesis of hamster buccal pouch. Cancer Res 26: 2218-2224
SHKLAR G, SONIS ST (1975): The effect of methotrexate on experimental salivary gland neoplasia in rats. Archs Oral Biol 20: 787-790
SILVER CE (1977): Surgical management of neoplasms of the larynx, hypopharynx and cervical esophagus. Curr Probl Surg 14: 2-69
SINCLAIR WK (1968): Cyclic-X-rays response in mammalian cells in vitro. Radiat Res 33: 620-643
SKOLNIK EM, SOBOROFF BJ, TENTA LT, SABERMAN MN, JONES HC (1968): Preoperative radiation of head and neck cancer. Trans Am Acad Ophthalmol Otolaryngol 72: 937-942
SKOLNIK EM, SOBOROFF BJ, TARDY ME, LEVIN RJ, TENTA LT (1970): Preoperative radiation of the larynx. Analysis of serial sections. Ann Otol Rhinol Laryngol 79: 1049-1056
SKOLNIK EM, MARTIN LD, WHEATLEY MA, YEE KF, KOTLER R (1975): Combined therapy in the management of laryngeal carcinoma. Can J Otolaryngol 4: 236-246
SNOW JB, GELBER RD, KRAMER S, DAVIS LW, MARCIAL VA, LOWRY LDVA, LOWRY LD (1980): Randomized preoperative and postoperative radiation therapy for patients with carcinoma of the head and neck: preliminary report. Laryngoscope 90: 930-945
SOM ML (1951): Hemilaryngectomy. A modified technique for cordal carcinoma with extension posteriorly. Arch Otolaryngol 54: 524-533
SOM ML (1975): Cordal cancer with extension to vocal process. Laryngoscope 85: 1298-1307
SOM ML, SILVER CE (1968): The anterior commissure technique of partial laryngectomy. Arch Otolaryngol 87: 138-145
SPRING E, SALMO M, RISSANON PM (1972): The effect of the treated volume and cell survival fractions on the recurrence of carcinoma of the larynx in radiotherapy. Strahlentherapie 144: 18-21
STEEL GG (1968): Cell loss from experimental tumours. Cell Tissue Kinet 1: 193-207
STEINER W, JAUMANN MP, PESCH H-J (1980): Endoskopische Laserchirurgie im Larynx. Ther Umsch 37: 1103-1109
STEINER W (1984): Transoral microsurgical CO2-laser resection of laryngeal carcinoma. In: WIGAND ME, STEINER W, STELL PM (eds), Functional partial laryngectomy. Conservation surgery for carcinoma of the larynx; pp 121-125. Springer, Berlin - Heidelberg - New York - Tokyo
STEINER W (1985): Krebsvorsorge- und Früherkennungsuntersuchungen der oberen Luft- und Speisewege bei Risikogruppen. W.Kohlhammer, Stuttgart - Berlin - Köln - Mainz
STELL PM (1981): Malignant tumours of the larynx and trachea. Wilson JSP (edr), Operative Surgery - Head and Neck. Butterworth, London - Boston, vol II p 700-705
STREFFER C (1969): Strahlen-Biochemie Springer, Berlin - Heidelberg - New York
STREFFER C (1980): Biologische Grundlagen der Strahlentherapie. In: SCHERER E (edr), Strahlentherapie, Radiologische Onkologie, 2nd edn. Springer, Berlin - Heidelberg - New York
STRONG MS (1975): Laser excision of carcinoma of the larynx. Laryngoscope 85: 1286
STUCKRAD H VON, LAKATOS I (1975): Über ein neues Lupenlaryngoskop (Epipharyngoskop). Laryngol Rhinol Otol 54: 336-343
SUAREZ O (1963): El problema de las metastasis linfatias y alejadas del cancer de laringe e hipofaringe. Rev Otorinolaringol 23: 83-99
TERRAHE K (1972): Die Indikationen zu Teilresektionen des Kehlkopfes beim Kehlkopfkarzinom. HNO 20: 65-73
THOMLINSON RH (1968): Changes in oxygenation in tumours in relation irradiation. In: VAETH JM: Frontiers of radiation therapy and oncology, Vol 3, p 109. Karger, Basel - München - Paris - London - New York - Sidney
THOMPSON LH, SUIT HD (1969): Proliferation kinetics of X-irradiated mouse L-cells studies with timelapse photography. Int J Radiat Oncol Biol Phys 15: 347-362
TUBIANA M (1970): The kinetics of tumor cell proliferation and radiotherapy. Br J Radiol 44: 325-347
UICC UNION INTERNATIONALE CONTRE LE CANCER (1978): Report of Committee on TNM Classification. Geneva
UICC UNION INTERNATIONALE CONTRE LE CANCER (1986): Report of Committee on TNM Classification. Geneva
VANDENBROUCK D (1977): Results of a randomized clinical trial of preoperative irradiation versus postoperative in treatment of tumors of the hypopharynx. Cancer 39: 1445-1449
VAUGHAN CW, STRONG MS, SHAPSHAY SM (1980): Treatment of T1 and in situ carcinoma: the transoral approach. Otolaryngol Clin N Amer 13: 459
VEGA MF (1984): Oncological and Functional Results of Horizontal Partial Laryngectomy. In: WIGAND ME, STEINER W, STELL PM (eds), Functional partial laryngectomy. Conservation surgery for carcinoma of the larynx; pp 226-228. Springer, Berlin - Heidelberg - New York - Tokyo
VIRAG M, KRAJINA Z, KOSOVIC F, KUBOVIC M, ZUNTER F, VOSKRESENSKY I, SMILJANIC B (1976): Die präoperative Bestrahlung von Patienten mit Larynx- und Hypopharynxkarzinom. Laryngol Rhinol Otol 55: 477-481
VOSTEEN KH, FRANKE H (1965): Über den Wert der präoperativen Strahlenbehandlung beim fortgeschrittenen Kehlkopfkarzinom. Arch Otorhinolaryngol 185: 673-677
WANG CC, SCHULZ MD (1963): Cancer of the larynx. Radiology 80: 963-972
WANG CC (1975): Radiation therapy for head and neck cancers. Cancer 36: 748-751
WELSH LW, WELSH JJ, BEHLKE FM (1961): Surgical alterations of the laryngeal lymphatics. Ann Otol Rhinol Laryngol 70: 52-63
WIGAND ME, STEINER W, STELL PM (eds) (1984): Conservation Surgery of the Larynx. Springer, Berlin - Heidelberg - New York - Tokyo
WHITTAM DE, WILKINSON KW (1981): Pharyngolaryngooesophagectomy and repair with mobilized stomach. In: WILSON JSP (edr), Operative Surgery - Head and Neck. Butterworth, London - Boston, vol II, p 769-778
ZUPPINGER A (1971): Die Vorbestrahlung - Einleitende Übersicht. In: HUG O (edr), Präoperative Tumorbestrahlung. Urban & Schwarzenberg, München - Berlin - Wien, p 49-51

References

7 Unusual Malignant Tumours

Abemajor E (1983): Metastatic cancer to the larynx. Cancer 52: 1944-1948

Abemajor E, Cochran AJ, Calcaterra TC (1983): Metastatic cancer to the larynx. Cancer 52: 1944-1948

Abramowsky CR, Witt WJ (1983): Sarcoma of the larynx in a newborn. Cancer 51: 1726-1730

Abramson AL, Brandsma J, Steinberg B, Winkler B (1985): Verrucous carcinoma of the larynx. Arch Otolaryngol 111: 709-715

Ackerman LV (1948): Verrucous carcinoma of the oral cavity. Surgery 23: 670-678

Adams GL, Duvall AJ (1971): Adenocarcinoma of the head and neck. Arch Otolaryngol 93: 261-270

Aird J, Johnson HD, Lennox B, Stansfeld AG (1954): Epithelioma cuniculatum. A variety of squamous carcinoma, peculiar to the foot. Br J Surg 42: 245-250

Alberti PW, Bryce DP (1976): Centennial conference of laryngeal cancer. Appleton-Century-Crofts, New York

Albertini A von, Roulet FC (1974): Histologische Geschwulstdiagnostik. 2nd edn. Thieme, Stuttgart

Alguacil-Garcia A, Alonso A, Pettigrew M (1984): Sarcomatoid carcinoma (so-called pseudosarcoma) of the larynx simulating malignant giant cell tumour of soft parts. Am J Clin Pathol 82: 340-343

Allsbrook WC, Harmon JD, Chongchitnant N, Erwin St (1985): Liposarcoma of the larynx. Arch Pathol Lab Med 109: 294-296

Al-Saleem T, Tucker GF, Peale AR, Norris CM (1970): Cartilaginous tumors of the larynx; clinical-pathologic study of ten cases. Ann Otol Rhinol Laryngol 79: 33-41

Amendola BE, Amendola A, McClatchey KD (1985): Radiation induced carcinoma of the larynx. Surg Gynecol Obstet 161: 30-32

Arlen M, Shah IC, Higinbotham N, Huvos A (1972): Osteogenic sarcoma of head and neck induced by radiation therapy. N Y State J Med 72: 929-934

Atkins JP, Sullivan RD, Jones R (1951): Endobronchial lymphoma and his simulation by bronchogenic carcinoma. Ann Otol Rhinol Laryngol 60: 849-863

Aubry M, Leroux-Robert J (1937): Dense cas de tumeurs pédiculées de l'endo-larynx. Ann Otolaryngol Chir Cervicofac 3: 207-214

Bak M, Erdös M (1975): Verrucous carcinoma of the larynx. Arch Otorhinolaryngol 209: 1522

Baker DC, Weissman B (1971): Postirradiation carcinoma of the larynx. Ann Otol Rhinol Laryngol 80: 634-637

Barsocchini LM, McCoy (1968): Cartilaginous tumors of the larynx; a review of the literature and a report of four cases. Ann Otol Rhinol Laryngol 77: 146-153

Batsakis JG (1979): Tumors of the Head and Neck. Clinical and Pathological Considerations. 2nd ed. Williams & Wilkins, Baltimore

Batsakis JG, Fox JE (1970): Supporting tissue neoplasms of the larynx. Surg Gynecol Obstet 131: 989-997

Batsakis JG, Regezi JA, Rice DH (1980): The pathology of head and neck tumors: fibroadipose tissue and skeletal muscle, part 8. Head Neck Surg 3: 145-168

Batsakis JG, Hybel R, Crissman JD (1982): The pathology of head and neck tumors: verrucous carcinoma. Head Neck Surg 5: 29-38

Batsakis JG, Luna MA, Byers RM (1985): Metastases to the larynx. Head Neck Surg 7: 458-460

Bewtra CH, Krishnan R, Lee S (1982): Malignant changes in nonirradiated juvenile laryngotracheal papillomatosis. Arch Otolaryngol 108: 114-116

Biller HF, Bergman JA (1976): Verrucous carcinoma of the larynx. In: Centennial Conference on Laryngeal Cancer; ed by Alberti PW, Bryce DP; p 462-465 Appleton-Century-Crofts, New York

Biller HF, Ogura JH, Bauer WC (1971): Verrucous cancer of the larynx. Laryngoscope 81: 1323-1329

Binder WJ, Kaneko M, Som P, Biller HF (1980): Mucoepidermoid carcinoma of the larynx. A case report and review of the literature. Ann Otol Rhinol Laryngol 89: 103-107

Blok PhHHM, Manni JJ, Vandenbroek P, Haelst U, Slooff JL (1985): Carcinoid of the larynx: a report of three cases and a review of the literature. Laryngoscope 95: 715-719

van den Bogaert W, Ostyn F, van der Schneren E (1983): The primary treatment of advanced vocal cord cancer: laryngectomy or radiotherapy. Int J Radiat Oncol Biol Phys 9: 329-334

Boswarth FH (1892): Sarcoma of the larynx. Diseases of the nose and throat. William Wood & Co., New York

Broughton-Barnes E, Duthie ES, Jolles B (1948): Case of sarcoma of larynx. Br Med J 1948: 1237

Brownstein MH, Shapiro L (1976): Verrucous carcinoma of skin-epithelioma cuniculatum planture. Cancer 38: 1710-1716

Burkhardt A (1980): Der Mundhöhlenkrebs und seine Vorstadien. Ultrastrukturelle und immunpathologische Aspekte. Fischer, Stuttgart - New York

Busuttil A (1976): Dentritic pigmented cell within human laryngeal mucosa. Arch Otolaryngol 102: 43-44

Busuttil A, Forbes J (1978): Chondrosarcoma of the thyroid cartilage. J Laryngol 92: 633-638

Cachin Y, Schwaab (1978): Association of broncho-pulmonary cancers and of cancers of the upper aero-digestive tract (43 cases). J Fr Otorhinolaryngol 27: 15-17

Cady B, Rippey JH, Frazell EL (1968): Non-epidermoid cancer of the larynx. Ann Surg 167: 116-120

Calvet I, Claux I, Birague C et al (1968): Les sarcomes du larynx. Etude génerale à propos de 7 observations. J Fr Otorhinolaryngol 17: 21-30

CANALIS RF, GREEN M, KONRAD HR, HIROSE FM, COOPER S (1975): Malignant fibrous xanthoma (xanthofibrosarcoma) of the larynx. Arch Otolaryngol 101: 135-137
CANTRELL RW, REIBEL JF, JAHRSDOERFER RA, JOHNS ME (1980): Conservative surgical treatment of chondrosarcoma of the larynx. Ann Otol Rhinol Laryngol 89: 567-571
CAPPER JWR, MICHAELS L, GREGOR RT (1981): A malignant carcinoid tumour of the supraglottic larynx. J Laryngol Otol 95: 963-971
CEFIS F, CATTANEO M, RICCI KMC, FRIGERIO B, USELLINI L, CAPELLA C (1983): Primary polypeptide hormones and mucin-producing malignant carcinoid of the larynx. Ultrastruct Pathol 5: 45-53
CELESTINO D (1963): Dei tumori mesenchimali maligni primitivi della larynge. Boll Mal Orecch 81: 305-364
CHATELLIER HP, GUERIN (1927): Maladie de Hodgkin avec localisation laryngée. Ann Otolaryngol Chir Cervicofac 46: 1136-1139
CITELLI S (1912): Su un caso molto raro di fibrosarcoma gigante laringo-tracheale guarito con cordectomia. Boll Mal Orecch 30: 205-212
COAKLEY JF (1985): Primary oat cell carcinoma of the larynx. J Laryngol Otol 99: 301-303
COAKLEY LP, SALE GG (1948): Fibrosarcoma in a foreign body giant cell tumor of the larynx. Ann Otol Rhinol Laryngol 57: 514-518
COHEN SR, LANDING BH, ISAACS H, KOSTER KING K, HANSON V (1978): Solitary plasmacytoma of the larynx and upper trachea associated with systemic lupus erythematosus. Ann Otol Rhinol Laryngol (Suppl) 87: 11-14
COHEN SR, LANDING BH, ISAACS H (1979): Neurofibroma of the larynx in a child. Ann Otol Rhinol Laryngol 87: 29-31
COHEN J, GUILLAMONDEGUI OM, BATSAKIS JG, MEDINA JE (1985): Cancer of the minor salivary glands of the larynx. Am J Surg 150: 513-518
COOKE RG (1931): Hodgkin's disease with unusual onset. Br Med J 1: 308-309
COYAS A, ANASTASSIADES OT, KYRIAKOS J (1974): Malignant giant cell tumor of the larynx. J Laryngol Otol 88: 799-803
COYAS A, ANASTASSIADES O, TZAGARAKIS M, KONTOGEORGOS G (1978): Chondrosarcoma of the larynx. J Laryngol Otol 92: 529-531
COYAS A, ELIADELLIS E, ANASTASSIADES O (1983): Kaposi's Sarcoma of the larynx. J Laryngol Otol 97: 647-649
CRISSMAN JD, ROSENBLATT A (1978): Acinous cell carcinoma of the larynx. Arch Pathol Lab Med 102: 233-236
DAHM LJ, SCHAEFER StD, CARDER HM, VELLIOS F (1978): Osteosarcoma of the soft tissue of the larynx. Report of a case with light and electron microscopic studies. Cancer 42, 2343-2351
DAMIANI JM, DAMIANI KK, HAUCH K, HYAMS VJ (1981): Mucoepidermoid-adenosquamous carcinoma of the larynx and hypopharynx: a report of 21 cases and a review of the literature. Otolaryngol Head Neck Surg 89: 235-243
DEGROOT TR, FRAZER JP, WOOD BP (1980): Combination therapy for laryngeal rhabdomyosarcoma. Am J Otolaryngol 1: 456-460
DEMIAN S, BUSHKIN R, ECHEVERIA R (1973): Perineural invasion and anapalstic transformation of verrucous carcinoma. Cancer 32: 395-401
DESHOTELS SJ, SARMA D, FAZIO F, RODRIGUEZ F (1982): Squamous cell carcinoma with sarcomatoid stroma. J Surg Oncol 19: 201-207
DIEHL KL (1953): Sarcoma of the larynx. Arch Otolaryngol 57: 40-43
DIEHN KW, HYAMS VJ, HARRIS AE (1984): Rhabdomyosarcoma of the larynx. Laryngoscope 94: 201-205
DITO WR, BATSAKIS JG (1962): Rhabdomyosarcoma of the head and neck. Arch Surg 84: 582-588
DOCKERTY MB, PARKHILL EM, DAHLIN DG, WOOLNER L, SOULE EH, HARRISON EG (1968): Tumors of the oral cavity and pharynx. In: Atlas of Tumor Pathology, Sect IV, Fasc 10. Washington DC, Armed Forces Institute of Pathology
DONALDSON J (1978): Fibrosarcoma in a previously irradiated larynx. J Laryngol Otol 92: 425-428
DONAT R (1959): Isolierte, tumorartige, polypöse Lymphogranulomatose des Stimmbandes bei allgemeiner Lymphogranulomatose. Zentralbl Allg Pathol 100: 7-11
DRAETTA G, PINTUS ML, SANTA-CRUZ G, PINTO G (1980): I tumori mesenchimali maligni della laringe. Pathologica 72: 821-832
DWYER GK (1953): Fibrosarcoma of the larynx. Arch Otolaryngol 58: 442-443
EBY LS, JOHNSON DS, BAKER HW (1972): Adenoid cystic carcinoma of the head and neck. Cancer 29: 1160-1168
EGGSTON AA, WOLFF D (1947): Histopathology of the ear, nose and throat. Williams & Wilkins Co., Baltimore
EHRLICH A (1954): Tumor involving the laryngeal cartilages. Arch Otolaryngol 59: 178-185
EIBLING DE, ROSNAGLE RS (1980): Pathological quiz case. 1. Chondrosarcoma of the larynx. Arch Otolaryngol 106: 134-136
ELLIOT GB, DOUGALL JA, ELLIOT JD (1973): Problems of verrucous squamous carcinoma. Ann Surg 177: 21-29
ESCHER A, ESCHER F, ZIMMERMANN A (1984): Zur Klinik und Pathologie chondromatöser Tumoren des Larynx. HNO 32: 269-285
EWING J (1928): Neoplastic diseases. 3rd ed. Saunders, Philadelphia - London
FECHNER RE (1976): Adenocarcinoma of the larynx. In: Centennial Conference on Laryngeal Cancer; ed by ALBERTI PW, BRYCE DP; p 466-471 Appleton-Century-Crofts, New York
FECHNER RE (1984): Spindle cell carcinoma of the larynx. Arch Otolaryngol 110: 554-555
FECHNER RE, MILLS StE (1982): Verruca vulgaris of the larynx. A distinct lesion of probable viral origin confused with verrucous carcinoma. Am J Surg Path 6: 357-362
FERLITO A (1976): Primary anaplastic giant cell adenocarcinoma of the larynx. J Laryngol Otol 90: 1053-1060
FERLITO A (1978): Histiocytic tumors of the larynx: a clinicopathological study with review of the literature. Cancer 42: 611-622
FERLITO A (1978): Primary malignant haemangiopericytoma of the larynx. A case report with autopsy. J Laryngol Otol 92: 511-519
FERLITO A (1980): Double primary synchronous and metachronous cancer of the larynx and hypopharynx with dissimilar histology. Arch Otorhinolaryngol 229: 107-119
FERLITO A (1985): Diagnosis and treatment of verrucous squamous cell carcinoma of the larynx: a critical review. Ann Otol Rhinol Laryngol 94: 575-579
FERLITO A, CARUSO G (1984): Secondary malignant melanoma of the larynx. ORL 46: 117-133
FERLITO A, RECHER G (1980): Ackerman's tumor (verrucous carcinoma) of the larynx. A clinicopathologic study of 77 cases. Cancer 46: 1617-1630
FERLITO A, RECHER G (1986): Laryngeal involvement by mycosis fungoides. Ann Otol Rhinol Laryngol 95: 275-277
FERLITO AG, ANTONUTTO G, SILVESTRI F (1976): Histological appearances and nuclear DNA content of verrucous squamous cell carcinoma of the larynx. ORL 38: 65-86
FERLITO A, RECHER G, POLIDARO F, ROSSI M (1979): Malig-

nant pleomorphic fibrous histiocytoma of the larynx. J Laryngol Otol 93: 1021-1029
FERLITO A, NICOLAI P, BARION U (1983): Critical comments on laryngeal fibrosarcoma. Acta Otorhinolaryngol Belg 37: 918-925
FERLITO A, NICOLAI P, RECHER G, NARNE S (1983): Primary laryngeal malignant fibrous histiocytoma: review of the literature and report of seven cases. Laryngoscope 93: 1351-1358
FERLITO A, FRIEDMANN J, RECHER G (1985): Primary giant cell carcinoma of the larynx. ORL 47: 105-112
FERLITO A, NICOLAI P, CARUSO G (1985): Angiosarcoma of the larynx. Case report. Ann Otol Rhinol Laryngol 94: 93-95
FIGI FA (1933): Sarcoma of the larynx. Arch Otolaryngol 18: 21-23
FISHER HR (1976): Verrucous carcinoma of the larynx - a study of its pathologic anatomy. In: ALBERTI PW, BRYCE DP (eds); Centennial Conference on Laryngeal Cancer; pp 452-459. Appleton-Century-Crofts, New York
FISH B, NUSSBAUM M, SMULEWICZ JJ (1982): Chondrosarcoma of larynx. Computerized tomographic study. N Y State J Med 82: 216-218
FISKER AV, PHILIPSEN HP (1984): Verrucous hyperplasia and verrucous carcinoma of the rat oral mucosa. Acta Pathol Microbiol Immunol Scand (A) 92: 437-445
FLANAGAN P, CROSS RM, LIBCKE JH (1965): Fibrosarcoma of the larynx. J Laryngol Otol 79: 1049-1056
FLEISCHER I, GLANZ H, KLEINSASSER O (1978): Kehlkopftumoren. Adenoidzystische Karzinome des Kehlkopfes. Laryngol Rhinol Otol 57: 218-224
FONTS EA, GREENLAW RH, RUSH BF, ROVIN S (1969): Verrucous squamous cell carcinoma of the oral cavity. Cancer 23: 152-160
FRANZ B (1979): The cytopathology of pleomorphic rhabdomyosarcomas of the larynx. Laryngol Rhinol Otol 58: 920-925
FRIEDEL W, CHAMBERS RG, ATKINS JP (1976): Pseudosarcomas of the pharynx and larynx. Arch Otolaryngol 102: 286-290
FRIEDMAN I (1976): Sarcomas of the larynx. In: ALBERTI PW, BRYCE DP (eds) Centennial Conference on Laryngeal Cancer. Appleton-Century-Crofts, New York, p 122-126.
FRUGONI P, FERLITO A (1976): Pleomorphic rhabdomyosarcoma of the larynx. J Laryngol Otol 90: 687-698
GALLE E, VOLLMAR F, RÜDIGER KD (1971): Beitrag zum Carcinosarkom des Larynx. HNO 19: 336-338
GALLOWAY TC, SOPER GR, ELSEN J (1960): Carcinoma of the larynx after irradiation for recurring papillomas. Arch Otolaryngol 72: 289-294
GATTI WM, ERKMAN-BALIS B (1980): Mucoepidermoid carcinoma of the larynx. Arch Otolaryngol 106: 52-53
GATTI WM, STROM CG, ORFEI E (1975): Synovial sarcoma of the laryngopharynx. Arch Otolaryngol 101: 633-636
GAYNOR EB, RAGHAUSAN V, WEISBROT JM (1984): Primary myxoid liposarcoma of the larynx. Otolaryngol Head Neck Surg 92: 476-480
GEAHCHAN NE, LAMBERT J, MICHEAU C, RICHARD JM (1983): Synovialome malin du larynx. Ann Otolaryngol Chir Cervicofac 100: 61-65
GERARD M, DE GANDT JB (1975): Un cas de cylindrome glottosous-glottique. Acta Otorhinolaryngol Belg 29: 692
GERUGHTY RM, HENNIGAR GR, BROWN FM (1968): Adenosqamous carcinoma of the nasal, oral, and laryngeal cavities. Cancer 22: 1140-1155
GIORDANO AM, EWING S, ADAMS G, MAISEL R (1983): Laryngeal pseudosarcoma. Laryngoscope 93: 735-740
GIRAUD I, LAMAS H, MAURIN R (1957): Un cas de sarcoma fibroblastique de la sous-glotte. J Fr Otorhinolaryngol 6: 1066-1069
GLANZ HK, KLEINSASSER O (1976): Radiogene Zweitkarzinome des Larynx. HNO 24: 48-59
GLANZ HK, KLEINSASSER O (1978): Verrucous acanthosis (verrucous carcinoma) of the larynx. Laryngol Rhinol Otol 57: 835-843
GLICK HN (1944): An unusual neoplasm in the larynx of a child. Rhabdomyosarcoma. Ann Otol Rhinol Laryngol 53: 699-704
GNEPP DR, FERLITO A, HYAMS V (1983): Primary anaplastic small cell (oat cell) carcinoma of the larynx. Cancer 51: 1731-1745
GODOY J, JACOBS JR, CRISSMAN J (1986): Malignant fibrous histiocytoma of the larynx. J Surg Oncol 31: 62-65
GOETHALS PL, DAHLIN DC, DEVINE KD (1963): Cartilaginous tumors of the larynx. Surg Gynecol Obstet 117: 77-82
GOLDMAN JL, LAWSON W, ZAK FG, ROFFMAN JD (1972): The presence of melanocytes in the human larynx. Laryngoscope 82: 824-835
GOOLDEN AWG (1951): Radiation cancer of the pharynx. Br Med J 2: 1110-1112
GOOLDEN AWG (1957): Radiation cancer. A review with special reference to radiation tumors in the pharynx, larynx and thyroid. Br J Radiol 30: 626-640
GORENSTEIN A, NEEL HB, DEVINE KD, WEILAND LH (1977): Solitary extramedullary plasmacytoma. Arch Otolaryngol 103: 159-161
GORENSTEIN A, NEEL B, WEILAND LH, DEVINE KD (1980): Sarcomas of the larynx. Arch Otolaryngol 106: 8-12
GOTO T, NAKASHIMA Y (1973): Giant cell tumor of the larynx. Otologia (Fukuoka) 19: 507
GRIEPENTROG F (1955): Ein Carzinosarkom des Taschenbandes. Arch Otorhinolaryngol 166: 350-354
GRIMAUD R, WERNER J (1954): Un cas de sarcome du larynx avec métastases cutanées multiples. Ann Otolaryngol Chir Cervicofac 72: 84
HAAR JG, CHAUDRY AP, KARANJIA MD, MILLEY PS (1978): Chondroblastic osteosarcoma of the larynx. Arch Otolaryngol 104: 477-481
HACIHANEFIOGLU U, ÖZTÜRK AS (1983): Sarcomas of the larynx. Report of ten cases. Ann Otol Rhinol Laryngol 92: 81-86
HALL LS (1958): Sarcoma of the larynx. J Laryngol Otol 72: 906-909
HALPHEN E (1927): Maladie de Hodgkin á localisation laryngée. Ann Otolaryngol Chir Cervicofac 46: 1140
HAMPERL H (1967): Early invasive growth as seen in uterine cancer and the role of the basal membrane. In: DENOIX P: Mechanisms of invasion in cancer. UICC Monography, vol 6. Springer, Berlin - Heidelberg - New York
HANSEN D, ARNDT HJ (1965): Das extramedulläre Plasmocytom. HNO 13: 306-308
HARRIS HH (1961): Rhabdomyosarcoma of the larynx. Report of a case. Arch Otolaryngol 74: 205-209
HART C, MAYER E (1928): Kehlkopf, Luftröhre und Bronchien. In: HENKE F, LUBARSCH O (eds), Handbuch der Speziellen Pathologischen Anatomie und Histologie, vol III.1, pp 288-530. Springer, Berlin
HEADINGTON JT (1978): Verrucous carinoma. Cutis 21: 207-211
HELLQUIST H, OLOFSSON J, GRÖNTOFT O (1979): Chondrosarcoma of the larynx. J Laryngol Otol 93: 1037-1047
HIGAZI MT (1979): Primary oat cell carcinoma of the larynx. J Laryngol Otol 93: 835-837

HOLINGER PH, JOHNSTON KC, ANISON GC (1950): Papilloma of the larynx. A review of 109 cases with a preliminary report of Aureomycin therapy. Ann Otol Rhinol Laryngol 59: 547-564

HOMMERICH CHP (1985): Zur Frage der primären Adenokarzinome des Larynx. Laryngol Rhinol Otol 64: 25-31

HOOD AF, MARK GJ, HUNT JV (1979): Laryngeal mycosis fungoides. Cancer 43: 1527-1532

HORN RC, ENTERLEIN HT (1958): Rhabdomyosarcoma - Clinical pathological study, classification of 39 cases. Cancer 2: 181-199

HUIZENGA CH, BALOGH K (1970): Cartilaginous tumors of the larynx. A clinicopathologic study of 10 cases and a review of the literature. Cancer 26: 201-210

HYAMS VJ (1976): Discussion to Biller HF, Bergman JA. In: ALBERTI PW, BRYCE DP (eds) Centennial Conference on Laryngeal Cancer. Appleton-Century-Crofts, New York. p 464

IWASAWA T, FUNASAKA S, ABE H (1978): A case of laryngeal rhabdomyosarcoma. Nippon Jibiinkoka Gakkai Kaiho 81: 437-447

IWASZKIEWICZ J, KAMIENIEC M (1966): Sarcomatous neurofibroma of the larynx. Otolaryngol Pol 20: 541-542

JACOBSON S, SHEAR M (1972): Verrucous carcinoma of the mouth. J Oral Pathol 1: 66-75

JOHNSTON KC (1957): Fibrosarcoma of the larynx. Laryngoscope 67: 1194-1207

JOSIPESCU A, MANOLESCU N (1965): About some rare localizations of cylindroma (Rom) Otorinolaring (Buc) 10: 63

KAHLER O (1908): Ein Karzinosarkom des Recessus piriformis bei Ekchondrose des Ringknorpels. Dtsch Med Wschr 34: 614-647

KAMADASS T (1984): Malignant pleomorphic fibrous histiocytoma of the larynx. J Laryngol Otol 98: 93-96

KAO GF, GRAHAM JH, HELWIG EB (1982): Carcinoma cuniculatum verrucous carcinoma of the skin. A clinicopathologic study of 46 cases with ultrastructural observations. Cancer 49: 2395-2403

KATHOLM M, KROGDAHL A, HAINAU B, BRETLAU P (1984): Spindle cell carcinoma of the larynx. Acta Otolaryngol (Stockh) 16: 163-166

KAWABE Y, KONDO T (1967): Laryngeal leiomyosarcoma. Evaluation of the authors case and observation of the literature. Otolaryngol 39: 427-443

KIM H (1982): Primary malignant laryngeal melanoma. Yonsei Med J 23: 118-122

KIM H, PARK CI (1982): Primary malignant laryngeal melanoma. Yonsei Med J 23: 118-122

KIMMELMAN CP (1983): Small cell carcinomas. Otolaryngol Head Neck Surg 91: 708-712

KLEINSASSER O (1958): Über die gut- und bösartigen Formen der Kehlkopfpapillome und deren histologisches und klinisches Bild. Arch Otorhinolaryngol 171: 44-69

KLEINSASSER O (1961): Kritische Betrachtung der Behandlungsergebnisse bei 410 Kehlkopfkarzinomen unter besonderer Berücksichtigung der Indikation zur Radical Neck Dissection. Laryngol Rhinol Otol 40: 652-674

KLEINSASSER O (1983): Bösartige Geschwülste des Kehlkopfes und des Hypopharynx. In: BERENDES J, LINK R, ZÖLLNER F (eds) Hals-Nasen-Ohrenheilkunde in Praxis und Klinik. Thieme, Stuttgart - New York; vol 4.2, Kehlkopf II

KLEINSASSER O, GLANZ H (1978): Sarkomähnliche Gewebsbilder in Larynxkarzinomen (Pseudosarkome, Karzinosarkome, Spindelzellkarzinome, pleomorphe Karzinome). Laryngol Rhinol Otol 57: 225-234

KLEINSASSER O, GLANZ H (1979): Myogenic Tumours of the Larynx. Arch Otorhinolaryngol 225: 107-119

KLEINSASSER O, SEBASTIAN B (1985): Einbruch von Schilddrüsentumoren in Larynx und Trachea. Laryngol Rhinol Otol 64: 128-132

KOEHN K (1969): Nase und Nasennebenhöhlen, Kehlkopf und Luftröhre. In: DOERR W, SEIFERT G, UEHLINGER E; Spezielle pathologische Anatomie; vol 4. Springer, Berlin - Heidelberg - New York

KOGELNIK HD (1977): Über die Häufigkeit von Zweittumoren nach chirurgischer und strahlentherapeutischer Behandlung. Strahlentherapie 153: 163-167

KOMORN RM, FECHNER RE, ALFORD BR el al (1973): Simultaneous squamous carcinoma and adenocarcinoma of the larynx. Arch Otolaryngol 97: 420-422

KRAJINA Z (1976): Laryngeal sarcoma. In: ALBERTI PW, BRYCE DP (eds) Centennial Conference on Laryngeal Cancer. Appleton-Century-Crofts, New York, p 485-487

KRATZ R, RITTERHOFFER (1961): Sarcoma of the larynx. Ann Otol Rhinol Laryngol 70: 239-250

KRAUSEN AS, GALL AM, GARZA R, SPECTOR GJ, ANSEL DG (1977): Liposarcoma of the larynx: a multicentric or a metastatic malignancy. Laryngoscope 87: 1116-1124

KRAUS FT, PEREZ-MESA C (1966): Verrucous carcinoma. Clinical and pathologic study of 105 cases involving oral cavity, larynx and genitalia. Cancer 19: 26-38

KÜPPER K (1976): Radiogenes Sarkom im Bereich der Schilddrüse. HNO 24: 89-93

KÜPPER K, BLESSING MH (1974): Carcinosarcoma of the larynx. HNO 22: 103-107

LACHMANN I (1951): Sarcoma of the larynx. Arch Otolaryngol 53: 299-307

LAGACE R, SCHURCH W, SEEMAYER TA (1981): Polypoid pseudosarcomatous carcinoma. Histogenesis with evidence of myofibroblastic response. Ann Pathol 1: 27-37

LAMBERT PR, WARD PH, BERCI G (1980): Pseudosarcoma of the larynx. A comprehensive analysis. Arch Otolaryngol 106: 700-708

LANE N (1957): Pseudosarcoma (Polypoid sarcoma-like masses) associated with squamous cell carcinoma of the mouth, fauces and larynx. Cancer 10: 19-41

LASSER KH, NAEIM F, HIGGINS J, COVE H, WAISMAN J (1979): "Pseudosarcoma" of the larynx. Am J Surg Pathol 3: 397-404

LAUTZ HA (1958): Nasal and laryngeal involvement in abdominal Hodgkin's disease. Arch Otolaryngol 67: 78-80

LAWSON SA, SOM M (1975): Second primary cancer after irradiation of laryngeal cancer. Ann Otol Rhinol Laryngol 84: 771-775

LEDRAZZINI A (1983): A case of metastasizing paraganglioma of the larynx. Schweiz Med Wochenschr 113: 1363-1366

LENNERT K (1981): Histopathology of non-Hodgkin's lymphomas (based on the Kiel classification). Springer, Berlin - Heidelberg - New York

LEUSZLER RW, SHAPSHAY SM, STRONG M (1981): Laryngeal pseudosarcoma. Otolaryngol Head Neck Surg 89: 210

LEVENTON GS, EVANS HL (1981): Sarcomatoid squamous cell carcinoma of the mucous membranes of the head and neck: a clinicopathologic study of 20 cases. Cancer 48: 994-1003

LICHTENSTEIN L, JAFFE H (1943): Chondrosarcoma of bone. Am J Pathol 19: 553-589

LICHTIGER B, MACKAY B, TESSMER CF (1970): Spindle cell variant of squamous carcinoma: a light and electron microscopic study of 13 cases. Cancer 26: 1311-1320

LINK R (1949): Chondroma and chondrosarcoma of the larynx. Ann Otol Rhinol Laryngol 58: 70-85

LORENTZ E (1979): Malignant melanoma of the larynx. HNO 27: 275-277

LUND V, SAWYER R, PAPAVASILIOM A (1982): Second respiratory tract carcinomas following radiotherapy to the larynx. Clin Oncol 8: 201-206

MAJOROS M, PARKHILL EM, DEVINE KD (1964): Papilloma in the larynx in children. Am J Surg 108: 470-475

MALLONEE MS (1979): Adenocarcinoma of the larynx. Ear Nose Throat J 58: 115-118

MARKEL SF, MAGIELSKI JE, BEALS TF (1980): Carcinoid tumor of the larynx. Arch Otolaryngol 106: 777-778

MASON DA (1972): Verrucous carcinoma of the mouth. Br J Oral Maxillofac Surg 10: 64-68

MAW AR, CULLEN RJ, BRADFIELD JWB (1982): Verrucous carcinoma of the larynx. Clin Otolaryngol 7: 305-311

MCCLURE BL (1984): Verrucous carinoma. J Otolaryngol 13: 7-12

MCDONALD JR, HAVENS FZ (1948): A study of malignant tumors of glandular nature found in the nose, throat and mouth. Surg Clin N Am 28: 1087-1106

MCDONALD JS, CRISSMAN JD, GLUCKMANN JL (1982): Verrucous carcinoma of the oral cavity. Head Neck Surg 5: 22-28

MCINTOSH WA, KASSNER GW, MURRAY JF (1985): Fibromatosis and fibrosarcoma of the larynx and pharynx in an infant. Arch Otolaryngol 111: 478-480

MCKEE PH, WILKINSON JD, CORBETT MF, DAVEY A, SAUVEN P, BLACK MM (1981): Carcinoma cuniculatum: a case metastasizing to skin and lymph nodes. Clin Exp Dermatol 6: 613-618

MCKEE PH, WILKINSON JD, BLACK MM, WHIMSTER IW (1981): Carcinoma (epithelioma) cuniculatum: a clinicopathological study of nineteen cases and review of the literature. Histopathology 5: 425-436

MEDINA JE, DICHTEL W, LUNA MA (1984): Verrucous-squamous carcinomas of the oral cavity. Arch Otolaryngol 110: 437-440

MEDINA JE, MORAN M, GOEPFERT H (1984): Oat cell carcinoma of the larynx and Eaton-Lambert syndrome. Arch Otolaryngol 110: 123-126

MERTENS J, GRIESSER GH, KAISERLING E, RUDERT H (1986): Papilläres Adenokarzinom des Stimmbandes - der erste Fall in der Literatur. HNO 34: 81-84

MEYER-BRETING E, ROSEMANN G (1977): Über seltene Malignome des Larynx. Gemeins Herbsttagung der Österr, Süddtsch und Wiener Ges der HNO-Ärzte. Salzburg

MEYER-BREITING P (1981): Katamnestische Untersuchungsergebnisse zur radiochirurgischen Kombinationstherapie fortgeschrittener innerer und äußerer Kehlkopfkarzinome. Inauguraldissertation, Frankfurt am Main

MEYER-BREITING E (1975): Lymphogranulomatose des Kehlkopfes. Laryngol Rhinol Otol 54: 897-904

MICHAELS L (1984): Pathology of the larynx. Springer, Berlin - Heidelberg - New York - Tokyo

MICHEAU C, LUBOINSKI B, SANCHO H, CACHIN Y (1976): Modes of invasion of cancer of the larynx. Cancer 38: 346-360

MICHEAU C, LUBOINSKI B, SCHWAAB G, RICHARD J, CACHIN Y (1979): Lymphoepitheliomas of the larynx (undifferentiated carcinomas of nasopharyngeal type). Clin Otolaryngol 4: 43-48

MILLER D (1950): Fibrosarcoma of the larynx. Report of a case in a child. Ann Otol Rhinol Laryngol 59: 246-253

MILLER D, GOODMAN M, WEBER A, GOLDSTEIN A (1975): Primary liposarcoma of the larynx. Trans Am Acad Ophthalmol Otolaryngol 80: 444-447

MILLS SE, JOHNS ME (1984): Atypical carcinoid tumor of the larynx. A light microscopic and ultrastructural study. Arch Otolaryngol 110: 58-62

MINCKLER DS, MELIGRO CH, NORRIS HT (1970): Carcino-Sarcoma of the larynx. Case-report with metastases of epidermoid and sarcomatous elements. Cancer 26: 195-200

MOHR RM, HUSSAIN M (1981): Extended vertical frontolateral laryngectomy for a low-grade chondrosarcoma. Otolaryngol Head Neck Surg 89: 213

MOHR W, PIRSIG W (1984): Synoviales Sarkom des Larynx. Laryngol Rhinol Otol 63: 453-456

MOHS FE, SAHL WJ (1979): Chemosurgery for verrucous carcinoma. J Dermatol Surg Oncol 5: 302-306

MORITSCH E, JARISCH R, KONRAD K (1978): Morbus Kaposi. Pharyngolaryngeale Manifestation, Therapie. Laryngol Rhinol Otol 57: 792-796

MORLEY AR, CAMERON DS, WATSON AJ (1973): Osteosarcoma of the larynx. J Laryngol Otol 87: 997-1005

MURRAY JF, LOTHE F (1962): The histopathology of Kaposi's sarcoma. Acta Int Congress 18: 413-428

MYEROWITZ RL, BARNES EL, MYERS E (1978): Small cell anaplastic (oat cell) carcinoma of the larynx: report of a case and review of the literature. Laryngoscope 88: 1697-1702

NABAR BV (1968): Plasmacytoma of the upper respiratory tract. J Laryngol Otol 82: 657-664

NEEL BH, UNNI KK (1982): Cartilaginous tumors of the larynx: A series of 33 patients. Otolaryngol Head Neck Surg 90: 201-207

NEW GB (1935): Sarcoma of the larynx. Report of two cases. Arch Otolaryngol 21: 648-652

NEW GB, ERICH JB (1941): Adenocarcinoma of the larynx. Ann Otol Rhinol Laryngol 50: 706-714

NONOMURA A (1983): Primary carcinoid tumor of the larynx. Acta Pathol Jpn 33: 1041-1049

NORRIS CM, PEALE AR (1961): Sarcoma of the larynx. Ann Otol Rhinol Laryngol 70: 894-909

VAN NOSTRAND AWP, OLOFSSON J (1972): Verrucous carcinoma of the larynx. A clinical and pathologic study of ten cases. Cancer 30: 691-702

ÖSTBERG Y, BOQUIST L, DIAMANT H (1979): Laryngeal chondrosarcoma in Sweden. Acta Otolaryngol (Stockh) 88: 142-147

OHSAWA M (1973): Malignant chemodectoma. Acta Pathol Jpn 33: 1279-1288

OLOFSSON J, VAN NOSTRAND AWP (1977): Adnoid cystic carcinoma of the larynx. A report of four cases and a review of the literature. Cancer 40: 1307-1313

OTTE T, KLEINSASSER O (1981): Liposarcoma of the head and neck. Arch Otorhinolaryngol 232: 285-291

PAGES A (1983): Carcinoid tumor of the larynx. Ann Pathol 3: 59-64

PAHOR AL (1978): Plasmacytoma of the larynx. J Laryngol Otol 92: 223-232

PALADUGU RR, NATHWEIN BN, GOODSTEIN J, BARDI LE, MEMOLI VE, GOULD VE (1982): Carcinoma of the larynx with mucosubstance-production and neuroendocrine differentiation. An ultrastructural and immunohistochemical study. Cancer 49: 343-349

PEDRAZZINI A, PEDRINIS E, LUSCIETI P, LOSA G, CAVALLI F (1983): Ein Fall von metastasierendem Paragangliom des Larynx. Schweiz Med Wochenschr 113: 1363-1366

PERILLI M, BAGNARIOL V (1969): I fibrosarcomi della laringe (contributo clinico-statistico sulla base di cinque osservazioni personali). Arch Ital Otol 80: 31-41

PORTMANN G (1964): Le plasmocytome du larynx. Rev Laryngol Otol Rhinol (Bord) 85: 1-9

PRIOLEAU PG, SANTA CRUZ DJ, MEYER JS, BAUER WC (1980): Verrucous carcinoma. A light and electron microscopic, autoradiographic, and immunofluorescence study. Cancer 45: 2849-2857

QUICK D, CUTLER M (1927): Transitional cell epidermoid carcinoma. Surg Gynec Obstet 45: 320-331

QUINN FB jr, MCCABE BF (1957): Laryngeal metastases from malignant tumors in distant organs. Ann Otol Rhinol Laryngol 66: 139-143

RAMADASS T, BALASUBRAMANIAM CVC, ANNAMALIA L (1984): Malignant pleomorphic fibrous histiocytoma of the larynx. J Laryngol Otol 98: 93-96

RANDALL G, ALONSO WA, OGURA JH (1975): Spindle cell carcinoma (pseudosarcoma) of the larynx. Arch Otolaryngol 101: 63-66

RASINGER G, ULRICH W (1983): Adenocarcinoma of the larynx as a recurrence. Laryngol Rhinol Otol 62: 363-365

RATZENHOFER M (1978): Karzinosarkom und Karzinom. Analogien und Unterschiede. Das primäre und das sekundäre Stroma im Karzinosarkom und Karzinom. Verh Dtsch Ges Pathol 62: 380

RATZENHOFER E (1982): Epithelioma cuniculatum: eine Sonderform eines verrukösen Karzinoms. Wien Klin Wochenschr 94: 118-120

REBOUL J, DELORME G, LUGAGNE J (1956): Localisation endocavitaires trachéobronchiques de la maladie de Hodgkin. Rev Laryngol Otol Rhinol (Bord) 77: 233

RECHER G (1985): Spindle cell squamous carcinoma of the larynx; clinico-pathological study of seven cases. J Laryngol Otol 99: 871-879

REGAUD C (1921): Lymphoépithéliome de l'hypopharynx traité par la roentgenthérapie. Bull Soc Fr Otorhinolaryngol 34: 209-214

REICH H (1982): Verruköses Karzinom. Z Hautkr 57: 1128-1136

REMAGEN W (1983): Osteosarcoma of the larynx. HNO 31: 366-368

REMAGEN W, LÖHR J, VON WESTERNHAGEN B (1983): Osteosarkom des Kehlkopfes. HNO 31: 366-368

REUTER VE, WOODRUFF JM (1986): Melanoma of the larynx. Laryngoscope 94: 389-393

RICHARDSON MA, KREUTNER AM, PUTNEY FJ, CLAIRMONT AA (1978): Carcinosarkoma and associated squamous cell carcinoma of the larynx. South Med J 71: 1034

RIDER WD (1976): Toronto experience of verrucous carcinoma of the larynx. In: ALBERTI PW, BRYCE DP (eds) Centennial Conference on Laryngeal Cancer; pp 460-461. Appleton-Century-Crofts, New York

RIGBY RC, HOLLINGER PA (1943): Fibrosarcoma of the larynx in an infant. Arch Otolaryngol 37: 421-428

ROHNER Y, WEY W (1977): Zur Diagnose und Therapie extramedullärer Plasmocytome. Arch Otorhinolaryngol 214: 263-270

SABRI JA, HAJJAR MA (1967): Malignant mixed tumor of the vocal cord, report of a case. Arch Otolaryngol 85: 332-334

SCEVOLA A (1968): Patologia rara della laringe: il plasmocitoma. Ann Laringol (Torino) 67: 638

SCHIMPF A, MÜSEBECK K, MOOTZ W (1969): Naevuszellnaevus (compound naevus) im Larynxbereich (Plica ventricularis). Z Hautkr 44: 137-144

SCHMIDT-BÄUMLER U, RUPP W (1975): Karzinosarkom des Stimmbandes. Laryngol Rhinol Otol 54: 772-777

SCHMINCKE A (1921): Über lymphoepitheliale Geschwülste. Beitr Pathol Anat 68: 161-170

SCHWADE JG, WARA WM, DEDO HH, PHILIPPS TL (1976): Radiotherapy of verrucous carcinoma. Radiology 120: 677-679

SEEHAFER JR, RAHAMAN D, SODERSTROM CW (1979): Epithelioma cuniculatum, verrucous carcinoma of the foot. Cutis 23: 287-290

SENIUKOV MV, ZUBOV OG (1979): Thrombosis of internal jugular veins in a patient with cancer of the larynx. Zh Ushn Nos Gorl Bolezn 3: 81-83

SEO IS, WARFEL KA, TOMICH CE, HULL MT (1980): Clear cell carcinoma of the larynx. A variant of mucoepidermoid carcinoma. Ann Otol Rhinol Laryngol 89: 168-172

SHAFER WG, HINE MK, LEVY BM (1983): A textbook of oral pathology. Saunders, Philadelphia-London

SHANMUGARATNAM K, SOBIN LH (1978): Histological typing of upper respiratory tract tumors. International histological classification of tumors, No. 19. WHO, Geneva

SHEAR M, PINDBORG JJ (1980): Verrucous hyperplasia of the oral mucosa. Cancer 46: 1855-1862

SIROTA HH, HURWITZ A (1952): Chondrosarcoma of the larynx. Arch Otolaryngol 56: 290-293

SLOOTWEG PJ, MÜLLER H (1983): Verrucous hyperplasia or verrucous carcinoma. An analysis of 27 patients. J Maxillofac Surg 11: 13-19

SMITH RRL, KUHAJDA FP, HARRIS AE (1985): Anaplastic transformation of verrucous carcinoma following radiotherapy. Am J Otolaryngol 6: 448-452

SPENCER MG, ELLIOTT RIK, WADSWORTH PV, DEUTSCH GP (1983): Pseudosarcoma of the pharynx and larynx. J Laryngol Otol 97: 85-91

SQUIRES JE, MILLS SE, COOPER PH, INNES DJ, MCLEAN WC (1981): Acinic cell carcinoma: its occurrence in the laryngotracheal junction after thyroid radiation. Arch Pathol Lab Med 105: 266-268

SRINIVASAN U, TALVALKAR GV (1979): True carcinosarcoma of the larynx: a case report. J Laryngol Otol 93: 1031-1035

STANKIEWICZ C, POPIEL L (1979): Rhabdomyosarcomas of the head and neck. Pol Tyg Lek 34: 1077-1079

STANLEY RJ, WEILAND LH, DESANTO LW, NEEL HB (1985): Lymphoepithelioma (undifferentiated carcinoma) of the laryngohypopharynx. Laryngoscope 95: 1077-1081

STANLEY RJ, DESANTO LW, WEILAND LH (1986): Oncocytic and oncocytoid carcinoid tumours (well-differentiated neuroendocrine carcinomas) of the larynx. Arch Otolaryngol 112: 529-535

STILLWAGON GB, SMITH RRL, HIGHSTEIN Ch, LEE D-J (1985): Adenoid cystic carcinoma of the supraglottic larynx. Am J Otolaryngol 6: 309-314

SUCCAVA I, SIMU G (1972): Sarcome du larynx. Ann Otolaryngol Chir Cervicofac 89: 137-140

SUEHS OW (1960): Cylindroma (adenoid cystic carcinoma) of the larynx and trachea. Texas State J Med 56: 934-944

SWERDLOW JB, MERL SA, DAVEY FR, GACE RR, GOTTLIEB A (1984): Non-Hodgkin's lymphoma limited to the larynx. Cancer 53: 2546-2549

TAMAI S, IRI H, MARUYAMA T, KASAHARA M, AKATSUKA S, SAKURAI S, MURAKAMI Y (1981): Laryngeal carcinoid tumor: light and electron microscopic studies. Cancer 48: 2256-2259

TANTURRI D (1927): Linfogranulomatosi maligna primitiva della trachea e vie superiori del respire. Rass Ital Otorinolaringol 1: 245

TAN C, ROSEN G, GHAVINI F (1975): Adriamycin (NSC-123127) in pediatric malignancies. Cancer Chemother Rep 6: 259-266

TAYLOR RF (1977): Late recurrence of cancer in the larynx and hypopharynx after irradiation. Orl 39: 251-256

THOMAS K (1971): Mucoepidermoid carcinoma of the larynx. J Laryngol Otol 85: 261-267

THOMPSON DH, KAO YH, KLOS J, FAY J, FETTER TW (1982): Primary small cell (oat cell) carcinoma of the larynx. Associated with an IgD multiple myeloma. Laryngoscope 92: 1239-1244

TOBEY DN, WHEELS RF, YARINGTON CT jr (1979): Electron microscopy in the diagnosis of liposarcoma and fibrosarcoma of the larynx. Ann Otol Rhinol Laryngol 88: 867-871

TOKER C, PETERSON DW (1978): Lymphoepithelioma of the vocal cord. Arch Otolaryngol 104: 161-162

TOM LW, WURZEL JM, WETMORE RF, LOWRY LD (1981): Mucoepidermoid carcinoma of the hypopharynx. Otolaryngol Head Neck Surg 89: 753-757

TOOMEY JM (1967): Adenocarcinoma of the larynx. Laryngoscope 77: 931-961

TRAVIS LW, SUTHERLAND C (1980): Coexisting lentigo of the larynx and melanoma of the oral cavity: report of a case. Otolaryngol Head Neck Surg 88: 218-220

ULLMANN H (1922): Ein echtes Karzinosarkom des Kehlkopfes. Z Hals-Nasen-Ohrenheilk 1: 130-147

UNGERECHT K (1951): Multiple Chondrome und Chondrosarkome des Larynx und der Trachea mit chondromyxosarkomatösen Rezidiven. Arch Otorhinolaryngol 160: 158-169

UNGERECHT K (1965): Das Zylindrom der Zunge. HNO 13: 185-197

VAN DISHOECK HAE (1968): Malignant tumors in the Leiden Ear-Nose-Throat-Clinic. Pract Otorhinolaryngol 30: 248-250

VELEK JP (1976): Liposarcoma of the larynx. Trans Am Acad Ophthalmol Otolaryngol 82: 569-570

VERHEST A, JORTAY A (1968): Carcinosarcome. Un cas d' épithélioma Malpighien du sinus piriforme accompagné d'une réaction pseudo-sarcomateuse du stroma. Bull Cancer (Paris) 55/3: 429-437

VLODYKA J (1962): The cancerogenic effect of x-ray on the larynx. Arch Otolaryngol 76: 372-376

VOLMER J (1985): Malignes fibröses Histiozytom des Larynx. Laryngol Rhinol Otol 64: 579-581

VON EICKEN C (1934): Larynxkarzinom nach alter Röntgenschädigung. Zentralbl Hals-Nasen-Ohrenheilk 21: 71

VYSLONZIL E (1956): Sarkom des Kehlkopfes. Monatsschr Ohrenheilkd 90: 246-247

WALLNER KE, LEIBEL StA, WARA (1985): Squamous cell carcinoma of the head and neck after radiation therapy for Hodgkin's disease. Cancer 56: 1052-1055

WALSH TE, BEAMER PR (1950): Epidermoid carcinoma of the larynx occuring in two children with papilloma of larynx. Laryngoscope 60: 1110-1124

WALTHER H (1962): Das Karzinosarkom des Larynx. Z Ärztl Fortbild (Jena) 56: 1171-1172

WATANABE S, OHATA T, KOBAYASHI T (1978): Reticulum cell carcinoma occurring primarily in the head and neck tumor. Soc Head Neck Tumor, Nagoya

WEBER AL, SHORTSLEEVE M, GOODMAN M, MONTGOMERY W, GRILLO HC (1978): Cartilaginous tumors of the larynx and trachea. Radiol Clin North Am 16: 261-271

WEIDAUER H, BLOBEL GA, NEMETSCHEK-GANSLER H, GOULD VE, MALL G (1985): Das neuro-endokrine Larynxkarzinom vom kleinzelligen (Oat-Cell) Typ. Laryngol Rhinol Otol 64: 121-127

WHICKER JH, CARDER GA, DEVINE KD (1972): Metastasis of the larynx. Report of a case and review of literature. Arch Otolaryngol 96: 182-184

WHICKER JH, NEEL B, WEILAND LH, DEVINE KD (1974): Adenocarcinoma of the larynx. Ann Otol Rhinol Laryngol 83: 487-490

WILBUR JR, SUTOW WW, SULLIVAN MP et al (1975): Chemotherapy of sarcomas. Cancer 36: 765-769

WILHELM HJ, DIETZ R, SCHÖNDORF J (1980): Diagnostik und Therapie seltener Tumoren im Larynx-Pharynx-Bereich. Laryngol Rhinol Otol 59: 137-143

WILTSHAW E (1976): The natural history of extramedullary plasmacytoma and its relation to solitary myeloma of bone and myelomatosis. Medicine (Baltimore) 55: 217-238

WINTHER LK, LORENTZEN M (1978): Rhabdomyosarcoma of the larynx. Report of two cases and a review of the literature. J Laryngol Otol 92: 417-424

WOLFOWITZ BL, SCHMAMANN A (1973): Smoothmuscle tumors of the upper respiratory tract. S Afr Med J 47: 1189-1191

WOODS GL, ESPINOZA CG, AZAR HA (1982): Carcinomas with spindle cell (sarcomatoid) component: an immunocytochemical and electron microscopic study. Meeting abstract of 71st Annual Meeting of the Intern Academy of Pathology; p 95. International Academy of Pathology, Boston

ZEIDLER R (1929): Lymphogranulomatose der oberen Luftwege. Monatsschr Ohrenheilkd 62: 604

References

8 Pseudotumours of Larynx

AVELLIS (1891): Tuberkulöse Larynxgeschwülste. Dtsch Med Wochenschr 973: 993

BARNES EL, ZAFAR T (1977): Laryngeal amyloidosis; clinicopathologic study of seven cases. Ann Otol Rhinol Laryngol 86: 856-863

BAUER E (1951): Über lokale Schäden nach Intubationsnarkose. Mschr Ohrenheilk 85: 108

BECKMANN G (1963): Akute und chronische Entzündungen des Kehlkopfes (mit Tuberkulose). In: BERENDES J, LINK R, ZÖLLNER F (eds), Hals-Nasen-Ohrenheilkunde, vol II.2, pp 851-930. Thieme, Stuttgart

BECKMANN G (1982): Akute und chronische Entzündungen des Kehlkopfes (mit Tuberkulose). In: BERENDES J, LINK R, ZÖLLNER F (eds), Hals-Nasen-Ohrenheilkunde in Praxis und Klinik; vol 4,1 Thieme, Stuttgart - New York

BOEHME G, ROSSE E (1969): Zur Häufigkeit, Altersverteilung, Therapie und Prognose von Stimmlippenknötchen. Folia phoniat (Basel) 21: 121-128

BOUCHAYER M, CORNUT G, LOIRE R, WITZIG E, ROCH JB (1985): Epidermoid cysts, sulci, and mucosal bridges of the true vocal cord: a report of 157 cases. Laryngoscope 95: 1087-1094

CHAMBERLAIN D (1970): Congenital subglottic cyst of the larynx. Laryngoscope 80: 254-259

CHÜDEN H, KOCHEM HG, NEUSSEL H, WEHMER W (1970): Über einen Fall von Sklerom. HNO 18: 276-279

CLAUSEN J (1932): Unsual sequela tracheal intubation. Proc roy Soc Med 25: 1507

COHEN AS, WEGELIUS O (1980): Classification of Amyloid: 1979-1980. Arthritis Rheum 23: 644-645

COPPO E (1935): Contributo anatomo-clinicomallo studio dei tumori tubercolari della laringe. Granuloma tubercolare laringeo gigante. Ann Laringol (Torino) 35: 63

CRIFO S (1973): Laryngeal idiopathic amyloidosis. ORL 35: 117-126

DENECKE HJ (1947): Zur Behandlung der kongenitalen Larynxcyste. HNO 1: 175

DEVINE KD (1965): Sarcoidosis and sarcoidosis of the larynx. Laryngoscope 75: 533-569

DOERING L (1973): Larynxzyste bei einem Neugeborenen. Monatsschr Kinderheilkd 121: 684-685

ELIACHAR J, LICHTIG C (1970): Local amyloid deposits of the larynx; electron microscopic studies of three cases. Arch Otolaryngol 92: 163-166

EMAMI-NOURI M (1977): Amyloidtumor im Larynx. Laryngol Rhinol Otol 56: 996-998

EPSTEIN SS, WINSTON P, FRIEDMANN J, ORMEROD FC (1957): The vocal cord polyp. J Laryngol Otol 71: 673-688

FALK P (1936): Über ortsfremde gutartige Gewebsbildungen. Arch Otorhinolaryngol 141: 118-132

FERNANDES CMC, PIRIE D, PUDIFIN DJ (1982): Laryngeal amyloidosis. J Laryngol Otol 96: 1165-1175

FRENZEL H, KLEINSASSER O, HORT W (1980): Light and electron microscopic observations on polyps of human vocal cords. Virchows Arch(A) 389: 189-204

FRENZEL H, SCHMITT-GRÄFF A, SEITZ RJ (1985): An immunohistochemical and electron-microscopic study of vascular endothelial cells in vocal fold polyps. Arch Otorhinolaryngol 241: 271-278

FRIEDMAN BA (1975): Rheumatoid nodules of the larynx. Arch Otolaryngol 102: 361-363

FRIEDMANN I (1976): Sarcomas of the larynx. In: ALBERTI PW, BRYCE DP (eds), pp 122-126. Centennial Conference on Laryngeal Cancer. Appleton-Century-Crofts, New York

GERTLER R, RAMAGES L (1985): Tuberculous laryngitis - a one year harvest. J Laryngol Otol 99: 1119-1125

GIANNI O (1933): Fibrotuberculoma della laringe. Valsalva 9: 450

GILMAN RH, KARMODY CS, FRIED MP, SPETH R (1982): Gigantic obstructing laryngeal polyp. J Laryngol Otol 96: 167-172

HAAS E (1967): Zur Genese der intralaryngealen Struma. Laryngol Rhinol Otol 46: 229-232

HAGUENAUER JP, GAILLARD J, DUFLOT C (1976): Pseudo-tumeur amyloide laryngo-trachéeale. J Fr Otorhinolaryngol 25: 233

HOFER G (1928): Die entzündlichen Erkrankungen der Luftröhre und der Bronchien. In: DENKER A, KAHLER O (eds), Handbuch der Hals-Nasen-Ohrenheilkunde; vol III. Springer, Berlin

HOMMERICH KW (1952): Über seröse Mesaortitis. Zugleich ein Beitrag zur Frage spontaner Aortenrupturen und ihrer Ursachen. Virchows Arch(A) 322, 282

HOWLAND W, LEWEIS S (1956): Mechanism in the development of post intubation granuloma. Ann Otol Rhinol Laryngol 65: 1006

KAMBIC CV, RADSEL Z, ZARGI M, ACKO M (1981): Vocal cord polyps: incidence, histology and pathogenesis. J Laryngol Otol 95: 609-618

KEEN M, CHO HT, SAVETSKY L (1986): Pseudotumor of the Larynx - an unusual cause of airway obstruction. Otolaryngol Head Neck Surg 94: 243-246

KHEIR SM, FLINT A, MOSS JA (1983): Primary aspergillosis of the larynx simulating carcinoma. Hum Pathol 14: 184-186

KLEIN P (1967): Die intratracheale Struma. In: Hals-Nasen- und Ohrenheilkunde, H. 18. Barth, Leipzig

KLEINSASSER O (1977): Histopathogenese der Stimmlippenpolypen. Arch Otorhinolaryng 216: 626

KLEINSASSER O (1982): Pathogenesis of vocal cord polyps. Ann Otol Rhinol Laryngol 91: 378-381

KLUMPP W (1938): Die Pathologie der sog. Sängerknötchen und Stimmbandpolypen. Inauguraldissertation, Tübingen

KÖHN K (1969): Zur Pathologie der gutartigen Stimmbandprozesse. HNO 8, 71

LAHOVARY A, REDLI M, BURKHARDT A (1986): La tuberculose du larynx aujourd'hui. Méd et Hyg 44: 2940-2944

LEROUX-ROBERT J (1962): Tumeurs amyloides du larynx. Ann Otolaryngol Chir Cervicofac 79: 249

MALAN (1933): Riesentuberkulom des Kehlkopfes. Arch ital Otol 44, 15

MANASSE P (1927): Anatomische Untersuchungen über die Tuberkulose der oberen Luftwege. Beih Beitr Klin Tuberk Berlin, Springer

MATZKER J (1953): Larynxschäden durch Intubationsnarkose. Z Laryngol Rhinol Otol 32: 563-568

MATZKER J (1957): Über große Zysten und Zellen des Larynxeinganges und seiner Umgebung. Laryngol Rhinol Otol 36, 318-329

MICHAELS L (1984): Pathology of the larynx. Springer, Berlin - Heidelberg - New York - Tokyo

MONDAY LA, CORNUT G, BOUCHAYER M, ROCH JB (1983): Epidermoid cysts of the vocal cords. Ann Otol Rhinol Laryngol 92, 124-127

NAGATA K, KURITA S, YASUMOTO S, MAEDA T, KAWASAKI H, HIRANO M (1983): Vocal fold polyps and nodules. A 10-year review of 1156 patients. Auris Nasus Larynx 10, 27-35

OLTERSDORF U (1949): Beitrag zur Genese der intralaryngotrachealen Strumen. Arch Otorhinolaryngol 157, 12-27

PAYNE J, KOOPMANN CF (1984): Laryngeal carcinoma - or is it laryngeal blastomycosis? Laryngoscope 94, 608-611

RANDOLPH J, GRUNT J, VAWTER GF (1963): The medical and surgical aspects of intratracheal goiter. N Engl J Med 268: 457-465

RAUCHFUSS A (1983): Die Fibroxanthomatose des Kehlkopfes. Laryngol Rhinol Otol 62, 33-34

RICHARDSON GM, ASSOR D (1971): Thyroid tissue within the larynx; case report. Laryngoscope 81, 120-125

ROESSLE R (1944): Seröse Entzündung. Verh Dtsch Ges Pathol (Breslau)

SCHAUER A, HERRMANN J, FISTERER H (1973): Zytologische Untersuchungen zur Erkennung praeneoplastischer und neoplastischer Larynxveränderungen. Verh Dtsch Ges Pathol 57, 370-373

STEINBERG D (1969): Die Struma intratrachealis. HNO 17, 139-147

TILLMANN B, WUSTROW D (1982): Kehlkopf. In: BERENDES J, LINK R, ZÖLLNER F (eds), Hals-Nasen-Ohrenheilkunde in Praxis und Klinik; 2nd edn, vol 4,1. Thieme, Stuttgart - New York

TRAUTMANN G (1902): Tuberkulöse Larynxtumoren. Arch Otorhinolaryngol 12, 26

ZIEGELMAN (1932): Tuberculoma of the laryngeal ventricel resembling prolaps of the mucous membrane. Arch Otolaryngol 15, 382

Subject Index

t

u

v

w

x

MIX
Papier aus verantwortungsvollen Quellen
Paper from responsible sources
FSC® C105338

If you have any concerns about our products,
you can contact us on
ProductSafety@springernature.com

In case Publisher is established outside the EU,
the EU authorized representative is:
Springer Nature Customer Service Center GmbH
Europaplatz 3, 69115 Heidelberg, Germany

Printed by Libri Plureos GmbH
in Hamburg, Germany